35.00

D1599304

BC

Impasse and Interpretation

The New Library of Psychoanalysis is published in association with the Institute of Psycho-Analysis. The New Library has been launched to facilitate a greater and more widespread appreciation of what psychoanalysis is really about and to provide a forum for increasing mutual understanding between psychoanalysts and those working in other disciplines like history, linguistics, literature, medicine, philosophy, psychology, and the social sciences. It is planned to publish a limited number of books each year in an accessible form and to select those contributions which deepen and develop psychoanalytic thinking and technique, contribute to psychoanalysis from outside, or contribute to other disciplines from a psychoanalytical perspective.

The Institute, together with the British Psycho-Analytical Society, runs a low-fee psychoanalytic clinic, organizes lectures and scientific events concerned with psychoanalysis, publishes the *International Journal of Psycho-Analysis* and the *International Review of Psycho-Analysis*, and runs the only training course in the UK in psychoanalysis leading to membership of the International Psychoanalytical Association – the body which preserves internationally-agreed standards of training, of professional entry, and of professional ethics and practice for psychoanalysis as initiated and developed by Sigmund Freud. Distinguished members of the Institute have included Wilfred Bion, Anna Freud, Ernest Jones, Melanie Klein, John Rickman, and Donald Winnicott.

NEW LIBRARY OF PSYCHOANALYSIS

1

General editor: David Tuckett

Impasse and Interpretation

Therapeutic and anti-therapeutic
factors in the psychoanalytic
treatment of psychotic,
borderline, and neurotic patients

HERBERT ROSENFELD

TAVISTOCK PUBLICATIONS
LONDON AND NEW YORK

First published in 1987 by
Tavistock Publications Ltd
11 New Fetter Lane, London EC4P 4EE

Published in the USA by
Tavistock Publications
in association with Methuen, Inc.
29 West 35th Street, New York NY 10001

Set by Hope Services, Abingdon
Printed in Great Britain by
Richard Clay (The Chaucer Press) Ltd
Bungay, Suffolk

British Library Cataloguing in Publication Data
Rosenfeld, Herbert A.
Impasse and interpretation: therapeutic and
anti-therapeutic factors in the psychoanalytic
treatment of psychotic, borderline, and neurotic patients. –
(The New library of psychoanalysis; 1)
1. Psychoanalysis
I. Title   II. Series
616.89'17   RC504
ISBN 0–422–61010–0

Library of Congress Cataloging in Publication Data
Rosenfeld, Herbert A.
Impasse and interpretation.
(New library of psychoanalysis; 1)
Bibliography: p.
Includes indexes.
1. Psychoanalysis.   2. Narcissism.   3. Projection (Psychology)
4. Impasse (Psychotherapy) I. Title.   II. Series.
[DNLM: 1. Psychoanalytic Therapy. WM460.6 R813i]
RC504.R59   1987   616.89'17   86–30081
ISBN 0–422–61010–0

Contents

Acknowledgements   vii

Part One: Introduction

1   A psychoanalytic approach to the treatment of psychosis   3

Part Two: The analyst's contribution to successful and unsuccessful treatment

2   Some therapeutic and anti-therapeutic factors in the
    functioning of the analyst   31
3   Breakdown of communication between patient and analyst   45

Part Three: The influence of narcissism on the analyst's task

4   The narcissistic omnipotent character structure: a case of
    chronic hypochondriasis   63
5   Narcissistic patients with negative therapeutic reactions   85
6   Destructive narcissism and the death instinct   105
7   The problem of impasse in psychoanalytic treatment   133

Part Four: The influence of projective identification on the analyst's task

8   Projective identification in clinical practice   157
9   Projective identification and the problem of containment
     in a borderline psychotic patient   191
10   Further difficulties in containing projective identification   209
11   Projective identification and the psychotic transference
     in schizophrenia   220

Contents

12 Projective identification and counter-transference
    difficulties in the course of an analysis with a schizophrenic
    patient   241

Part Five: Conclusion

13 Afterthought: changing theories and changing techniques
    in psychoanalysis   265

Appendix: on the treatment of psychotic states by
psychoanalysis – an historical approach   281

    References   312
    Indexes   319

Acknowledgements

I want here to thank particularly the members of the Publications Committee of the British Psycho–Analytical Society; Dr Ron Britton and afterwards Mr David Tuckett who helped me to reshape the chapters of the book and encouraged me to add the concluding paper, Afterthought, in which I focus attention on the development of my ideas. Mrs Elizabeth Spillius assisted with careful criticism and Mrs Jane Temperly with reading and correcting the drafts.

I also want to thank all the colleagues who contributed to the book by presenting to me case material of difficult patients, mainly in seminars, and all those patients whose analytical material I have used in this book.

I am indebted to my secretary, Mrs Willans, whose devoted typing from dictation was essential to my working; Ms Jackie Craisatti, who typed chapters on to the word processor and made the final shaping and correction of the book possible; and Ms Jill Duncan who helped with the bibliography.

PART ONE

Introduction

1

A psychoanalytic approach to the treatment of psychosis

Patients who suffer from severe psychotic illness, those who are severely narcissistic, and those who do not get better or even get worse as psychotherapeutic treatment progresses have always been a special focus of my interest. In this book, drawing on material from my own practice and from those of psychoanalysts and psycho-therapists whom I have supervised over the last twenty years, I want to give an outline of the ideas I have developed about such patients. In Part Two of the book, I shall present my ideas about the specific contribution the analyst or therapist can make towards influencing the patient for better or worse. In Part Three, I will outline how I think a correct understanding and approach to the problems created by what we have come to term 'narcissism' are essential if the analyst is to function therapeutically. In Part Four, I shall discuss the complex ways in which aspects of projective identification can both assist and undermine the therapeutic relationship.

It is central to my thinking that analytic psychotherapy can be an enormous influence on very disturbed patients, but this influence can be for both good and ill. Some of the treatments I shall discuss did not end well, although not, I think, because the patients were beyond help. What happened was that an impasse developed in the relationship between patient and analyst, something which can happen very easily with a psychotic patient, and this could not be overcome. I believe that such impasses are often created by the therapist's response to the patient's communications and can be avoided by paying careful attention to what the patient is saying. It is my conviction that the psychotic patient's speech and behaviour (particularly in sessions) invariably make a statement about his relationships to the therapist. In this context it is important for the therapist to pay minute attention to the patient's communications and to seek to conceptualize and understand what these communications mean in the transference relationship. However, to provide some background for these views, I want to use this first chapter to say something about the development of my own thinking and therapeutic technique and the clinical experiences that prompted it.

Beginnings

My interest in psychological medicine began during my medical training in Germany, and my MD thesis dealt with the influence of 'Multiple Absences in Childhood'. However, I had no chance to pursue the study of disturbed children or adults in the Germany of 1933 and '34. The Hitler regime forbade non-Aryan doctors to have personal contact with their patients. On coming to England I had intended to practise general medicine for several years before following my psychological interest. But I was catapulted into becoming a psychotherapist after passing my qualifying examination to practise medicine in Britain in the autumn of 1936. At that time the Home Office was prepared to allow only experienced foreign doctors, generally specialists, to stay in Britain to practise, and so I was among those who were asked to leave once I was qualified. However, on closer investigation into the possibility of becoming a psychotherapist, for whom there were openings in Britain, I found that the Tavistock Clinic had a two-year course for training psychotherapists and I immediately applied and was accepted for it.

In the waiting period of nine months before I began at the Tavistock I succeeded in getting first a locum job in a mental hospital near Oxford and later one at the Maudsley Hospital, London. At the mental hospital near Oxford I had to look after 350 patients, half the patient population. There were only three doctors to look after about seven hundred patients: the Superintendent in charge of the hospital and its administration, a senior colleague, and myself. My senior colleague, who had been working in the psychiatric hospital service for many years, introduced me to my job by explaining that there was very little work to do. After occasionally seeing a new admission, my task was to do rounds of the wards. Altogether I would work no more than one and a half hours in the morning and I would then generally be free for the rest of the morning and the afternoon. In fact, apart from their being looked after in the hospital physically, no treatment was given to the patients.

I decided to look among the new admissions for patients who might be suitable for psychotherapy. I selected a patient diagnosed as having catatonic schizophrenia. He had severe attacks of catatonic excitement every four weeks which always lasted one week. The patient, Edgar, had been in the hospital for more than a year, and the staff complained that he was uncooperative, would not do any work in the wards, and was at times violent. However, he seemed to be quite friendly to me. I asked the Superintendent whether he would agree that I could practise some simple psychotherapy with Edgar. At the same time I inquired whether he would agree, if an improvement was to take place, that such an outcome had been achieved by psychotherapy. Few in England believed that psychotherapy could have an appreciable effect, and so any improvement was called a 'remission'. Although I did not doubt that remissions were common, there was obviously a difference between a spontaneous remission and one which was due to some external positive influence, such as a psychotherapeutic approach. Such a hypothesis would imply that schizophrenia might have a psychogenic basis, which at that time was not acceptable to psychiatrists in Britain – apart perhaps from R. D. Gillespie and one or two others, such as Clifford Scott, whom I had not then met. In any case the Superintendent agreed with me that Edgar appeared chronic, and therefore that any improvement would have to be attributed to my work with the patient.

When I talked to Edgar, he explained to me that he had to endure electric shocks every night when he was going to bed. This occurred about every few weeks and made him feel very disturbed. I realized that what he was describing was a delusion of being influenced by a machine, a condition Tausk described in 1919 (Tausk 1919). Edgar asked me many questions and was friendly. He readily listened to my explanations about the physical sensations that were troubling him, which I thought were mainly sexual feelings. He seemed to be completely ignorant about sex. When I informed him about it, it seemed to enable him to become less frightened of his sexual feelings and more accepting of them. He was very appreciative and asked me what he could do for me. I told him that it would be useful if he could show his appreciation by co-operating in the ward and so make it easier for everybody. He proceeded to do so. From this time onwards Edgar's periodic excitement ceased, and I saw him only occasionally. When I left the mental hospital a month or two later he had not been discharged. However, when I returned six months later I asked the Superintendent about him and what the Superintendent now thought of psychological treatment. He was surprised by my question. He said the patient had been discharged. It had been an unexpected remission!

This kind of response to psychological treatment was something I had to get used to when later that year I worked at the Maudsley Hospital for a few months. There, I had the opportunity to have talks with Doctors Slater and Gutman, two well known psychiatrists of the day. I explained to Dr Gutman that I was interested not only in taking detailed case histories but also in following up the patients for a while and in talking to them regularly. He did not object to what I wanted but considered that talking to patients for any purpose other than to make a diagnosis was a complete waste of time. I had to realize that schizophrenia was an organic illness, and talking could have no causal effect on its appearance and disappearance.

While I was working at the Maudsley I kept an open mind. Eliza, one patient I observed, was a schizophrenic girl of sixteen who was severely withdrawn and refused to talk to anybody or to take part in any occupation. She explained to me that it was impossible for her to be part of a world where horrible things were going on. She said that she had been born through a hole in her mother's body which disgusted her to the extent that she felt life was unacceptable. Eliza said that she had discovered this fact just a short time before her illness began and that the knowledge had turned her violently against her mother. Eliza seemed to me a similar case to Edgar, the young catatonic who had responded to the very simple psychological approach to discussing his sexuality, which I had attempted in the hospital near Oxford; but unfortunately I was not allowed to treat her.

In fact, I saw only a few patients regularly at the Maudsley. One of them, whom I shall call Edward, was highly intelligent, suffered from paranoid delusions, and was very withdrawn. He had had two or three schizophrenic attacks which lasted a few months and from which there had always been a spontaneous remission. He seemed to take very little notice of me when I spoke to him, and when I left the Maudsley he did not seem to have improved. However, two years later when I was working privately, I was contacted by the patient's father. Edward had apparently been talking to his father about my visits to him in the hospital and during the intervening years he had asked the father again and again to try to find out whether he could come to see me. Since my leaving the Maudsley, Edward had had several more quite severe schizophrenic attacks of a paranoid kind. I saw him for a consultation, and he was very pleased to see me. He asked to come regularly, and I arranged to see him twice a week.

Edward was generally very carelessly dressed and unshaven but he

6

would always come on time and report some problems relating to himself. I do not now remember the details of my talks with him but I recognized at the time that many of the stories he told me had some symbolic meaning, and this I would explain to him. At that time I did not know anything about transference analysis, and very little of that would have entered into this treatment. However, after about six months Edward started to dress very much better and appeared in the consulting room cleanly shaven. He had not been able to work for many years and was now keen to do some. Therefore, when his boarding-school, which he had left about seven years before, asked to have him as a teacher, he felt eager to accept. This seemed rather risky, but in fact he decided without any hesitation to do so, and the job was a great success. However, from this time onwards he was reluctant to see me, saying he was afraid that returning to me would remind him of his previous illness. His father reported to me from time to time that he was getting on well, but I had to accept Edward's need to keep his split-off schizophrenic state in control by avoiding me. I later came to realize that this is a typical response of patients who achieve an improvement in psychotherapy but who do not sufficiently work through the process in a transference analysis. My view now is that it is only when the psychotic process, particularly the splitting mechanisms, is thoroughly worked through in psychoanalytic treatment that returning to visit the therapist reminds the patient not only of the previous illness but also of the help he has been able to get.

My experiences with Edgar, Eliza, and Edward all made me optimistic about treating schizophrenic patients – or at the very least about communicating with them – and this was a considerable influence on my career.[1] My approach in those days was very simple as I had little knowledge of psychotherapy or psychoanalysis nor of analysing the transference relationship between patient and therapist. However, some features of what I did then remain a central part of my approach. I always felt at ease with the idea that the patient was trying to communicate something and so I tried to adopt a very open attitude with the hope that this would help him to do so. In this I was almost always successful, and even persistently mute patients often talked to me. I also tried to adopt an empathic attitude, attempting to put myself as much as possible into the patient's state of mind. Looking back, I think the few patients who responded well to this simple treatment probably felt helped by their experience of me as close to them and as able to hold them together. Of course, the improvements that took place were superficial. Moreover, the 'mechanics' of the 'cure' were based most likely on the idealization of

7

the therapist and the idealization of the patient–therapist relationship.[2] At this early time I was unaware of the dangers of an unskilled therapeutic approach to the psychosis, as the importance of analysing the transference and the detailed psychotic mechanisms I and others came to formulate were a closed book to me. However, the experiences themselves were very powerful ones that I remember and which helped me to formulate my views later. As I hope to show in later chapters, unskilled psychotherapy of the psychosis is a danger to the therapist's personality because it inevitably stimulates his feelings of omnipotence and helplessness. Fortunately, it was obvious to me in those days that there were only very few schizophrenic patients who were able to respond to the simple empathic understanding I was offering with temporary, even less so with lasting, improvement.

After working at the Maudsley Hospital I began my psychothera-peutic course at the Tavistock Clinic. Training at the Tavistock in psychotherapy then consisted of some form of analysis by somebody on the staff or outside the Clinic, treatment of several patients, who were seen three times a week, and supervision once a week by a member of the staff. In those days one could not choose who supervised one's work, and this, together with the fact that my analyst at that time gave me very little understanding, was frustrating. Nevertheless I went on for some time, and several further experiences were, I think, formative to my later thinking.

One of my patients at the Tavistock Clinic, Thomas, had been diagnosed as suffering from obsessions. Most patients were treated on the couch, but Thomas refused to lie down. However, he formed a strong positive transference and had little difficulty in talking. He was fascinated by cancer and cancer research and he was also very interested in experimenting with death. For example, he would describe how he would turn on the gas at his home and estimate the time it would take before he might be overcome by the fumes and lose consciousness. He would try to turn off the gas just before this event occurred. Obviously this was a very dangerous way of behaving, and it also became apparent that he was not suffering simply from obsessional thoughts and behaviour. Behind this was a real psychotic thought disorder. My senior colleagues at the Tavistock Clinic were convinced that the patient was schizophrenic and they were probably right. As a result they asked me to discontinue the treatment.

Stopping Thomas's treatment was painful for both the patient and myself. At that time I was not very clear whether I could help him or how I could prevent one of his experiments from going wrong, so I reluctantly persuaded him to go to a mental hospital for treatment. He eventually agreed but wrote me pathetic letters from the hospital telling me that he was not better and that he felt deserted by me. He did not return to me for treatment after leaving the hospital – something for which I do not blame him. I clearly had a very meagre knowledge of psychopathology and offered a rather primitive form of treatment. Moreover, I had let him down.

My feeling that I had let Thomas down decided me that whenever possible in future I would try to treat any schizophrenic patient who was offered to me for treatment, and would continue with them whenever possible. In the event, when I qualified to do private work with patients in autumn 1938, a senior colleague, Dr B.B. of the Tavistock Clinic, sent me a schizophrenic patient whom he had treated for many years. The patient came from a Quaker family and as a young man had been very ignorant and frightened about sex. When he was about twenty-five he had developed a delusion that to teach him sex his mother wanted him to have sexual intercourse with her. When he had proceeded to creep into bed with her one night she had abruptly rejected him, and soon afterwards he had attempted suicide and had to be hospitalized. He was sent to Bowden House, a private hospital near London, where Dr B.B. had worked as an assistant to the Director, Dr Crighton–Miller. The patient had paranoid delusions of reference for many years after the acute schizophrenic episode had passed, and Dr B.B. attempted to treat the patient mainly by re-education, encouragement, and friendly social relations. Dr B.B. had recognized that the schizophrenic breakdown had a psychogenic origin, but his own approach was purely intuitive. Over a period of more than ten years there had been some improvement, but when Dr B.B. referred him to me the treatment had got stuck. I treated this patient from 1938 onwards, when he discussed in great detail the ambivalent relationship existing with Dr B.B. Fundamentally the patient felt not understood and rejected by his too active treatment, which he experienced as intrusive and seductive. My non-intrusive approach, with which he felt more comfortable, was also idealized. During the first years of the Second World War the patient attended only occasionally but then he came regularly for more than ten years and occasionally thereafter. Over the course of treatment he gradually became more able to work as a caretaker in a psychiatric nursing home, and his relationships with other people improved. He even had a woman friend for many years although he never achieved a really close relationship with her.

My experience with Dr B.B.'s patient directed my attention to the dangers if the therapist becomes idealized or appears to be seductive or intrusive. A second patient, seen for a short period during 1939, emphasized the problem. She was a young girl who had sexual delusions of people wanting to marry her. During the treatment the delusions could be seen very clearly within an Oedipal framework, and I interpreted her only too obvious incestuous sexual wishes in relation to myself. For example, after she had told me that a voice had just told her that she was going to get married in a month's time I pointed out to her that she had begun to care for me and hoped that I would marry her. To my surprise these transference interpretations unfortunately made her very much worse; her delusions increased, and she had to go into a mental hospital for a long time. I felt very bad about this result, but it eventually helped me to realize that interpretations of openly Oedipal material were very dangerous in schizophrenia. This was an important discovery which eventually enabled me to formulate ideas about the concrete nature of psychotic thinking and feeling and its influence on the way the analyst's interpretations can be distorted so that they are misheard as actual suggestions. For this reason interpretation of sexual material in the transference was experienced by the patient as seduction. However disturbing this worsening of the patient's condition had been, it also convinced me that the psychological approach was very powerful; if psychotherapy was able to make a patient so much worse it should also be able to make him or her better. This was probably the first time that I attempted to analyse sexual delusions in a woman patient by interpreting the delusions both in relationship to her father and in the transference. In other words, I treated her as if she were one of the neurotic patients about whom I had supervisions at the Tavistock Clinic. My earlier treatments of schizophrenic patients had been much simpler, and in one way this had been an advantage, because I did not stir up problems which I could not deal with at the time.

The Influence of Melanie Klein

At the beginning of the war I was working at the Tavistock Clinic as a psychotherapist, and in my discussions with colleagues there the name of Melanie Klein and her way of thinking and interpreting were generally admiringly discussed. It seemed accepted that she had made very important contributions to psychoanalysis and psycho-pathology, but in spite of using her terminology none of the therapists at the Tavistock Clinic had yet had an analysis from her or from her closest colleagues. In those days I felt very dissatisfied with my work, particularly with my very difficult patients. My wife needed treatment at that time, and one of the doctors at the Tavistock Clinic recommended Dr Paula Heimann, who was a co-worker of Melanie Klein's. My wife frequently discussed her analysis with me, and I was astonished by the understanding and insight which she gained very quickly. I also found that I could apply much of what she told me to my difficult patients and I realized even more forcefully how limited my own knowledge was. During this period I heard that Melanie Klein was returning to London from Pitlochry, Scotland, where she had been evacuated for a while. As it was not likely that I would be called up to the Forces as an enemy alien, even if I was a friendly alien, I decided to apply for training at the Institute of Psychoanalysis. I then saw Melanie Klein, who accepted me for analysis, and members of the Training Committee of the British Psycho-Analytic Society, who accepted me for training. The analysis with Melanie Klein was a revelation to me from the beginning. I felt particularly receptive to analysis, and Melanie Klein had the capacity to understand immediately the anxieties and problems which were preoccupying me and to interpret them to me in a very direct way. However, I experienced the benefits of the analysis not only in myself. Many of my patients improved with the widening of my personal psychoanalytic experience. My contact with Melanie Klein as a therapist and thinker inaugurated a new phase of work.

My second training case at the Institute turned out to be a patient suffering from a schizophrenic state with depersonalization. I have published my experience with this patient in the first chapter of my book on *Psychotic States* (Rosenfeld 1965). When I first saw her, Mildred had been suffering from what she called *influenze* for four to five months. She said she felt tired and ill and could not get up in the morning. She also had difficulty in feeling and thinking because her head felt so heavy. During the early stages of the analysis she described her sensations and feelings in great detail. She said she felt dim and sleepy, half unconscious, and could hardly keep awake. At times there was something like a blanket separating her from the world, and she felt dead, 'not here', cut off from herself. She also indicated her awareness of the danger of insanity because she frequently said that if she tried to join up with this self it might force her mind completely out of joint. My supervisor for this patient was Dr Sylvia Payne, who was very experienced diagnostically and psychoanalytically. She warned me that the patient was suffering from a latent psychosis and thought the analysis would mobilize an acute schizophrenic state, so that I would very likely find myself with an acute schizophrenic patient who would need hospitalization. For this reason she tried to persuade me to stop the analysis. I fully agreed with Dr Payne about the danger of mobilizing the schizophrenic state and the responsibility I had towards the patient. But I also remembered vividly Thomas, my first patient at the Tavistock Clinic. I felt I had let him down and strongly believed that I could not repeat the experience. Terminating a treatment might have even more severe consequences, driving the patient deeper into her illness, than if I were to continue seeing her. Mildred presented me frequently with the experience of a sort of barrier or stone wall of the kind Freud (1916) described as characteristic of the experience of treating psychotic and narcissistic patients. This time I hoped that with more experience and better understanding, and with the help of my own analysis, I would find a way to make contact with this patient's psychotic state. So I decided that I would continue the treatment of Mildred, and Mr Payne agreed that this patient could remain my training case for the time being. I continued to report to her.

A prerequisite of psychoanalytic treatment is that it is necessary to make enough contact with the patient's feelings and thoughts to feel and experience oneself what is going on in the patient. These processes have been examined very sensitively by Money-Kyrle (1956). He stressed that the analyst's empathy and insight, as distinct from his theoretical knowledge, depend on his capacity to identify himself with aspects of the patient's self: for example, his infantile self. He also described the unconscious interplay between the patient's and the analyst's mental processes and the need of the analyst to be able to be conscious of what is going on in the patient and in himself, in order to disentangle and interpret to the patient the aspects belonging to the patient. Such success as I had achieved in treating psychotic patients so far had probably been due to my capacity to make enough contact with them to make some interaction between them and me possible. However, with a patient as emotionally blocked and negativistic as Mildred this was extremely difficult. In the first year of Mildred's analysis I found it very hard to understand her relationship to me. Put more theoretically, her transference reactions were so peculiar that I could not recognize them. However, as I realized that my own mind and my own responses to the patient could be a guide to reaching a better understanding, I examined my own 'counter-transference' to the patient much more fully. My analysis helped me to understand my own reactions to the patient and it also mobilized in me those areas which corresponded to the infantile levels at which the patient was functioning. This could then be worked through in my own analysis. Gradually, I began to experience in myself a number of the defence mechanisms which were particularly prominent in Mildred: namely, the schizoid mechanisms in which the self is split and both the good and bad aspects of it are projected into other people, particularly into the analyst, a process which Melanie Klein (1946) described as 'projective identification'. In this way I realized that many of my difficulties with Mildred were related to her intense projection of parts of herself into me and to her persecutory fears of retaliation. As I myself became aware of feeling blocked and defensive in the sessions, two things happened. Not only could I understand Mildred better, but also she seemed more able to show her feelings openly to me – presumably because she noticed that I was more receptive to what was going on in her.

Melanie Klein's paper on 'schizoid mechanisms', which I have just mentioned, was read to the British Society in 1946 and was a further important milestone. In it she elaborated the ideas in her paper 'A Contribution to the Psychogenesis of Manic-Depressive States' (Klein 1935) in an important way. In 1935 she had described in some detail various aspects of the early infantile object relations, experiences, ego mechanisms, and defences which she viewed as characteristic of certain phases of infantile development. The earliest phase, lasting approximately four to six months, she had named 'the paranoid position', because of the quality of the anxieties predominating at that early time. A later phase, which she thought started somewhere between the fourth and sixth month, she had named 'the depressive position', as during this time infantile anxieties and object relations assumed a depressive quality. She felt that the early anxieties of the infant had similarities to the psychotic illnesses developing later on in life and actually referred to the early infantile anxieties as 'psychotic anxieties', which she believed were regressively revived in the later psychotic illnesses. Now, in 1946, she emphasized in much greater detail the earliest infantile anxieties and the defences against them – focusing on mechanisms such as the splitting of the ego, projective identification, denial, and omnipotence. She took the view that these were characteristic of the earliest infantile phase, which she now renamed 'the paranoid schizoid position' to emphasize the importance of the schizoid or splitting mechanisms she had discovered. She stressed that, if the early paranoid anxieties and schizoid mechanisms continued to persist and were not sufficiently modified during the later depressive position, there was a danger that schizoid or schizophrenic illnesses could develop in later life.

The paper in which I reported my experiences with Mildred (Rosenfeld 1947) was a rigorous application of Melanie Klein's ideas to my experience and understanding of the treatment of Mildred's psychotic illness. The paper can be regarded as a fundamental one in the history of the treatment of schizophrenia as it describes the importance of analysing, in the *transference psychosis* which patients like Mildred develop in their treatment, the infantile object relations and mechanisms which persist within them and are constantly enacted. The importance of recognizing and analysing such psychotic transference phenomena during the analysis of psychotic patients remains a crucial aspect of my work with them which I will stress in later chapters. I have found that, once these phenomena are recognized by those trying to treat psychotic patients, some of the anxiety and mystery about helping them by psychotherapy and psychoanalysis disappears. The insights I gained with Mildred provided a sound basis for the development of my work and for teaching other analysts how to treat patients psychoanalytically, and since 1947 I have always had at least one psychotic patient in analysis. There has also been a growing community of those trying to treat psychotics by psychoanalytically influenced therapy, and an expanding literature describing their efforts – especially in North and South America.[3]

The recognition of the psychotic transference and how to become aware of it, based on Melanie Klein's 1946 paper, opened the way for me to a much greater understanding of psychotic patients and the nature of the relationships they create in treatment. Some of the important general problems they present to the therapist and their implications for training and technique are worth describing.

First, one of the most important aspects of the treatment of psychotic patients, which became very clear to me in the experiences I have described so far, is the need to recognize that they communicate with the analyst in very primitive ways, not only by verbal but also by non-verbal means. Non-verbal communication takes place in a great number of ways, for example through simple behaviour, posture, and other actions such as bodily movements and facial expressions. In addition to the tone of voice, then, such expressions of different feelings or of lack of feelings are often made. There are, however, a further number of non-verbal communications that are conveyed by the patient's projection of his own feelings into the analyst or the analytic setting. These are often difficult to define or to observe by visual or auditory means. None the less, it is easy to notice the power such patients have to create an emotionally charged atmosphere. Some of their projections are accompanied by phantasies that have strong dynamic force, and these phantasies are often experienced by the patient as so real that they acquire a delusional character. Such delusional projections seem to exert a strong

14

hypnotic influence on the analyst, which may interfere with his functions. They may lead to collusion and acting out by the analyst or to the analyst feeling intruded on and overwhelmed by the projection. In other words, not only the patient but the analyst feels that the projection has a realistic element: for example, when an analyst feels something is being forced into him by the patient. Such disturbing experiences created by the patient in the analyst should disappear as soon as the analyst becomes able to realize what has been going on. Lasting disturbances in the analyst take place only if his own feelings become inextricably entangled with those of the patient. Over the years, probably through the development of my own inner self and personality and a great deal of experience, feelings of entanglement with my patients have fortunately become the exception rather than the rule. Patients often fear that by their projection they can damage the analyst, and these fears become true if the analyst is not able to cope well with the patient's projections.

In receiving the non-verbal communications, particularly those feelings communicated by projection, the analyst has to be fairly certain that he can differentiate between his own feelings and the patient's projected emotions and experiences. It often takes some time to diagnose the situation. At first one may be aware only that an inner tension arises. Then one can notice that something is going on inside one which is difficult to understand. At such moments one may have to remain quiet and allow oneself to open further so that the projection of the patient does not get blocked by one's personal defensive reaction. One may then become aware, for example, of feeling small, hurt, helpless, and powerless to deal with any situation. In these situations the patient may outwardly have been talking in an aggressive or assertive voice accompanied by similar behaviour when he has in fact been projecting an infantile helpless part into one. The only way the analyst notices this projection is by a sudden experience of the emotional situation, representing an aspect of the patient in his own inner experience. For this reason the capacity to pick up the patient's non-verbal projections is essential in the treatment of psychotic patients.

A second general issue in the treatment of psychotic patients is that the analyst must consider how much of his perceptive experience should be communicated to the patient, in what form, and at what time. I have already mentioned the problems of interpretations at the wrong level – as when sexual wishes are interpreted but then experienced as a seduction by the patient. Another pressing issue is the matter of timing. In some situations one can interpret *too* quickly what one has recognized, with the result that the patient experiences what is said as a rejection of him. What has happened in these situations is that through projective identification the analyst has been experienced concretely as expelling the projected feelings and so expelling the patient as well. For this reason the analyst must learn to contain the feelings which the patient creates in him for a considerable time before he can interpret them to the patient. Such containment should not be confused with inaction. The analyst has still to identify the patient's projections and *to verbalize them to himself as quickly as possible*, otherwise he will not be able to understand the details of the patient's communication or know when and what to interpret. As some of my earlier examples have illustrated, psychotic patients think very concretely, engage in overwhelming projections, and very easily get confused. As a result the transference relationship with such patients is constantly shifting, with a very considerable danger that communications can break down and a severe misunder-standing, leading to increased anxiety and impasse, can set in. For this reason an important part of technique is to try to understand carefully and specifically what the patient wants to project. When one begins to realize what is going on in detail, one can then attempt to bring a number of different aspects or parts of the patient's personality meaningfully together. These parts often exist in a split-off form which prevents the patient from understanding and thinking about himself. This integrative form of interpretation seems both to help the patient to regain his mental functioning and to strengthen his ego, whereas a piecemeal interpretation of the various aspects which are projected into the analyst may simply add to the confusion.

As well as the issue of timing, there is the question of how to give interpretations which make emotional sense to the patient. Some analysts, such as Searles (1965), have tried a number of different techniques for reaching psychotic patients. For example, the projections being made can be clarified to the patient by trying to act out and play the role of another person in order to make the relationship more vivid. I myself do not feel that it is useful for me to act out any particular role which has been assigned to me by a psychotic patient, because of the risk of confusion. However, when the material of a patient appears particularly distant and dead, I do feel that it is important to make the interpretations lively and meaningful and so to illustrate what has really been going on. This has often proved very useful, but many psychotic and particularly also borderline patients, who are frozen because they are covering up their terror by deadness, become terrified when one tries to dramatize the inter-pretations. This is similar with young children. Some babies enjoy a

16

make-believe game quite early on, while others become easily stiff and frightened. Re-enactment by dramatization can be experienced by the patient as an attack or rejection by the analyst, for it can produce states of disintegration which are often experienced by the patient as anxiety that he will fall to pieces. The anxieties and sensations of falling, or of falling to pieces, are central with psychotic patients. They are probably related to the earliest infantile anxiety experiences of the birth situation where the infant has to relinquish the state of being held safely in the mother's womb. It is therefore understandable that the early mother–infant relationship must be looked upon as a situation which is dominated by the infant's need to be treated by the mother in a way that resembles as much as possible the pre-birth experience. Winnicott's (1956, 1960) work on the holding environment and Bion's (1963) work on the mother as a container for the infant are related to these experiences. Most psychotic patients either experience overwhelming anxiety of falling or falling into pieces or defend themselves in different ways against the emergence of these anxieties.

Given the nature of psychotic anxieties about falling to bits it is understandable that in the treatment of psychotic patients the analyst's attitude and empathy towards his patient must play a particularly significant role. As I have pointed out, the psychotic patient communicates his anxieties and needs predominantly in a non-verbal or pre-verbal form, to which the analyst has to be receptive. For this reason analysts such as Fromm-Reichmann (1954), Winnicottt (1956, 1960), and Searles (1965) have argued that the needs of the psychotic patient have often to be satisfied by the analyst's behaviour rather than by verbal interpretations, which may actually be harmful. For example, Searles (1965) stresses the importance of recognizing the infant's symbiotic needs by creating a long period of symbiotic oneness with the patient in which the analyst's capacity to remain silent with the patient is of central importance. Similarly, Nacht (1962) has emphasized how the analyst's silence is needed to try to re-create for the patient an ideal mother–infant experience.

On this question of the role of verbal interpretations I agree that most patients, particularly psychotic ones, often experience the use of words in a way that makes them acutely aware of being separate from the analyst. Sometimes, the analyst's verbal interpretations may be experienced by the patient as a rejection of his wish for non-verbal oneness with the analyst/mother, and it is the persistent silence of the patient which draws attention to his resentment of verbal communication. On the other hand, I have found that most

17

psychotic patients understand and value verbal communications from the analyst, when the analyst succeeds in conveying in a precise way to the patient what he has understood. In this way the analyst's intuitive and receptive empathy is expressed in a verbal form, which has the advantage that the patient is not infantilized, i.e. is not treated as if he were in fact an infant. An important part of the technique is that the analyst should acknowledge fully what the patient feels and needs but should not leave out the equally significant fact that the patient is also a separate being and an adult. It needs tact and sensitivity to interpret this to the patient so that he feels helped and held together through the analyst's words. But I have sometimes been told by patients that when interpretations fit into their own experience they actually feel a kind of physical contact and holding conveyed by my interpretations. This has convinced me that verbal interpretations can create a holding experience, and this has always been my aim. I have found that psychotic patients rarely experience correct verbal interpretations as rejection if the analyst's whole attitude, behaviour, and way of communicating also convey to the patient acceptance and understanding.

I have said enough to indicate how important I believe it to be that the analyst has the capacity to use his own feelings to recognize his patient's non-verbal communications. I have also argued the need for him to follow the patient's communications carefully so that he can time his interpretations appropriately and enable words to make emotional sense to the patient. In this way the psychotic transference can be worked through. In the last few years I have been encouraged and interested to see how (in many places in the world) so many young doctors and residents are attempting to treat psycho-therapeutically, sometimes successfully, very ill psychotic patients. But this brings me to a fourth general point about the treatment of psychosis by psychoanalytic methods: the crucial role of a personal analysis. As I have mentioned in describing my own development, contact with one's own hidden psychotic areas is an essential part of being in touch with the patient and the psychotic transference relationship. Such anxieties must become activated during the treatment of psychotic patients but, if they are not thoroughly dealt with through personal psychoanalysis, can create confusion and impasse in the therapy as well as severe strain and even disaster for the therapist. The psychotic patient often projects his feelings and problems quite violently, and any analyst who is afraid of such contact with his patient might himself become severely disturbed in attempting to treat psychotics. The most frequent but often unconscious anxiety is the fear of being driven mad by the patient. It is for this reason that the analysis of the analyst should be particularly thorough, and this of course includes the exposure of the psychotic areas in the analyst, so that the psychotic anxieties and defences can be worked through sufficiently during the training period. Occasionally a second analysis might be necessary. Even if the analyst feels consciously quite well but has split off or suppressed psychotic conflicts, he will tend to be insensitive or defensive; and it is inevitable that the patient consciously or unconsciously perceives the disturbances in the analyst and reacts or interacts with them. There is also the danger that the latent conflict of the analyst becomes stimulated and activated in contact with psychotic patients. For example, the tendencies to omnipotent and omniscient function can become greatly increased. We have to realize that in treating psychotic patients (even more so than ordinarily) both the analyst's personality and his intellect are his tools in the treatment, and therefore his mental health is an extremely important factor. Only in this way can he respond to the patient with empathy without too much involvement and also show sensitivity and receptiveness without being overwhelmed by the patient's projection.

Theoretical developments

My attempts to analyse the psychotic transference as a way of helping psychotic patients have led me since 1947 to understand a great deal more about it and to be able to conceptualize some of the processes underlying it and the difficulties it presents to the analyst. To be able to function therapeutically, I have come to believe, it is important for the analyst to understand two highly interrelated theoretical processes: narcissism and projective identification.

From the beginning of my career I was strongly influenced by Melanie Klein's suggestion to me that narcissism was related to introjective processes, a view which seemed to derive from Freud's (1914) theory of 'secondary narcissism', although she later contradicted this with the development of her theory of projective identification as a primitive narcissistic object relationship. Melanie Klein herself did not develop the theory of narcissism any further, but my experience in analysing schizophrenic and manic-depressive disorders impressed on me the importance of the processes of projective identification and their relation to severe narcissistic conditions. After *Envy and Gratitude* (1957), in which Melanie Klein described the early envy of the breast and her clinical experiences of the way envy in the transference situation created intense negative therapeutic reactions, I became increasingly aware of the close relation of envy and narcissistic attitudes and object relations.

In 1963 I described my clinical experiences and the way I had come to formulate narcissism in a manner very different to Freud (Rosenfeld 1963). In his paper on narcissism Freud (1914) argued that in psychotic conditions, such as schizophrenia and paranoia, the libido becomes detached from the object and the outside world and withdraws into the ego. In more ordinary language he was suggesting that such patients were so preoccupied with themselves and their security (so narcissistic) that they could not form dependent or meaningful relationships with anybody else. One consequence for psychoanalytic therapy, if this was correct, was that such patients could not form a transference relationship and could not, therefore, use the main instrument of the therapeutic setting to get better. Much of my early experience with schizophrenic patients suggested to me a different view to that of Freud. I have already described that despite apparent indifference or deadness I found that psychotic patients in fact formed very powerful transferences, albeit different from those found with neurotic patients. This was proof to me that Freud had been mistaken. As time went by I also noticed that narcissistic attitudes and transferences were described by other analytic authors dealing with such patients (Abraham 1924b, Stern 1938 and 1948, Federn 1943, Stone 1954). Psychotic patients seemed typically to show omnipotent attitudes to others and particularly to their therapists. In phantasy they seemed to make insatiable demands on their objects, to confuse self and others, to take others into themselves, and to put themselves into others.

To formulate what I observed about narcissim, I introduced the term 'narcissistic object relations' to emphasize that it was not generally an objectless state. In fact, I suggested, psychotic patients had a particular relationship to objects; they were able to relate to them only for narcissistic purposes and only in a highly omnipotent way. Eventually I coined the phrase *'narcissistic omnipotent object relations'*. I had in mind the way psychotic patients use others (objects) as containers into which, feeling all powerful, they project those parts of themselves which are felt to be undesirable or which cause pain and anxiety. Another feature of the process is that the patient identifies (by projection or introjection) with the object, to the extent that he feels he is the object or the object is himself. In the case of introjection the object becomes part of the self to such a degree that any separate identity or boundary between self and object is felt not to exist. In the case of projective identification parts of the self become so much part of the object, for example the mother, that

20

the patient has the idea he possesses all the desirable qualities of the object – in fact that he is the object in these respects. I took the view that identification by introjection and by projection usually occurs simultaneously and emphasized that narcissistic omnipotent object relations are partly defensive against the recognition of the separateness of self and object. Such modes of relating obviate both the aggressive and ambivalent feelings aroused by frustration as well as any awareness of envious or aggressive feelings. One cannot be envious or aggressive towards someone any more than one can love them or be dependent on them if one is one and the same with them. It seemed likely, therefore, that the strength and persistence of narcissistic omnipotent object relations were closely related to the strength of the infant's envious or aggressive feelings which are revived, and therefore can be studied, in the analytic transference relationship. The more envious a patient's wishes, for example, the more difficult it is to face separateness and to give up narcissistic omnipotent object relations.

A problem to which I drew attention in the analysis of the psychotic patient is that when narcissistic self-idealization diminishes, the patient becomes aware of his need and dependency on the object, the analyst. This creates pain and anxiety as well as envy and threatens to rekindle the process of narcissistic omnipotent object relating all over again – perhaps leading to a negative therapeutic reaction. With some therapeutic progress the patient begins to feel that the analyst has qualities and understanding which he wants to possess himself. It is in this situation that envy not only motivates the patient to expropriate the good qualities of the analyst and obliterate him as a separate person, but also motivates his devaluation. In this situation an analysis can reach impasse, and both analyst and patient become very frustrated. One defence against this kind of enactment in the transference, therefore, is that both analyst and patient seek to preserve their relationship as ideal and desirable and so resist anything interfering with this picture, such as the reality of their separateness or the progress of the patient's illness.[4]

In 1971 in a paper which was pre-published for the International Psycho-Analytic Congress of that year I made a substantial addition to my theory of narcissism by discriminating more formally between several groups of patients with a narcissistic omnipotent character structure.[5] Among those patients I had treated of this type there were a number who were consciously intensely destructive and sadistic and proud of it. They had often had one or more analyses previously but had been very little touched by them. To understand and to make progress with these patients I argued that it was essential to differentiate libidinal from destructive aspects of narcissism, something which had been completely neglected in both psychoanalytic theory and practice. Putting forward a theory of destructive narcissism, I suggested that in some cases, such as those I have just mentioned, there was an enormous idealization of the destructive parts of the self which were felt to be attractive because they made the patient feel so omnipotent. When destructive narcissism of this kind is a feature of a patient's character structure, libidinal (that is to say loving, caring, interdependent) object relationships and any wish on the part of the self to experience the need for an object and to depend on it are devalued, attacked, and destroyed *with pleasure*.[6] It was part of my thesis that such destructive and omnipotent wishes are often difficult to recognize in what a patient does and says because the patient unconsciously experiences them as protective and even benevolent, but very secretly. Secrecy is part of feeling omnipotent destructive superiority. Because the existence of omnipotent destructive wishes on the part of the self is obscured, patients dominated by destructive narcissism give the impression that they have no relationship to the external world. They appear not to care a jot. In fact, of course, they depend on constantly attacking anything and everything which might be likely to satisfy their libidinal needs, and their state can never be stable. Such patients may need to go on in analysis partly in order to have a libidinal relationship to attack.

In my experience the successful analysis of many psychotic (and indeed other) patients depends on understanding the psychopathology of destructive narcissism, and I have given clinical examples of this in Part Three of this book.[7] In particular, I have come to the view that the hidden and hypnotic power of destructive narcissism is a particularly significant factor in the negative therapeutic reaction and in the genesis of psychosis as such. In this connection, although some analysts, like Kernberg (1977), emphasize the importance of aggression and envy in narcissistic disorders, what I had in mind (and still adhere to) is far more thoroughgoing. To my mind Kernberg has not spelt out to what extent destructive and narcissistic but defused aggressiveness tends to take over the whole of the psychotic patient's personality. Other analysts, on the other hand, have tended to neglect destructive narcissism completely, Kohut (1972), for example, has described narcissistic rage. But this has very little to do with what I am trying to describe with the term 'destructive narcissism'. Narcissistic rage arises when a patient reacts to a narcissistic hurt and feels humiliated, looked down on, and misunderstood. It often improves when the patient feels well understood in analysis. In contrast, the destructive narcissistic patient enjoys hurting, has contempt when he finds somebody loving, understanding, and kind, and puts all his energies into remaining sadistically strong – regarding any love in himself as weakness. Such patients show prolonged resistance to treatment and often have a history of many failed attempts at it.

A second, very closely related line of thinking which I have developed to guide my clinical work, especially with psychotic patients, concerns projective identification. I have already referred in this chapter to the general role of projective and introjective processes of identification in creating a phantasy of oneness and so denying separateness, love, aggression, need, envy, and dependence. Projective identification is, therefore, an integral part of narcissistic omnipotent object relations.

Since 1946 the understanding of projective identification has become an enormously important aspect of many analysts' work. In her paper on 'schizoid mechanisms', Melanie Klein (1946) described the process of projective identification and regarded it as essential to understanding infantile development. She explained that there are patients who split off good and bad parts of themselves and project these parts into external objects in such a way that these objects become identified with their projected parts. One problem related to this mechanism of defence is that the objects containing the patient's projected self can be felt as persecuting, to a degree that the entire self is under threat of invasion. Other people are felt to have stolen parts of the patient or to be implicated in aggressive attempts to take him over. Persecutory anxieties of this type were particularly common in the psychotic patients I saw, who would often complain that people (including myself as their analyst) were trying to take over their personalities and dominate them. This is very important. However, I have also emphasized how projective identification is also a method of communication. By projecting their confused feelings and anxieties into the analyst, patients not only get rid of them. They also provide (just as they did in infancy with their parents) the opportunity for the analyst (parent) to become aware of their feelings. A major part of my theory was that psychotic patients project their feelings because they are too frightened to cope with them or to think about them themselves. The analyst, however, like the parents in more normal development, has the potential both to face the feelings and to think about them, and it is this capacity which he gradually offers the patient to develop for himself. The nature of the psychotic transference is that it provides the opportunity to demonstrate that unbearable feelings can be contained and thought about creatively.

In Part Three of this book I discuss several detailed aspects of projective identification and formulate my views about their impact on the kind of psychotic transference which can occur. While many negative therapeutic reactions which occur in psychotherapy and psychoanalysis arise from the difficulties introduced by destructive narcissism, and more generally the narcissistic omnipotent character structure, problems on the part of the analyst in diagnosing projective identification correctly can prevent an analysis from getting started or even give rise to a worsening of the patient's state. I have formulated several different types of projective process in the psychotic transference, which can be referred to as projective identification, and which must be clearly differentiated from one another. There are many analysts who, because they have not been able to diagnose and conceptualize the projective identification manifest in the transference for a long time, have become overwhelmed by feelings which they do not understand and cannot cope with. Ways of differentiating and diagnosing projective identification and the consequences when this is not done are discussed in Part Four.

Notes

1 As many may doubt the diagnosis of schizophrenia in the cases which I treated at that time I want to stress that all the cases reported here were typical schizophrenias regarded from the psychiatric point of view. The patients suffered from delusions and hallucinations and had typical schizophrenic thought disorders.

2 In addition there was most certainly a deepening of the split between the saner and the psychotic part of the patient's self, leading to an isolation of the psychotic process. This means that there was a great danger that the split–off psychosis might suddenly re-emerge, which would no doubt have overwhelmed the non–psychotic part of the patient.

3 During the very early period of my attempts at treating psychotic patients I felt naturally very isolated and alone, as there was nobody who could give me advice on how to proceed, and I was left almost entirely to my own resources. From 1950 onwards Hanna Segal and Wilfred Bion started treatment with psychotic patients, but at first we did not share our experiences because we all wanted to pursue and establish our own findings until they became sufficiently clarified to become convictions we could use for publication. After that the sharing of our experiences was most useful, and I also began to conduct seminars and supervisions to help all those interested in the treatment of psychotic patients. It seemed to me essential to give support and advice to analysts who attempted to

treat psychotic patients and that there was a possibility that we might gradually create a more established form of psychoanalytic treatment of the psychosis, one which would be recognized by the English school of Psychiatry.

The resistance of English psychiatrists to psychoanalytic treatment of the psychoses has lessened a little over the years, but even today it is far from being accepted by English psychiatrists as a whole. Psychiatric co-operation in establishing more fully the psychotherapeutic and psycho-analytic treatment of psychosis in hospital is still very limited. So far only in the Maudsley Hospital and in Shenley Hospital (outside London) have in-patient and out-patient units been established where patients can be treated with analytic psychotherapy by the staff. However, there has been an increase in the number of well trained psychiatrists who apply for psychoanalytic training. There is some hope that some change will occur over the years. My own appeal in papers and elsewhere for research funds to enable further work on schizophrenia has not been successful, so I have persisted in continuing with my own research with those cases which were sent to me privately. The supervisory work of the psychotic patients of colleagues seems to have also been a considerable help.

After my paper on 'Notes on the Superego Conflict' (Rosenfeld 1952a), American psychiatrists and analysts became increasingly interested in my work. In 1953 at the London Congress of Psychoanalysis I had the opportunity to discuss the treatment of the psychosis with a number of American analysts, for example with Bychowski (1953). Bychowski and I agreed that psychotics could be analysed, and he agreed with many of my findings. He was, however, surprised that I suggested that some of the problems which were encountered in our psychotic patients could also be found in our ordinary psychoanalytic patients who were at times merely neurotic or borderline. He did not agree that it was necessary to analyse psychoanalytic candidates more deeply. More recently some of the American analysts have changed their opinion. For example, when I was working for a few days in Topeka in 1969 some training analysts confided to me that many of the candidates in training had severe narcissistic disturbances, and they were worried as to whether this could be altered by analysis. So there was at least a recognition that narcissistic problems are as common in psychiatrists as in other people – and need analysis. There is evidence that some candidates in psychoanalytic training turn out to have borderline problems, and occasionally psychotic illnesses have been discovered. However, at the time of talking with Bychowski in 1953 I was convinced, not only from my own experience but also from my analytic experience with patients, that there were psychotic anxieties in everyone, though the degree and the intensity of the problem naturally varied from person to person.

25

From 1962 onwards the American Psychiatric Association (Rosenfeld 1963a, 1963b, 1964a) became interested in my work with psychotic patients. In 1962 they invited me to discuss the treatment of depressive patients at a meeting of American psychiatrists in Montreal. They repeated this invitation in 1964 when they asked me to talk in Boston about recent research into the psychoanalytic treatment of schizophrenic patients (1964a) (see Chapter 11). At the Boston meeting I was stimulated by the great interest shown to me by the large American audience, which was composed of psychiatrists, psychologists, social workers, and psychoanalysts. I was given more than one hour to deliver my paper, which was followed by a lively discussion. The Maclean Hospital in Boston, which was looking after 150 schizophrenic in- and out-patients, asked me at the same time to talk about 'Problems of dealing with the erotic transference in schizophrenic patients' (see Chapter 11). The choice of the title for this lecture showed the psychotherapeutic approach to psychotic patients was relatively well established in the hospital, but it was not possible at that visit to contact individual therapists to offer to supervise their work with schizophrenic patients. Therefore I could not judge the general standard or skill of the therapeutic work that was going on.

However, the interest in the psychological approach to the psychoses is very much wider in the United States than in Britain. The opposition to the psychological approach to the psychoses in Britain is mainly related to the continuing emphasis on the organic factors in schizophrenia and manic–depressive states. This discouraged and still discourages any psychotherapeutic interest. In the United States the situation is rather different. Probably through the influence of Adolf Meyer, Harry Stack Sullivan, Robert Knight, Frieda Fromm-Reichmann, Harold Searles, and possibly John Rosen, there was a general awareness that psychotic illness is largely determined by psychogenic factors, and this awareness encourages many psychiatrists to treat psychotic patients psychotherapeutically.

4 Kernberg's work on the narcissistic personality disorders is, I think, based predominantly on Melanie Klein's view of internal objects. I described in my 1963 paper my observations on the close relation of envy and narcissim. The earlier work of Federn on healthy and pathological narcissism, although influential, was difficult to use clinically, as he saw narcissism in a non-object-related way. Kernberg has spelt out the differences between normal and pathological narcissism in much greater detail than I have done so far. I believe that we have extended our understanding of narcissism a great deal during the last twenty years. None the less, much more work might be necessary in order to bring together the many different theories of narcissism which exist today.

5 I mean patients whose character is dominated by narcissistic omnipotent object relations.

6 André Green (1984), in the recent symposium on the death instinct held in Marseilles, talked about 'negative' narcissim, which in his view has a 'de-objectalizing' function to reach zero level in destroying object relations by attacking the process of objectalizing rather than the object itself. The process he describes is almost identical with my observation on the way destructive narcissism works – namely, it is directed against the libidinal and dependent ties or bonds of the self to the object, including to primary objects.

7 There are few analysts who have yet discussed patients with destructive narcissism as I have observed it. An exception was Meltzer, who described a tricky and foxy part of the self which for several years in a hidden split-off way dominated an analysis until gradually a powerful perverse structure appeared, which had even more destructive addictive omnipotent features which controlled the patient's personality for many years (Meltzer 1968). Meltzer tries to differentiate clearly between two narcissistic structures of the self and the severe persecuting anxieties created by dead objects who overwhelmed the patient with terror. The description of the 'tricky and foxy' parts of the self has a great deal in common with the tricky, envious parts of the patient I described in the common narcissistic organization, while his 'destructive addictive omni-potent' self has similarities with the powerful omipotent self in destructive narcissism which has such hypnotizing, sadistic control over all parts of the self.

PART TWO

The analyst's contribution to successful and unsuccessful treatment

2

Some therapeutic and anti-therapeutic factors in the functioning of the analyst

As the analyst's capacity to function is mainly expressed by his ability to convey understanding through the way he gives interpretations and what he selects for interpretation, one may say that the patient's feeling of being accepted and cared for depends to a large extent on the interpretative function of the analyst. Like others, I have found that patients respond to our interpretations not only as tools which make them aware of the meaning of the unconscious and conscious processes, but also as reflections of the analyst's state of mind (Segal 1962a, Loewald 1970, Langs 1976, Sandler 1976) – particularly his capacity to retain quietness and peacefulness and to focus on the central aspects of the patient's conscious and unconscious preoccupations and anxieties. The patient is also aware of the analyst's mind and memory through the way he holds together important external and internal factors and brings them together at the right time. The analyst's state of mind, his capacity to function well, is an essential therapeutic factor in analytic therapy. It plays an important part in the introjective processes, increasing the patient's capacity for object relations and strengthening his ego in its functions and in its capacity for integration and particularly for mental growth.

I indicated in Chapter 1 my belief that the principal therapeutic function of a psychoanalyst is to help the patient put into words and conscious thoughts the unconscious feelings and wishful phantasies which preoccupy him. In this way the patient's repetitions of early object relations and the omnipotent defences built up in the infantile period can be modified. Gradually, the patient can tolerate more feelings (and particularly the anxiety they provoke), recognize conflicts, and become able to think about them. As this becomes more possible the need for the gross distortion of inner and outer functioning which occurs in narcissistic omnipotent object relations is reduced. As I have said, the primary means by which the analyst achieves these aims is by precise verbal interpretation of the patient's phantasies of the transference relationship, focusing on the most pressing unconscious anxiety experienced by the patient at any time.

A corner-stone of my view about therapeutic change is my belief that even the most disturbed and tricky patients, whose pathology may cause them time and time again to defend themselves against anxiety by distorting and undermining the analytic process, not only seek to communicate their predicament but also have a considerable capacity for co-operating with the therapeutic endeavour, if the analyst can recognize it.

Some patients have a vivid and lively capacity to bring relevant material into analysis, through both their verbal and non-verbal communications. I have noticed in supervisions, for example, that if what a patient says is not understood by the analyst it will frequently be repeated two, three, or even four times in a session, in many different ways. Such attempts to communicate (even in the unfavourable circumstances in which an analyst has difficulty understanding the patient) are remarkable. Such patients seem to try to make the material more and more easy to understand with very little resentment about the failure of the analyst. They are particularly likely to communicate what they feel and think about the analyst, and, as others have noticed, their understanding of the analyst's problems is often vivid and precise (Searles 1965 and 1975, Langs 1976). I have observed psychotic patients with this capacity, not only neurotic ones. They seem to have much tolerance for the analyst's weakness and to have a great capacity to live and to look for object relations. Other patients, particularly schizoid ones, of course, are much more easily discouraged and quickly withdraw when they feel snubbed or not understood. Even so, I have noticed that psychotically regressed patients belonging to this group often have an amazing capacity for communicating their needs and observations, particularly by non-verbal means – although when non-verbal means predominate I do not mean to imply that the patient is silent and unable to use words. It is rather that their language sometimes sounds as if they are in a dream. Such language is common with schizophrenic patients and it takes some time to learn. It exemplifies my contention that careful consideration of even the most disturbed psychotic behaviour can be rewarded by finding that it communicates something meaningful.

Analytic material from several of my patients indicates that from very early on infants not only relate to the breast and the way the mother handles the feeding situation but also seem to be acutely aware of some aspects of the mental state of the mother as a whole person and of her capacity, or incapacity, to feel related to the infant. Such patients can sometimes be openly critical of the analyst's failure in understanding. If the analyst misinterprets such criticisms as sadistic attacks, then the patients often have great guilty feelings about their capacity to understand the situation better than the analyst himself. This guilt increases if they realize that the analyst seems unable to bear their correct observations. If the analyst continues to ignore the patients' criticism and insists on interpreting their observations as attacks on him, they feel they are being made stupid and infantilized. Some of these patients are at times capable of misusing their capacities and becoming omnipotent, destructive, and triumphant. They then have difficulty differentiating between their capacity for critical perception and such aggressive feelings as envy derived from infantile dependence; their helplessness is revived in the analytic situation. Probably this confusion developed during the traumatic experience of the infant–mother relationship, creating in these patients a sense of guilt which forces them to destroy their unusually sensitive capacities to function and to present themselves in analysis as severely disturbed in their mental functioning. Nevertheless, I have found that such patients, even if they are clinically psychotic or borderline, have a good prognosis if they are carefully and sensitively handled by the analyst.

Anti-therapeutic factors in the analyst

To function carefully and sensitively, and so to be therapeutic, an analyst depends to a crucial extent on the functioning of his personality as an important instrument or tool. For that reason we are trained not only clinically and theoretically through lectures and supervision, but also through personal analysis. As I mentioned in Chapter 1, in his analysis the candidate's character structure and character disturbance, his known and unknown problems, have to be located, gradually brought into the open, and integrated into his personality to help him withstand the wear and tear of analytic work and to be receptive to a multitude of patient problems, including psychotic and borderline problems. The analysis of the analyst's defensive structure must include his defences against deep-seated early infantile anxieties, which often hide unconscious psychotic anxieties or problems. Although our training forces us to be more sane, it must temporarily make us more disturbed and anxious in order to gain the knowledge and experience about ourselves necessary for us to function. I think we all realize that some of our problems remain unsolved and that we must strive to develop, and to remain in contact with, ourselves. We serve our patients best if we are honest with ourselves and thus open to accept fully what the patient is. Unless we help our patients to realize fully who they are, no real change in their personality can take place.

We must also accept that each analyst is different and works differently with his patients, but this does not mean that we should deny our own or our colleagues' shortcomings or achievements. Discrimination, a capacity for criticism, is one of the most important ego functions that we need in our work. Klauber (1972) had the courage to describe details of the analyst's pathology and how this interferes with his therapeutic role. His aim was to draw attention to the great difficulties in doing analytic work, although he was rather uncertain about them. I fully agree with him about how difficult it is to face up to the truth about ourselves and to maintain our concern with this problem. However, I think that more can be done about the problem than he envisaged by spelling out and making conscious the way an analyst can be anti-therapeutic. In this respect there are three issues which have particularly preoccupied me. They are the tendency of analysts to adopt particular directive roles towards their patients, the tendency to offer badly timed and vague interpretations, and the tendency too rigidly and restrictively to pursue a particular line of interpretation. Some of these tendencies arise from theoretical controversies and confusions about the nature of the analyst's therapeutic role but they are also compounded by unrecognized unconscious demands from the transference relationship with which the analyst can all too easily collude.

The analyst's attitude and role

In trying to clarify the role and attitude of the analyst towards his patient two views have tended to be advanced. On the one hand there is Freud's (1916–17) dictum that we should regard analysis simply as an investigation and should not approach it with any therapeutic expectancy or desire. This view was at least partly supported by Bion (1970) when he spoke of the need for the analyst to approach his patient without desire. On the other hand several analysts have pointed out that the attitude often adopted towards the patient is frequently a motherly one (Money-Kyrle 1956, Gitelson 1962, Langs 1976, Sandler 1976). Bion's (1962a) recommendation about the attitude of reverie and Winnicott's (1956) primary maternal preoccupation are also related to the role which a mother intuitively takes up towards her infant.

I have always felt that both the surgical approach described by Freud and the preoccupation with the analyst as substitute mother are inappropriate. There is a danger that we become caught up in a particular directive role towards the patient instead of taking care that this is left completely open throughout the analysis. The analyst will be placed via the transference in many roles, not just the role of mother or infant – good, bad, or indifferent. I therefore agree with Pearl King (1962: 225), who, when discussing the Symposium on the Curative Factors in Psychoanalysis in 1961 at the Edinburgh Congress, said that

> 'The attitude that an analyst adopts towards the curative process in psycho-analysis will determine his attitude to his patient, and his handling of the analytical relationship. . . . The relationship of the analyst to the patient is in my view unique. . . . It is not meant to be a parent–child relationship.'

She went on to say that 'I sometimes think of the analytic relationship as a psychological stage on which I as an analyst am committed to take whatever role my patient may unconsciously assign to me.' She makes it clear that it is not her wish to play exactly any original role but to make the patient aware of the role he is making her inhabit. I am in full agreement with this formulation. By contrast, if the patient successfuly provokes the analyst to take on a certain role, to act out, it will bring the therapeutic function of analysis to an impasse.

If I am doubtful about assuming any fixed role I am also dubious about an attitude of detachment. It seems to me impossible to destroy our desire and intention without severely damaging the relationship with our patient. When we accept a patient for analysis, or a candidate for training, we are in fact expected to concern ourselves with that particular patient very thoroughly, and we intend to try to understand and to help him. However, it is essential that we thoroughly analyse our attitudes and intentions. The desire or expectancy which interferes in analysis and which is felt to be disturbing by our patients is our narcissistic desire to do well with or to have a patient who gives us satisfaction in our work and so indirectly increases our satisfaction with our therapeutic capacities. We all know that even normal satisfaction with our patient's improvement is often very suspect to that patient and is an important factor in negative therapeutic reactions. Although it is sometimes extremely difficult to differentiate between the patient's projections and true perception of the remnants of the analyst's narcissistic attitude, we do know that these narcissistic needs make the analyst liable to act out with the patient and become personally involved. This experience creates a feeling in the patient, not of being accepted or cared for, but of being seduced by the analyst, and on a deeper level it creates a feeling of loneliness and rejection or of being misunderstood. It leads to impasse or worse.

The analyst's intentions exert a particular danger, I believe, in those situations where the nature of the patient's psychopathology is particularly likely to create strain in the counter-transference. Severely traumatized patients, who are often driven to repeat past traumatic situations in the analytic situation, are particularly likely to draw the analyst into unconscious collusion with them. They insist that the analyst must know exactly what conscious and unconscious terrors they have suffered in the past, projecting these experiences violently into him. These situations are, of course, extremely painful for the analyst. If they are unbearable to him, the analyst may collude with certain idealized patient phantasies by creating 'corrective therapeutic experiences', rationalizing these as assisting the patient in the search for a much better environment or a more comforting object than he had in the past. Such efforts destroy the analytic process and the process of trying to verbalize what is happening and to help the patient to face it.

In my experience a misunderstanding of the reason why the traumatized patient feels so compelled to repeat his past experiences goes along with the enormous transference demand felt by the analyst. As I see it, one of the most important facts which has to be considered about the traumatic experience is that the patient has had to cope all on his own, sometimes for a considerable time. Often he has survived only through such severe defensive reactions as denial, splitting, and depersonalization. Thus, when the patient dares to turn to an analyst for help, he expects him to share the terrifying experiences which are quite unbearable for him. Unconsciously he often tries to involve the analyst in his experiences by very forceful projections, sometimes so violent that they appear to be attacks on the analyst and his work. This is a painful and difficult situation for any analyst to bear, and, if he does not err on the side of providing corrective experience, a second anti-therapeutic response to which the analyst can so easily resort is to interpret the projections as sadistic attacks on his noble efforts to help. In this case the patient also feels rejected and withdraws. He fears that the analyst wants to retreat and cannot stand being involved with him. In consequence the violent projections can increase and make the situation all the worse. Only if the analyst succeeds in the difficult task of interpreting the patient's anxieties correctly, as well as pointing out his need to share his experiences with the analyst by making the analyst experience them, can the violence of the patient's projections gradually diminish.[1]

Vague or badly timed interpretations

A second way in which an analyst can very easily be anti-therapeutic is if his interpretations are not sufficiently precisely orientated towards the patient's immediate anxieties or are badly timed. Sometimes an analyst will be aware that there is something about himself that is worrying the patient but be unable to interpret accurately enough about it.

Many patients react very strongly to the analyst's timing of interpretations – for example, to prolonged silence or to his interpreting too quickly. The patient may feel left alone too long, or may feel criticized or rejected by the analyst's silence. If some problems are not taken up by the analyst, the patient may react as if the analyst does not want to know about these problems because they are unacceptable. Consequently the patient will feel that he must keep these problems to himself. The analyst's capacity to respond with sensitive timing of his interpretations, and through assisting the patient to face those areas of his mind which are unacceptable to him, has an important therapeutic function. However, if we interpret material too precipitately before it is possible to know the full significance of the patient's communication, the patient may suspect we are too anxious. The patient will realize that we are uncertain and afraid that we may not know and understand. This will not just be felt as a rejection; it can also be perceived as an omnipotent defence, on the part of the analyst, against experiencing anxiety or uncertainty with which the patient may feel he has to collude (Langs 1976). There are many patients who are afraid to get into full contact with their deepest anxieties, so instead of feeling and knowing who and what they are, they pretend to know. If the analyst joins with them in this activity, the therapeutic function of analysis comes to a halt.

Other patients, however, like those mentioned a little earlier, will often do a very great deal to try to communicate to the analyst an anxiety such as that the analyst is frightened of them or the kind of feeling they experience. One analytic session I have encountered illustrates this phenomenon particularly clearly.

At the beginning of the session, which took place on a Wednesday, the patient, Sylvia, seemed to the analyst to talk about a mental state of remoteness, indefiniteness, and timelessness which worried her. The analyst related Sylvia's state to the weekend, when the analyst had of course not seen her. To this Sylvia responded by saying, 'It is important for people I am with', explaining that she functioned 'on the level of feeling'. The analyst told me that she had difficulty understanding what this might mean but commented to Sylvia that she thought she might be talking about how influenced she is by her ideas about what other people are feeling. Sylvia replied that she agreed, she must be very careful when other people get flustered. At this point her analyst made a third comment suggesting that Sylvia was frightened of being left alone. This time Sylvia replied by talking about how she had rung the bell at the beginning of the session but had to wait for the analyst to use the buzzer to let her in. This comment confused the analyst, but subsequently Sylvia repeated how she felt unreal, stating that, as she was waiting at the door, she had tried to look at the analyst's name-tag under the bell. This time the analyst interpreted that the patient was trying to express how much she needed evidence that the analyst existed. The analyst emphasized that she was actually there with the patient at that moment. The patient responded to this communication with silence. Later she talked about a car that had cut right across in front of her, but was reluctant to say any more.

This interchange between Sylvia and her analyst will be described and discussed in much greater detail in Chapter 3. I quote it now to illustrate how patients try very hard to communicate with their analysts and how in the absence of an accurate understanding they can get more and more confused, leading to an impasse in the therapeutic relationship. I suggest that on various occasions during the session Sylvia tried to indicate to her analyst that something was going wrong. The problem which developed in the session and became more and more frightening was her feeling that her analyst did not understand her, could not cope with her feelings, and therefore absented herself not just at the prearranged weekends but more crucially in the sessions themselves. First, Sylvia responded to the weekend interpretation by gently correcting the analyst – saying the problem was not at the weekend but now, with 'the people I am with'. When this is not understood she begins to be frightened because she fears that her analyst is 'flustered' by her. Next, growing more worried, she employed strong symbolic language to suggest that she felt the analyst was out of touch with her, that she didn't ring a bell in the analyst's mind. Then, worried by the time it is taking for the bell to work in the analyst, she repeats how she feels unreal and implies she is getting confused about where she is and who she is talking to, referring to the name-tag. Finally, exasperated in her own way, she still tries to communicate about what is happening by talking about how the analyst (car) is dangerously cutting her up. The remarkable thing about this interchange, understood from this point of view, is how tenaciously the patient keeps trying to communicate her ideas about what is happening with her analyst. Instead of being able to help her understand her anxiety and to explore the basis of it (no doubt in her infantile sadistic and omnipotent wishes), the analyst misses the chance to be therapeutic, grows more and more anxious herself, and actually contributes to the patient's anxieties about how dangerous she is. A patient who is able to communicate forcibly needs desperately an analyst who is receptive to her communication, and there is a great danger that the patient will deteriorate if she cannot find this particularly close contact and understanding which psychotic patients depend on.

I shall not explore the disturbed interaction between Sylvia and her analyst any further here, as the case is discussed in detail in Chapter 3.

Rigidity and inflexibility

Areas in which the analyst functions badly and which lead him rather too rigidly and inflexibly to pursue a line of interpretation without noting its harmful effects (as in the example just given) may be the result of only temporary blockages activated by internal or external conflicts. If these problems interfere with the analysis for only a short length of time, the therapeutic co-operation of the patient will generally return. However, if the analyst has many areas which can be described as 'private: no entry' – as Heimann (1975) has recently so perceptively described them – then the analyst and patient may collude unconsciously to keep those areas out of the analysis and so create a therapeutic impasse. The patient may criticize the analyst quite violently in many different ways, but nevertheless avoid the area and the situation where the traumatic experience of feeling rejected by the analyst's behaviour occurs. The attacks of such a patient are often misinterpreted by the analyst, who may try to relate this behaviour to past experiences. This may lead to acute anxiety and increased critical or contemptuous attacks on the analyst, augmenting feelings of hopelessness in the patient because it nourishes his fears that it will be forever impossible for him to be understood and accepted. If the analyst is able to diagnose the patient's behaviour and recognize his own mistakes along with the detailed causes of the failure, the patient can generally bring his observations to the notice of the analyst. When in fact the analyst is able to take the observations of the patient seriously and is able to succeed in verifying both in himself and in the patient the various areas of blocking, the impasse in the analysis will clear.

The most common blockages in the patient–analyst interaction relate to the analyst's unconscious, infantile anxieties. One defensive manoeuvre through which the analyst deals with his anxieties is to collude excessively with one aspect of the patient's personality in order to keep other unwelcome problems out of the analysis. If the analyst is open and receptive to the patient's early infantile anxieties, the patient is generally aware of this, and if these anxieties are urgent, he will be able to follow his need to project his anxieties into the analyst for communication, help, and understanding. It is generally only when the analyst is defensive and disturbed by the violence of the patient's reactions that arguments and battles between patient and analyst occur. There is then the danger that long-lasting psychotic transference manifestations may become fixed.

Battles and long-lasting psychotic transference reactions can often be shortened if the analyst understands the most prominent immediate anxiety. In these states the predominant patient anxiety is often the fear that he will drive the analyst mad or that the analyst will drive him mad (Searles 1959a). One can readily understand that in such situations the patient becomes acutely panicky and defensive. It is very reassuring for the patient if the analyst can succeed both in functioning well in his interpretative role and in retaining his quiet, thoughtful state of mind.

I think in all cases of impasse or deadlock in analysis it is essential, first of all, for the analyst to examine very carefully his own feelings and behaviour towards the patient. It is equally important to scrutinize carefully the patient's communications and dreams both for any information that may throw some light on the picture of the analyst which the patient has incorporated and for any hint about collusion between analyst and patient. It is only by the analyst's recognition of his own mistakes and a change in his emotional orientation towards his patient that the patient is allowed to feel freer. It is then that the patient is released from the collusive trap. The impasse can then be lifted fairly quickly.

An analyst stuck in a collusive counter-transference may need

40

some discussion with an uninvolved colleague; such an observer often has a chance to diagnose the problem much more easily. An example of the way an uninvolved observer can help comes from the work of a female analyst, Dr T., who some years ago consulted me about an eighteen-year-old female patient, Lucy. She reported that she was concerned about the discrepancy between Lucy's frequent emphasis that she needed a great deal of help and her simultaneous appearance of being unresponsive and dead, unable to take in more than the minimum of interpretation. It seemed that after any interpretation she became silent, and she generally gave only a few associations to dreams. Dr T. felt very dissatisfied with the progress of the analysis and believed that it had reached an impasse.

Dr T. reported a session after a weekend. Lucy said she had had a very upsetting dream. In the dream she was in a car, her boyfriend was driving, and she sat beside him; on the back seat were two friends – a couple. It was night, and they drove through fields. There were cherry trees full of ripe cherries near the road, and she picked some of them. They soon came to the farm to which the field belonged, and there was a girl of ten. They stopped, and the girl said, 'You should not take the cherries.' 'To taste only,' said Lucy. 'Not even to taste,' answered the girl. Lucy ran to the car, and they drove away. The girl shouted for help, and several people pursued the car. In the end, Lucy found herself in a big country house where she and her boyfriend were caught. A woman dressed in black said prayers as if Lucy were condemned to death. She and her boyfriend were brought to a church, where again there was some kind of ceremony of punishment. This time there were high priests with their mitres.

In a second dream Lucy knew that she had died in a car accident. She rushed home to tell her mother that she was still alive and that she should not worry. At home she found that people were crying, and her corpse lay in state. The people suggested dressing the corpse, and Lucy said she could give some dresses to it. She associated that there had been talk over the weekend of breaking off the relationship with her boyfriend because it had no future. She also discussed a meeting with other friends.

She then reported a third dream. In this dream she was with a man with whom she had more communication than with her boyfriend. She would have liked to be amorous with him but thought she did not know how to go on with it. She was probably 'too little expressive'. There were no associations to this dream. Dr T. interpreted in some detail that she felt that Lucy was secretly stealing from the analysis and using this for other relationships. This was causing here severe guilt and feelings of persecution, making contact with Dr T. impossible.

In listening to the presentation of the material I was impressed that Dr T. had given interpretations which had an accusing and guilt-provoking character. She had not really used the three dreams, although they were vivid and lively as well as revealing. There seemed at that time some collusive relationship going on between patient and analyst which was creating a picture of Dr T. as a woman in black, making funeral speeches. Lucy colluded with this, as in the dream she contributed material – the dress – to the corpse. However, the condemning attitude of Dr T. was reinforced by her not taking up the information tht Lucy had visited the mother – standing for Dr T. – to tell her that she should not worry and that Lucy was alive.

In listening to the details of the dream I had the impression that the secret stealing and the desire to taste the cherries referred to secret sexual wishes, as did her associations to the dream in which she felt sexually attracted to a man-friend but unable to express this to him (as in the analysis). In this way the dreams gave evidence of Lucy's difficulties in expressing her secret lesbian desires in the transference – evidence only slightly obscured by making the analyst into a man. The detailed examination of Lucy's history revealed that her mother had not been able to feed her as a baby, and her father had immediately engaged a wet-nurse, a sensuous woman, who fed the child for at least one year. The father had died in a car accident when Lucy was thirteen, and Lucy had dreamt about a car accident. After her father died, it was revealed that he had had a secret love affair with a woman for the past three years. (The age of the girl in the dream, ten, could thus represent the beginning of the father's love affair.) When the mother found out about this, she became severely depressed. The positive feature in the analysis seemed to be the very open revelation of the whole situation through the dream. Even the lack of associations contributed to the better understanding of the dream. However, it seemed that the analyst considerably colluded with Lucy in repeating the behaviour of the left-out and depressed mother when the secret love affair was revealed. Lucy's secrecy about her attraction to Dr T., which repeated her attraction to the breast of the wet-nurse, contributed to the collusive creation of the deadly punishment situation, in identification with the dead father in the transference.

I have chosen this material to clarify an impasse in the analysis caused by a collusive relationship between analyst and patient. I also wanted to illustrate how it is essential during the analysis to be able to observe one's own tendency to make interpretations which sound accusatory or super-egoish to the patient. Dr T. in this case reported that her discussion with me helped her to understand her critical counter-transference better, and that she was able to feel much better about Lucy. This is, of course, easier when one arrives at a fuller understanding of the patient's history and mental organization. In cases of impasse the detailed examination of analytic material, in order to find possible evidence for a collusive relationship between analyst and patient, seems to be especially important. The re-enactment of the history in the transference impasse is rather common. In this connection it is interesting that Dr T. chose to report the session with the three dreams in which the crucial problems she was having with the patient were so astonishingly clearly highlighted.

Summary

In this chapter I have tried to develop the investigation of transference and counter-transference begun in Chapter 1. The therapeutic function depends on the analyst's openness and sensitivity and his capacity for detailed observation which enables him to follow the patient's material in detail in order to establish the main anxiety at any moment. The analyst has also to know that there is a healthier, sane part in every patient that, if understood, consistently tries to communicate to the therapist the predicament the patient finds himself in.

Briefly to repeat the main points:

1 The analyst will be placed via the transference in many roles by the patient, not just the role of father or mother or good or bad person or infantile parts of the self. The analyst should perceive the changing role which is often indicated by his projection but not act this role out with the patient.
2 Analysts tend at times to get caught up in a certain way of thinking which really implies a not thinking. This leads to interpreting, for example, envy all the time when something else is more pressing. The persistent interpretation of weekend or separation anxiety, when the problem for the patient is the analyst's existence or non-existence in the sessions, is another example.
3 Sometimes analysts will be insensitive to criticism from their patients and in so being will miss significant communications.
4 Sometimes analysts will be blind to the patient's tendency to get them to collude with their ways of thinking and being.

These four points, summarized here, are illustrated at least once in later chapters, beginning with Chapter 3.

Note

1 Freud has said that traumatized patients respond better to treatment than those with constitutionally determined conditions. My own experience confirms Freud's statement. It is, however, inevitable that the severely traumatized patient who has to relive early infantile states in the transference will have to get in touch with severe psychotic anxieties which tend occasionally to get out of control. This may temporarily cause a confusion that is difficult to deal with. In the traumatized, deprived patient, psychotic anxieties often continue to exist in their original form. The early infantile anxieties were often severely exaggerated by the traumatic situation, particularly if it involved early childhood separation lasting for years, starvation, illness, or maltreatment.

3

Breakdown of communication between patient and analyst

In Chapter 2 I briefly drew attention to some of the things which can go wrong to undermine the analyst's therapeutic efforts. In this chapter I want to illustrate some of these difficulties more thoroughly by examining in more detail some of the material about the patient, Sylvia, mentioned in Chapter 2 and presented in one of my seminars. The analyst presenting the case had previous psychiatric hospital experience but had not previously attempted a psychoanalysis of a psychotic patient. She got into considerable difficulties with Sylvia's treatment, and the patient eventually broke it off. In the seminar we came to be aware that this outcome occurred partly because the analyst had not obtained a clear enough assessment of the patient and so had not arranged adequate support for herself and her patient, but also because the analyst was not able to bring the therapeutic factors in the treatment into effect. Specifically she became preoccupied with her own line of thinking and was unable to hear the patient's warnings that she was pursuing a wrong line. To illustrate what I think happened I shall interpose reports about Sylvia's sessions (made by her analyst, Dr M., and printed in italic type) with my own comments printed in roman type.

'In May 1974 Sylvia was twenty-seven and had come five years ago, with her husband and first child, who was then six months old, to England. In the first consultation she told me that one month before Christmas 1973 she mentally collapsed and could not do anything. She suddenly had a feeling that she was never going to see her parents again and there would be no more aeroplanes, so that she felt it was like "dealing with the dead". She first attributed her breakdown to the fuel crisis in England. Only later on did she *remember that her husband had gone away on business for one day, and this had disturbed her to such an extent that it precipitated her breakdown. Apparently her husband had never been away from her for one whole day before this crisis arose. This short separation from her husband made her aware of her incapacity to keep a good ir.ner picture of the parents alive; her inner world was dead and empty; there was nothing at all that she could do in life.*

'In the first analytic session Sylvia seemed to feel rather better. She was lying on the couch and she talked quite well. However, in the second week she had a disturbing experience after seeing a sad African play. She and her husband had gone to a restaurant after the play and she described how the paintings all around the wall had represented starving people, and everybody in the rest~urant was starving also. She felt she ought to do more about starving people. She reported a dream which was full of people starving and then she was stabbed from behind.'

- Sylvia was clearly hallucinating in the restaurant. The dream also communicates severe psychotic anxieties. It sometimes takes quite a time before one knows how to interpret a psychotic dream to a patient. Both the account about the restaurant and the dream indicate that Sylvia is communicating psychotic experiences. They also indicate the extent to which Sylvia feels not only guilty but persecuted by her psychotic state. The complete inability to deal with separation and her obsession about starvation imply that Sylvia functions on a very early infantile level. Her terrible emptiness and starvation are projected into the external environment, which then is highly distorted. Her severe paranoid anxiety indicates that she is constantly threatened by the deathly return of her projections.

Dr M. discussed her counter-transference in those early sessions and reported that she found it difficult to remember or record the sessions. She felt that the material was too fragmented. She also described that she had a feeling that she had to bring the patient into the consulting room with her eyes and watch her go out of the room as if there was some need to maintain contact through the eyes. Sylvia lay on the coach and looked at Dr M. after the session. She then went towards the door, turned round, and looked at Dr M. again.

- In listening to the report one receives the impression that Sylvia feels in a very precarious state. She makes Dr M. feel aware that she needs Dr M.'s perception (i.e. her eyes), not only to perceive

46

her own actions but to guide them and to provide the perception of what is going on in her mind. She is unable to see it herself.

First seminar: session A

One session reported by the analyst and discussed in the first seminar will now be described in some detail. Although I have given part of this session in Chapter 2, I want to describe it in more detail here because of the clarity of Sylvia's communication. It highlights Dr M.'s difficulty in understanding her language and form of communication. Another problem we notice is that Sylvia functions on an early infantile level and, therefore, cannot deal with time in the manner her analyst expects. Although she cannot apparently think clearly, Sylvia is aware that she can communicate with feelings. Her language is highly personal and communicates her non-verbal experiences.

Dr M.: 'In the second week of the analysis Sylvia was suddenly unable to open the door of my flat. This is done by pushing open the door after I have used an electric buzzer in response to Sylvia's ringing the bell. The patient did not come in. I had to go to the door to let her in. During the session I was also preoccupied with the fact that my car was absent, and feared this could cause anxiety to Sylvia. It was a Wednesday, my car was not in front of the house, and I wondered if Sylvia knew what my car looked like and whether its absence might provoke her overwhelming fear of being left.

'In the session Sylvia came about five minutes early. There was a very short silence, and then she started to talk: "A thing that still worries me is my husband going away. I do not know where it will be, or how long it will be, it may be somewhere very remote, there is nothing definite – and there is nothing definite." Here she makes a long pause and then she says, "Anyway, this is what I am worrying about." I responded, "You appear to be living in a state of uncertainty with a feeling of dread hanging over you."'

- This is a straightforward acknowledgement by Dr M. of the patient's emotional state and does not introduce any misunderstanding. Sylvia said that she actually agreed with her.

'Sylvia replied with something which I do not recall, but I remember my interpretation, namely that Sylvia's anxiety seems to join up in her mind with the weekend.'

- In other words the analyst interprets Sylvia's anxieties as if she had

47

wanted to say, 'It is Wednesday today and it is already in my mind that the weekend is approaching and then on Saturday what will it be, where will Dr M. be, what will Dr M. be doing, and when will she come back to me?'

'Sylvia then said, "It is important for people I am with, whereas at one time I used to make comparisons about how people coped. Now it is the way things feel and how I feel." I interpreted that this meant that Sylvia was very much influenced by her feelings of what she believes other people to be feeling. Sylvia reported, "Yes, I must be very careful if somebody gets flustered. Then I have to be calm."'

- It seems to me that from the beginning of the session Sylvia attempted to bring her feelings of being at a loss and emotionally remote from Dr M. right into the session. First there was the non-verbal communication about the doorbell. Then, when Dr M. started to talk about her fear of the analyst's absence over the weekend. Sylvia immediately corrected her as if she wanted to say, 'No, I am not talking about actual separations now but I am talking about the feeling of loss and distance which occurs when I am actually with you. Dr M.' I would say that she tries to make clear that she is competitive about Dr M.'s difficulties in coping with her. She has observed the difficulties which Dr M. has in understanding those of her feelings which disturb her, and reports this. When Dr M. replies to the patient's very personal statement without relating it to herself, however, Sylvia becomes more explicit, attempting to say, 'Yes, I am influenced by your feelings. I must be very careful to keep calm if somebody gets disturbed [i.e. flustered]. Like you. Dr M.'

Dr M. reported that she was unclear what Sylvia meant and so she asked Sylvia, how did she feel now? Sylvia gave a little laugh and said, 'Well, actually I am feeling rather flustered.' She gave another little laugh and said, 'I do not want to annihilate you.' Dr M. replied to this interchange by saying that it seemed as if the interpretation (that she might have been worried that Dr M. might not be here over the weekend) had upset Sylvia. Sylvia replied to this, 'This takes me back to Monday, today, and wearing black.' (Dr M. explained to the seminar that Sylvia had reported in the Tuesday session that she had been rather disconcerted by the fact that Dr M. was wearing a black blouse on Monday. In fact Dr M. had been wearing a white shirt.) Dr M. therefore interpreted that it seemed that if she interpreted anything to Sylvia about her being absent it immediately recalled to Sylvia's mind the anxiety about the analyst dying. Sylvia feels confused when she comes to the session and she is not sure if Dr M. will be there. Dr M. added, 'Perhaps you are not quite sure if my car is here or not.' Sylvia answered, 'Oh no, I have given up about the car.' Then she said emphatically, 'It is when I ring the bell I feel a bit worried; the time between ringing the bell and you pressing the buzzer to let me in, that is when I feel a bit worried.'

- Dr M. missed the meaning of Sylvia's statement that she has to keep calm if Dr M. gets flustered. Sylvia is frank enough to admit that she is now getting flustered. She tries to reassure Dr M., however, that she does not want to destroy (annihilate) her with her critical observations. At this point Dr M. seems to have perceived that she has upset Sylvia. But she still interprets that Sylvia cannot stand being reminded of weekend separations. In fact in the session what is disturbing Sylvia is her analyst's state of mind. Sylvia's reference to her analyst wearing a black blouse could convey that she saw her analyst as being in a black, depressed state of mind today as well as on Monday. However, Dr M. continues to talk about separations and about the absent car. At this point Sylvia seems to get fed up: 'I have given up about the car.' She then makes a touching statement about the anxiety she experiences when she tries to communicate her feelings to Dr M. and has to wait until she is open to her communication. She has verbalized the non-verbal content of the beginning of the session: 'Will what I say ring a bell to Dr M.'s mind, or not?' In this session, as sometimes happens, the analyst could not respond to Sylvia.

Dr M. reported that at this stage she felt somewhat confused. She was aware that she had made a mistake by introducing the car because Sylvia suddenly talked about another car, a Citroën, which was not the analyst's car. Sylvia had said that she was sure that the Citroën was there that day. (In fact it was not.)

- In other words, in response to the analyst talking about problems which the patient experiences as non-existent, the patient now talks about problems which do not exist.

Sylvia now started to talk about her anxiety that she might wipe Dr M. out. She said, 'I used to be very complaining about having a bad memory, and it seems that having a bad memory is really wiping things out. That worries me and therefore I put it out of my mind.' She continued, 'This has something to do with my mother. I do not know if she wipes me out or my problems or it is I who wipe out my mother and my mother's problems.'

49

After a pause she continued, 'Or, is it my problem?' Dr M. interpreted, 'It is my presence and my absence which seems to be the problem for you and when it gets too worrying you have to wipe it out.' Sylvia then spoke about it having to do with getting old. She said that her age showed in her face and she worried about that very much. She mentioned that she thought she was already twenty-eight now and that her husband had questioned her about making a mistake in her own age. Dr M. felt these ideas were related to the patient's fear of Dr M. getting old and dying, and interpreted on these lines.

- Making herself a year older may have to do with the fear of the analyst's death but it also probably has to do with Dr M.'s persistently interpreting separation. Separation must be an anxiety of an older child (perhaps at one year of age), but at this moment in the session Sylvia probably experiences herself feeling much smaller. She is lost and unable to deal with time. She is anxious about something to do with Dr M.'s incapacity to understand her because she talks again about wiping out Dr M., albeit by talking about her mother: 'I do not know whether my mother wipes me out or my problems or whether I am the one who wipes out my mother and my mother's problems.' She now seems to fear that Dr M. is causing her (Sylvia's) incapacity to deal with problems by attacking her state of mind with her problems. But Sylvia also wonders whether she is attacking Dr M.'s mind with her problems. In the end she leaves it open: 'Or is it my problem?' In this entire communication one is struck that the patient's capacity to consider and to think is still present, but Dr M. continues having difficulties in following. One realizes that it is not Dr M.'s physical presence but her simultaneous mental absence which causes worry to the patient. It is this which makes her concerned about Dr M. getting senile or too old; she therefore becomes afraid of identifying with the old and senile analyst. But I think that the question as to whether she is maybe a year older than she in fact is has another meaning as well. In this whole session Sylvia has to be more reasonable and understanding than Dr M. She has to be more grown up, and I think this is being expressed in the fact that she calls herself twenty–eight instead of twenty–seven. She tries to convey. 'I can't be a baby, I have to try to be a bit older.'

  Dr M. seemed certain that Sylvia's anxiety was created by her physical absence (the coming weekend and the missing car), and this made Sylvia afraid that Dr M. might die. So, when Dr M. interprets this anxiety, Sylvia again very desperately tries to bring Dr M. back to the point. She says, as it were. 'I feel unreal, I am waiting at the door and I have to look at your [the analyst's] name-tag under the bell.' Dr M. interprets that Sylvia needs evidence that her analyst really exists, that she is here with Sylvia at this moment. This misunderstanding seems to be too much for Sylvia; she becomes silent. Dr M.'s suggestion that Sylvia needs evidence that she exists and that she is really there with her provokes silence because there is no evidence that Dr M. is mentally present. This is what Sylvia is worried about.

Dr M. broke the silence to ask Sylvia what she was thinking about. She replied she was thinking about the car. A car had cut in front of her one day and had parked across the drive. 'It must belong to somebody in here [Dr M.'s house]. Somebody who owns a garage.' Dr M. interpreted this to mean that Sylvia thought she would really like to be in the position of possessing Dr M., which would enable her to go in and out of her without any difficulty.

• In talking about the car which cuts right across her path Sylvia is communicating that it is Dr M. who today constantly cuts right across her way of thinking and feeling. When she says this car is parked in 'your' – the analyst's – garage she says the problem belongs to Dr M. This communication is again misunderstood by Dr M., who makes a symbolic interpretation about Sylvia intruding into Dr M. and possessing her.

The most striking feature in this session is the persistence of Sylvia's capacity to communicate repeatedly some of the problems which interfere in the patient–analyst relationship. One suspects from her reference to her mother that this problem may well repeat certain difficulties the patient and her mother had. Most psychotic patients project their feelings and anxieties very intensely into the analyst when they verbally or non-verbally communicate. This generally helps the analyst to understand the patient better. But if the analyst cannot cope with the patient's projections, she tends to get out of touch. This can happen in spite of the fact that in each session Dr M. has reported very sensitively about the patient–analyst interaction. In this session she was clearly out of touch and did not notice Sylvia's efforts to help to re-establish an understanding.

First seminar: Session B

Turning now to the next session, reported in the same seminar, one wonders whether the patient will become withdrawn or whether she will be able to continue to make her communication to Dr M. still clearer.

Sylvia started the next session by complaining that her mother rang her up but did not speak directly to her but to the au pair girl. Dr M. replied that it seems Sylvia thinks that there is no proper communication between the two of them and is complaining that the analyst is not in touch with her. Dr M., like her mother, is the one who is talking to somebody else, not to her. It is Dr M. who does not seem to be aware of her so she cannot feel that she matters to Dr M. Dr M. also interpreted that Sylvia is saying that Dr M. should put herself out sufficiently to understand and really to know what she is feeling.

• The patient's communication about her mother seem suddenly to have brought Dr M. into full contact with Sylvia, and she interprets sensitively and beautifully. The interpretation is particularly interesting, because, without any supervision, Dr M. fully sees and interprets what she missed the day before. However, there is no evidence that she relates Sylvia's complaint to the previous session, in which Sylvia had good reason for complaining. In my view such a link would be essential.

Sylvia went on to complain about her mother, who did not tell her that she was going away. Sylvia also said, 'I myself have been spending quite a lot of time with the baby but not so much with the older girl and it is from the baby that the jealousy seems to come.' Dr M. said that she felt confused about this statement.

• It seems to me that in the above Sylvia states that she has experienced herself over the weekend as the baby. Her problem of jealousy comes from her baby self, and this is why she cannot use her adult mind and feels just left and lost over the weekend. She does not understand, as a baby, that Dr M. has told her that she is leaving her over the weekend. She describes the awful experience of being suddenly left as a baby. What disturbs her most is that being left seems to come completely out of the blue. Neither her mother nor her analyst ever tell her that they are going away. This is the experience which Sylvia wanted to get across to Dr M., and I think she conveys her early infantile experiences about her mother's (and her analyst's) presence and absence very clearly. It is interesting that this experience is mainly conveyed through words, but the words convey feelings rather than verbal thought. In this connection I believe that it is essential that the analyst's interpretations convey, very clearly, the feelings which the patient communicates and also the state of the patient's self. It is necessary to convey to such a patient that she has communicated that she is a baby who does not know about time and therefore cannot think about time. The analyst's acknowledgement and understanding of such communications by the patient can diminish the patient's feeling of being isolated and lost so that gradually some restructuring of the personality can take place.

Third seminar: session C

I shall now discuss some material from the third seminar about this patient, which took place after the summer holidays. In the summer term Sylvia's mental state deteriorated, and during the last week of the holidays she almost completely retreated to bed. She found it virtually impossible to cope with looking after her children and her home. In the second seminar, immediately after the summer holidays, it became clear that Dr M. could not cope with the situation without the help of a psychiatrist. Luckily a member of the seminar, who was a consultant at a psychiatric hospital in London, offered to help, by seeing Sylvia and making her an in-patient. This did not solve the problem, but at least some continuity was possible. At first Sylvia did not want to go into hospital; but soon her husband insisted that, as she refused to get up and look after anything or anybody at home, she should. So when the seminar met for the third time to discuss her case (after the summer holidays) we had a very detailed report from the consultant about the management problem as well as the analytic material of the sessions.

Before the holidays, as I have mentioned, Sylvia presented a very early infantile transference, largely based on her desire for Dr M. to be in touch with her and to hold her together. During the holidays it seems that her self or ego fragmented, and the fragments of the various parts of her personality were projected into different objects in her environment. After the holidays, therefore, her previous difficulties in coping with her inner state had changed into difficulties in being able to function at all. This was accompanied by an almost complete lack of concern about the problem. Through the fragmentation of her ego she had lost her capacity to perceive what was happening to her and also her capacity to think. She was therefore, almost entirely dependent on Dr M. to bring her fragmented self together. Her complaint before the holiday had been that she could not cope with having to be an adult. Now the predominant anxiety was that she did not have a functioning ego. Her anxiety about this was projected almost entirely into her environment. This was the reason why her husband could not cope when his wife retreated from reality and withdrew into bed. She could not come to the analysis from her home, and so hospitalization was arranged. However, from the hospital she came by herself to her analysis and missed sessions only occasionally.

The hospital consultant present in the session reported that it was amazing how gay and active this patient had appeared when she was in hospital, as if there was nothing wrong with her. His observations confirmed how completely she denied or projected her awareness of illness. Indeed the hospital staff felt that she was just a spoilt child who should be smacked, and reacted to her with resentment. The consultant commented that he was impressed by Sylvia's lack of insight and any relationship to the analysis. He felt that there seemed to be an enormous destructive power expressed by Sylvia's behaviour, because the gaiety had a very manic and destructive character and seemed to lack any concern for anybody but herself. He had also had an interview with Sylvia's father and he was impressed by the omnipotent attitude which the father adopted. He seemed to blame Sylvia's difficulties entirely on her husband. I shall now discuss Dr M.'s report of a session during this period of the analysis.

Dr M. reported first that at the beginning of the last week Sylvia had been making a number of bitter accusations against her husband and her marriage. In the session Sylvia had come from the hospital arriving fifteen minutes early. She said that she had planned previously that she might go home for a while after the session. She then continued, 'I don't feel very positively about it. I don't feel positive about anything. My father and Peter [her husband] were at the hospital yesterday and my father told Peter that he blames him entirely for what has happened. He simply would not hear that I had any problems before.' Dr M. replied, 'There is now open antagonism between your father and your husband.'

● In other words, Dr M. responds to Sylvia's communication as a factual statement about reality. Any deeper meaning in Sylvia's communication is ignored.

Sylvia said, 'Yes, my father is determined that Peter must change his attitude towards me. He says if I cannot manage here [in England] without my parents then they will come and live here. It makes me want to scream.' Dr M. replied, 'It seems you feel that it would not help you. You feel

54

overwhelmed either by what is going on inside you or by being taken over by people outside you.' Dr M. did not remember how Sylvia replied.

- I think that Sylvia here makes it clear that her denial and omnipotent destructiveness are projected into her father. He acts as if he were her destructive omnipotent self who attacks and blames her husband entirely for the failure of the marriage. In fact the husband had supported and arranged the treatment – something not appreciated or defended by Sylvia, or the father, at this moment. In my view it was essential for Dr M. to interpret the splitting and projection of Sylvia's destructive omnipotent attitude at this point. She had made her father the omnipotent destroyer, and this reinforced her own omnipotent state and in no way supported a sane dependent self and her need for treatment. Dr M. is warned that the violent attack which threatens to break up the marriage, the connection between her and her husband, is also threatening to break up her perceptive capacity. Her perception is the link which could help her to find a way about the struggle inside herself: between her destructive madness and her sanity. This would explain why Sylvia feels she wants to scream if her parents are determined to come to England. If her husband, who represents her own insight, is destroyed by the attack of her parents (who stand for her destructive self), then the patient feels entirely alone. She becomes a completely helpless baby who can only scream in fear and anger. If my perception of this process is correct it would have been essential to look in the material for any evidence of the infantile relationship and how this was experienced by Sylvia, at that moment.

After a pause Sylvia said 'A few weeks ago when I went to the hospital, Erica [the previous au pair] had come back to us for a few weeks from Germany to look after the children. She has gone now. There is someone else there now. My father said he hated Erica. I suppose it's got something to do with Erica being German, but they [the parents] have been back and forth to Germany often. What is the point of him saying that? He should be able to control himself. It makes me very angry.'

- Now at this moment Erica, who helped Sylvia to look after her children (who in their turn represent Sylvia's infantile self), stands for Dr M., who has returned from her holiday. Sylvia recognizes the irrationality of the attack on Erica, standing for Dr M., and she is angry with the omnipotent father who attacks her husband and also Dr M. Both have to look after her infantile self (the children)

55

at this moment. Had Dr M. interpreted along these lines it would have been possible for her to strengthen the sane part of the patient defending Dr M. and the analytic situation against the omnipotent attack. However, Dr M. did not interpret very clearly.

Sylvia continued, 'I am worried that things have become too bad between Peter and myself. I seem to repeat what my parents did. It is no good for the children.'

- I think that this statement of Sylvia's is simply a confirmation that her parents' quarrels represent an attack on the analysis. This is no good for her infantile self or for her sanity.

After some other communications Sylvia explained further: 'When I met Peter he seemed to belong to a family that got on well with each other and it seemed I wanted to belong to it and to feel secure. I am the one weak link in the chain. The children are going to see other mothers cope. I turned away from my mother, and that caused her pain.'

- This communication is perhaps rather more difficult to understand. It seems that Sylvia may have been thinking of her originally united family as a way of expressing something about her lost coherent self. A coherent self was something she envied and wanted to be part of. But in trying to achieve such coherence she aggressively turned against her husband, who now stands for her own mother. Now she wants to turn away from Dr M., and this, she admits, is causing her husband and Dr M. pain. In other words, she is able to indicate that her positive self is unfortunately the weak link in her ego. This material is very touching and demonstrates, I feel, how clearly in such a destructive manic patient the awareness of her fundamental problems are presented, if one listens to her very carefully.

In her next communication Sylvia says, 'I feel guilty about hurting everyone and then I do not seem to be able to take in what is good. There seems to be so much good and it all turns bad.'

- In other words, Sylvia admits her anxiety about her destructive self and says that it is not so much Dr M. leaving her which worries her but the fact that she is distressed about being so destructive and evil. She hurts everybody so that the good things given to her turn bad. She has begun to realize that it is this she feels guilty about. In the material which followed Sylvia

56

complained that she had never been able to think. In other words, she became aware that her destructive attacks on her objects and her sane self had not only weakened her capacity to take things in but had also interfered with her capacity for thinking.

Dr M. acknowledged Sylvia's anxiety about her difficulties in thinking, but Sylvia then burst out, 'I must find some kind of logic.'

• At that moment, after her awareness of her aggressive attacks and the weakness of her positive links, Sylvia herself stresses that she has lost her capacity for common sense and logical thinking. She appeals to Dr M. to provide or restore to her the parts of herself which can think clearly and have common sense.

In the remaining sessions that we discussed in the seminars Sylvia continued to communicate very clearly in spite of the deterioration of her condition and the severe increase of splitting of the self, which occurred when she got rid of her anxious state of mind and projected it into her husband. However, when she did not improve in the analysis after many months, her husband left her. This was most unfortunate, because he had been the most stable influence in her life. With this deterioration in her environment eventually the patient stopped the analysis.[1]

Discussion

I hope, despite the truncation of the material I have been able to present, to have illustrated how, if the analyst is watching and listening carefully to the patient's material, he can visualize the structure of the psychotic patient's self and her object relations. It would then be possible for him to bring together in his interpretations the different aspects of the self which it is essential for the patient to understand.

I believe that it is the analyst's function with patients like Sylvia to interpret in such a way that the patient realizes, through the analyst's communications, the logic of her anxieties and conflicts. The treatment of psychotic patients is difficult but often rewarding for the patient and also for the analyst. I have tried to illustrate how the patient communicates but also to show the difficulties an analyst is faced with in understanding the communications of a psychotic patient during analysis. I have argued none the less, that this psychotic patient was able to bring her problems clearly to the analysis, and therefore hope that the example will help all of us understand and learn how psychotic patients can express themselves clearly in spite of the severity of their illness.

The analyst's main mistakes were, initially, her insensitivity to the patient's primitive anxiety of feeling utterly lost and unable to cope. The patient conveys these feelings again and again, but the analyst holds on to her belief that the patient suffers from separation anxiety, in spite of the patient's energetic protests and criticisms that this is wrong. This is expressed by the patient in symbolic language but very powerfully. Sylvia, who suffered from primitive anxieties about being lost, was particularly in need of being helped and understood by her analyst; it cannot therefore be surprising that her condition deteriorated.

During the long summer holiday Sylvia's self disintegrated, and she projected her anxieties and inability to cope into her husband, who then was overwhelmed with anxiety and could not cope himself. In the last session which I selected Sylvia illustrated the various aspects of her broken-up self and indicated where they were located. For example, the omnipotent destructive self was projected into her father, who laid all the blame for the patient's illness on her husband. The good analyst/mother whom the patient had lost appeared again as the au pair Erica, who had returned from Germany. She was obviously welcome to the patient but was utterly rejected by the omnipotent destructive father. Sylvia herself was left depleted as being only a weak link who could not integrate anything, while the husband presented the united family she wanted to be part of but which she enviously attacked. She made a strong appeal in the session for the analyst to link the split-up parts of herself together to re-establish her mind and acquire a self which might cope again with life, her marriage, her children, and her problems. The analyst failed to understand this important appeal by the patient to serve as a container and to help integrate her split-up self.

It was therefore inevitable that Sylvia would sooner or later stop treatment, which was very sad for Dr M. There are so many psychotic patients who need analysis or analytic-orientated psycho-therapy and there are only very few analysts sufficiently trained to treat them. In spite of Dr M.'s lack of experience in treating psychotic patients she presented the material of Sylvia very clearly in the seminar and was aware of her difficulties in understanding the patient. She obviously wanted to help the patient as much as she could. She had been landed with her and she had not felt it right to send Sylvia to somebody else too quickly. However, this patient needed a very special holding environment which could be created only by an analyst who could hold the material of the patient very clearly and logically in his or her mind. The analyst would also need to give it back to the patient in such a way that she could follow the logic of her own way of thinking and feeling and also understand the anxiety preventing her from holding on to the logical state of mind. An analyst wanting to treat psychotic patients needs additional training, and sometimes this may take several years. There are few analysts who find it easy to understand the psychotic patient.

Dr M.'s report is so interesting and useful to all learning to understand psychotic patients that we must be very grateful to her for allowing us to include it in this book. The difficulties illustrate how analysts who want to treat psychotic patients may need considerable help in understanding the peculiarities of the psychotic transference and the special way of talking which these patients use. Psychotic patients do sometimes talk in a very obscure way and hide much of what is going on in them. But this was not the case in the sessions presented in this chapter. Sylvia's communications were, to my mind, illustrative of the characteristic way psychotic patients try to make themselves understood. A sensitive counter-transference often helps the analyst to get quickly in touch with such patients, and this type of patient is generally happy when the analyst understands what they mean, which allows the theme of the analysis to develop. When the analyst makes some mistakes by misunderstanding the patient's appeal they quickly show what was wrong once, or even twice, but then they may get confused, much more than the patient who is presented here. Even supervision can be difficult when a severe confusion has arisen, until the supervisor can trace the point where things went wrong. The inexperienced therapist generally cannot find his own mistake, and the confusion may go on for many months with only from time to time a reminder in a word or sentence of the session where the confusion has occurred. In order to remedy a mistake, *one generally has to go back* to the point where the confusion or mistake by the analyst occurred, even when the analysis has been stuck for three to six months. Many psychotic patients do not bear a grudge if the mistake is remedied.

There is a great deal of difference between a patient communicating clearly with symbolic language and the confused way of talking of a psychotic patient who has lost his way in the analysis. This has to be carefully studied and observed. It is also very important to differentiate that part of a patient's confusion which is part of a negative therapeutic reaction following on progress, from the confusion which follows from the analyst's failure to understand. Dr M. had made brave efforts to cope with Sylvia, but the task was too difficult for her. It generally takes a long time for analysts to become effective in the treatment of psychotic patients; but there are, of course, analysts or therapists who are particularly gifted in treating psychotic patients, and we have also to admit that there are limits to what one can teach. Thus we can sometimes learn more from the mistakes of a carefully reported case, which reveals the mistakes in the analysis, than from a brilliant report of an analyst who implies that he has understood almost everything.

Note

1 It is in my experience important and necessary, before treatment starts, to make arrangements for hospitalization in all cases where there is some suspicion that one is dealing with a borderline psychotic patient. This will save a great deal of unnecessary anxiety and hardship, and difficulties in looking after the patient at home if a psychotic state becomes manifest. At the very least, some arrangements or contact with the patient's doctor must be made as soon as possible. This is necessary not only for the sake of the patient but also to preserve the analyst's peace of mind. He cannot devote himself fully to treatment if he has to worry unduly about what happens to the patient after he leaves the analyst's consulting room.

In my experience it is also important and necessary in treating psychotic patients to have as detailed a history as possible before the patient starts his analysis. This is because acute psychotic patients generally do not report historical factors, and their past and present can become easily confused.

I also try to assess at the beginning how the patient deals with the external environment, how this is perceived, and how external stimuli are reacted to, distorted, or denied. Even if the patient has a family who look after him he is often unable to cope with everyday experiences during certain phases of his illness, and severe anxiety may be aroused in those who are close to the patient. As we have seen in Sylvia, we can often notice a shift of the patient's anxiety about not being able to cope with problems of everyday life to it being the patient's relatives who become severely anxious and who then feel that they cannot cope with the patient at home any more. This frequently leads to demands for hospitalization, which is often difficult to arrange satisfactorily at short notice.

PART THREE

The influence of narcissism
on the analyst's task

4

The narcissistic omnipotent character structure: a case of chronic hypochondriasis

I described in Chapter 1 how I came to identify a mode of relating which I called narcissistic omnipotent object relations. To try to make this concept more accessible I want to use this chapter to give a detailed report of a patient, Adam, whom I treated many years ago. His life history and personality structure were deeply influenced by narcissistic omnipotent object relations which apparently originated in earliest infancy in the feeding relationship to his mother. Adam could, therefore, be described as a patient with a narcissistic omnipotent character structure. The material from his analysis which I shall set out demonstrates the way narcissistic omnipotent object relations function in analysis, the influence of envy and defences against it, and its relationships to the formation of negative therapeutic reactions, hypochondriacal anxieties, and delusions about sexual identity, all of which were particularly pronounced with this patient.[1]

Adam's history

Before he began treatment with me, Adam had received many years of psychotherapeutic, mainly psychoanalytical, treatment with several analysts in his own country. He suffered particularly from hypochondriacal anxieties related to fears of cancer of the throat, stomach, rectum, penis, and heart. Two years before he started treatment with me he had an acute intestinal obstruction and was hospitalized for about a fortnight. He had psychotherapy at that time, but nevertheless for several days it was feared that he might need an operation. Eventually his bowels started to function again. Adam reported that the intestinal obstruction followed a separation from a girlfriend on whom he was sexually very dependent. During the third year of analysis with me, after a long hypochondriacal preoccupation with his stomach and constant speculations about what food agreed or disagreed with him, his pains in his abdomen became so severe that his general practitioner sent him to be X-rayed. A duodenal ulcer was diagnosed by a specialist after a very thorough examination (which is particularly important in the treatment of hypochondriacal patients) and subsequently treated. The specialist managed to treat Adam with a minimum of fuss; he ordered a light diet and frequent meals, and under this scheme the severe pains improved fairly quickly. However, his hypochondriacal preoccupations with the ulcer and his fear of stomach cancer would return from time to time.

Adam was born on the Continent. An important feature was that he seemed to have been very much attached to his mother as a baby. She appears to have been a good but anxious mother. He cried very insistently as a baby when he had to sleep in his cot. Eventually, the only way his mother could find to satisfy him was to take him into her bed, where he went to sleep happily next to her skin. His father had to travel a great deal and so was frequently absent from home. However, even when he was present he was apparently not able to help his wife to cope with this very determined but also anxious baby. Adam was breast-fed, but when his mother tried to wean him after one year she was unsuccessful. He was at least two years old before she succeeded.

Between the ages of eight and twelve, Adam seemed to have been periodically severely mentally ill, suffering from visual hallucinations and delusions. He remembered that for a long time he believed that he was a train. During the treatment, he occasionally had visual hallucinations. When he was eighteen he developed severe hypo-chondriacal anxieties about cancer in his throat. Very soon afterwards his father, who had a good singing voice, started to develop cancer of the throat, was operated on, but died several months later. His father's death from a disease which was identical with Adam's hypochondriacal fears greatly increased his idea that he had projected his own fears of cancer into his father's throat.

Adam had one brother, two years older, to whom he was very much attached. In his dreams, there were many references to a homosexual relationship with him, but there was no evidence that this sexual relationship was ever manifest.

64

Working through oral envy by analysing the transference

Adam had innumerable relationships with girls but only rarely did he fall in love. Generally speaking it seemed that his constant sexual relations represented a projection of his anxiety, madness, and sexuality as well as a repetition of his early erotic relationship to his mother's body. During the analysis Adam had many girlfriends and changed them frequently. After about two years' treatment he gave up an intense relationship with a schizoid girl who had similarities to him and became interested in a girl who seemed to him to be more beautiful, pure, and lovable than any other he had met before. He wanted to approach her slowly, to allow feelings of love to develop, but then he lost control and tried to seduce her very quickly. She became afraid and withdrew from him, and he realized that his physically and mentally seductive and overpowering attempts had been the cause of her becoming frightened and wanting to turn away from him. He felt guilty and depressed about the possibility of losing her, but eventually after writing several urgent letters, to which she did not reply, he managed to get in touch with her again and felt relieved. He said that at times he was very concerned that she did not respond as much to him as other girls had done. He feared she could not show enough feelings and he described her as dead. During this time his bowel symptoms, pains, and severe constipation, which would flare up from time to time, grew very much worse. During one session Adam became convinced that he was suffering from cancer of the bowel. He gradually worked himself up to a state of absolute terror and panic and then felt hopeless. He almost screamed that he had to run away from everything, from where he lived and from the analysis. He felt convinced he would break down mentally and physically and that he would be driven mad. He was intensely restless on the couch. This panic was very impressive, and I felt in my counter-transference that something very overpowering was happening. I realized that I had to understand something fundamental, and quickly, because the situation seemed to be getting out of hand, and he was becoming deluded. I therefore interpreted then that Adam believed that he had really devoured and killed his girlfriend through his greedy, sexually overpowering approach and as a result he believed that she was concretely dead inside him. I related to this his fear of cancer, namely that he feared that he had her dead body inside him which now became terribly frightening and persecuting and which he could not expel. I suggested that the same conviction was also related to me. He felt I was swallowed up by him as well and thus no longer able to move and function. Adam responded to these ideas with silence, but the restlessness almost completely disappeared. I had a strong feeling that the interpretation had touched him, a sign that I was experienced as still alive and functioning.

The day after this very stormy session he admitted he felt a little better. He realized that he had been overwhelmed by his panic. Then he told me a dream. He was travelling with a girl in a train. Suddenly the train left the rails and it was violently shaking, swaying from right to left and left to right; he was aware that the train could tumble over any second. However, he kept the balance, and nothing frightful happened, apart from the train being derailed. Adam then described how during the last few days he had been running up- and downstairs in his home, stopping and starting again. Somebody living next to him had become concerned about his sanity, and this had increased his own anxiety.

Adam told me that the train and the problem connected with it must have something to do with his bowels because he still felt that they did not move and that something very disturbing was going on inside him – as if, like the train in the dream, he had brought his bowels to a standstill. He explained that some years before he had had a complete stoppage of the bowels and at that time there was a danger that he would have to be operated on. Adam was sure that during his childhood, particularly from the age of eight to twelve, he must at times have been psychotic. He remembered that he often felt he was a train and ran round the house stopping and starting again and making noises like a train. He then associated to ideas about how he felt he could put both his stomach and bowels out of action by making his food pass through his stomach and bowels either too quickly or too slowly so that the food could not be properly digested.

I tried to show him the consequences of his feeling that he could omnipotently control entirely what was going on inside him. It interfered with the working not only of his bowels but of his mind. He was then no longer able to think and function, and felt he could be mad. Moreover, I said, this process was linked with what he felt he had done to his girlfriend and to me inside him. He felt he controlled her as well as me, and this meant we were dead inside him. Also, in the dream, he claimed that he had re-established the balance (his sanity) single-handed. There had been only a slight deviation (derailment), which he felt as not dangerous. However, it seemed clear from what had occurred yesterday that it was in fact my interpretation of his dangerous way of incorporating (devouring) me and his girlfriend that had saved his sanity. He had, apparently, been amazed that in spite of his overwhelming behaviour I could keep my balance; but, as so frequently before, he had then denied it. He did this by taking over my identity as an understanding and balanced person, enabling him to believe that he had done all the balancing and life-saving work himself. I suggested that he had found it particularly humiliating and frightening when, during the panic, he completely lost both his capacity to think and his peace of mind, that he had become entirely dependent on me to save him from disaster – a situation which seemed to have aroused once again a great deal of envy rather than any feeling of affection or gratitude for being helped to get over his acute psychotic state so quickly.

Adam's envious take-over of my capacity to function had a number of significant consequences for him, which it was essential to understand and analyse. We must remember, first, that we are confronted in these situations with the basic problem of taking in food. Adam had never seemed able to digest his food as a normal baby does and even as an adult he always took over the function of the food supplier instead of acknowledging that he had been given it. This disturbing envy lay behind his constant indigestion.

In the following session Adam complained how he had difficulties in working and he continued to suffer from indigestion. He could not listen to me, and it seemed that he still had to insist that he could balance everything out by himself. A great deal of his inability to listen and his desire to do all the talking and giving were acted out with his girlfriend. She had pointed this out to him. Gradually, he became aware of how difficult it was for him to accept listening to her and to take in important interpretations from me, and also to show any appreciation for what I had given him. Throughout the analysis he had sometimes reacted quickly to something I had shown him with appreciation but just as quickly had found that it was more important to think of something he had contributed or something he could write about. He would stress that he had already thought of something similar to what I had said. I interpreted to him that at the moment when I told him something he felt he always knew it already and I related this to his insistence that when his mother was feeding him he believed that he had her breast already inside him and was feeding himself. Given that he possessed the food there was no need fully to take in and digest what was given to him. He had explained to me before that to this day he could never cook a meal for himself but that even when somebody cooked for him very well he still reacted with indigestion. I pointed out that he seemed repetitively to need to restore the 'true' feeding situation and to enact it. He had not himself owned his mother's breast to feed himself.

However, as soon as he recognizes this and allows himself to be fed he again steals the food and robs the person who is feeding him. Immediately he feels bad inside himself and gets indigestion. In reply he mentioned that he had such severe constipation that his writing production had stopped. I said that it seemed that writing now had the meaning of appreciating and digesting the food which I as mother had given him. I also said that his wish to produce something which could give me satisfaction was very limited. His constipation made it apparent that it was very important to him to give a stool as a gift (related to the capacity to take in food with love and gratitude), but I realized that it had been very difficult for him to make use of the interpretations I had given him about his overwhelming anxiety of dying of cancer and his difficulties in taking them. This was why he had a compulsion to act out his infantile problems of endlessly possessing the breast again and again. My interpretation, therefore, could not be digested.

A few sessions afterwards he told me that he had been invited over by a friend of his and his wife. They gave him some fried food to eat which gave him indigestion, so he did not feel well again. He then told me a dream. In the dream he joined a party of others going up to the moon in a rocket, but instead of landing on the moon this rocket landed on an island which had very similar structures to the moon. He felt that there was some kind of trick connected with the fact that the rocket went the wrong way. I felt that Adam was rather uncertain in his way of talking and associating. He did not know what was relevant or not and also did not know how to take in food. I therefore suggested that, since the day when he felt better in the session and when he had seemed more on the road to getting better, he had lost his way again. He was not satisfied with my interpretation and went rambling on in an uncertain way. I reminded him again that he had apparently lost his way soon after the session in which he had felt he was saved from the overwhelming anxiety of having cancer. He replied that he could not remember any important session. He then associated that the moon had something to do with the idealization of his girlfriend. He always wanted to love somebody. I interpreted that the rocket to the moon was related to his wish to lose himself in an ideal object, and going there with so many people implied that other people who were in love were doing the same thing. But in the dream this did not come off. He came down to earth and fell on an island which looked very similar to the moon. I suggested that this island was his own self (I-land), to which he returned; this implied that he realised that he was loving only him-self. The dream illustrated that his intention to grow up and love somebody else had failed. The main point, however, seemed to be that in the dream he attributed the failure to a trick. But now he had difficulty in investigating with me how this failure, or trick, arose.

The trickiness appeared again in the next session. Adam expressed envious feelings about a colleague of his who had seduced the analyst who treated Adam before he came to me. Obviously he now wanted to seduce me away from the truth. By this trick I said he wanted to turn away from all that he had been understanding here because it was too painful and difficult to admit that, just when I was able to help him, his envy interfered in the relationship to me and was forcing him to turn back to himself again. This spoiled his desire to become a more loving person. There was also trickiness in that he expressed envy of a colleague who succeeded in spoiling his analysis by seducing his analyst. There was a danger that I could be seduced by him, like he had seduced his mother. But his only hope to be analysed successfully was if he had an analyst who would remain firm in spite of his constant attempts at seduction. It seemed he was angry and envious of the firmness he needed from me to enable him to give up his narcissistic omnipotence. Yet it was this narcissistic omnipotence which kept him locked in the severe narcissistic neurosis or psychosis.

Adam did not acknowledge that I was right. But the next day he came with a very heavy cold. He said he was keen to come in order not to lose the session. He then told me a dream. In it a colleague of his, who is in analysis with me, had six holes drilled into his bones because I as a surgeon tried to find cysts there. No cysts could be found, but the patient, although near collapse, was very brave. There were no associations to this dream. The dream seemed another clarification to show the tricks Adam was playing at that time. The dream seemed to involve a wishful transformation of the truth. It recognized that I had been touching very precisely on some of Adam's more serious problems, and this he wanted to deny. In the dream he was proud and brave because he was coping so well with the suffering caused for him by a bad analysis. In fact he behaved much more as if he was avoiding the pain of realizing that I was locating his problems precisely.

Working through the envious devaluation of admired objects

After intense work on Adam's constant envious reaction to any progress, producing negative therapeutic reactions again and again, he eventually had a period in the analysis and in his life where he felt

69

distinctly better. He then decided to visit his home country (Italy) during the summer holidays. However, this proposed visit again stimulated a great deal of uncertainty and anxiety, and his hypochondriasis briefly flared up acutely. I could show him at that time how difficult it was for him to accept that he was much better, because accepting the improvement implied an acknowledgement of all that he had received in the analysis. In fact Adam overcame the crisis in a very short time, and his physical symptoms, which he feared would bring him into hospital, almost subsided. He had been particularly afraid of meeting colleagues in his own country. He came back from the summer holidays reporting an extremely successful trip. Just before the holidays he had acknowledged that he wanted to come back appearing extremely successful and important but then, having accepted the reality of having just got better through the treatment, he was able to feel much more real towards his family and also towards colleagues in his own country who were interested in his work and friendly towards him.

During the first week of his return he felt extremely peculiar. He felt lonely, miserable, and rejected by everybody in England. In his dreams incestuous relations were constantly emphasized. He seemed to praise the people in his own country and constantly wondered whether their analytic treatment was not much better than the one applied over here. It seemed that feeling so much better and successful during the holidays he had again felt overwhelmingly envious and had devalued me. As a result of this he lost me and feared that I would have nothing to do with him. This threw him back into the old 'incestuous' phantasies of his mother, when he had slept in bed with her. In the good relationship to me he had been able to develop a more normal relationship to me as both father and mother.

The set-back did not last long. Before the holidays he had often felt very jealous and excluded by his colleagues in this country. Now he suddenly got on better with them, and they took more notice of him. But now he had dreams of being robbed and cheated by other men, with whom he felt he had very friendly relations. He himself realized that these dreams were related to his own homosexual feelings. We had seen previously that he used to project his own feminine self into many easily excitable girls. He had begun to realize he was exploiting these girls in order to diminish his own homosexual excitement. He now had a dream that one of his earlier girlfriends with whom he had been identified slept with his landlord. He also had a dream of being in bed with his father. His father was concerned and friendly. But the next day Adam was again rather paranoid. I tried to show him that when I was experienced by him as a friendly, helpful father he felt afraid of his greedy, envious homosexual feelings towards me because in his feminine role he felt very sexy and exploiting. I reminded him how often he had accused women of sexually exploiting him.

At this time he had an opportunity to have some instruction from a woman about child care, which he knew very little about, and he immediately had a dream where a professor in Italy invited him to give a lecture on this subject. So when he had the opportunity of learning about children he immediately phantasized taking over the role of his instructor: her knowledge and capacity to look after children. During this time he also had a dream that his mother was reciting poetry to him. At first he did not listen to his mother, thinking that she could not possibly say anything of any consequence, but then he gradually started listening to her. In the end he felt it was rather beautiful and he started to admire her. Interestingly enough, all Adam's associations to the dream referred to poets who were men. I said to him that he had great difficulty in valuing his mother, or women, or the analyst in a feminine creative role. This was the first time that anything like that had been revealed in a dream. He had attempted several times to admire a woman, but this had always been extremely difficult. He had failed and then turned again to the sexually exploiting women with whom he had surrounded himself.

This dream did not, however, lead to any development in his capacity to appreciate women; on the contrary, he felt suddenly very bored, mainly in relation to food. Food seemed to become terribly uninteresting, so that he did not know what to eat. He also admitted that while he was studying and reading very voraciously there was really a wish to take more and more in, but he could not enjoy his reading. By way of interpretation I just acknowledged how I had heard how deeply his pleasure in taking things in, originally food from his mother, had been interfered with. I suggested that what prevented his feeling of pleasure seemed mainly to be his envy of the feminine creative capacity. Greed seemed to have replaced real pleasurable relationships, and on top of this he always tried to eroticize the relationship to his mother in order to overcome feelings of boredom.

It seemed very striking that it was out of a sense of boredom that the wish for exciting sexual relationships had become so prominent. So it became clear that some of Adam's constant eroticization was a defence against boredom, related to the devaluation of this early oral relationship with his mother. He made constant attempts to take things in but was not able to respond with strong emotions to my interpretations. The transference relationship during this time was mainly of a positive nature. The negative feelings were mainly displaced. His greed was expressed by his wish for many different relationships, mainly with women, but also for activities in other fields of his life. At this time he had a dream that he was travelling from his own country in a kind of tramp ship which was stopping in many different places and took a long time. It was a kind of round trip. In another dream there was a famous painter who came from the Continent to England and looked at a number of exhibitions but he seemed to get fed up with all of them and devalued them all, returning disillusioned to his own country. In this last dream he was obviously identified with the famous creative artist who came to England, was bored and fed up, and devalued everything including his analysis. So he predicted that he would return to his home country completely disillusioned after finishing his analysis. The dream exposed Adam's grandiosity and superiority, which related to his constant wish to claim that everything creative was his own possession. To the dream about the tramp steamer he associated that there was probably a *tramp* travelling in a famous ship, like the *Queen Elizabeth*. Here, he seemed to admit that he felt really like a tramp, but his being in England, or in analysis, had changed me from a famous ship into a tramp ship. He said that travelling round in the ship implied a very slow trip and stopping in many different places, so that his getting to his destination was very delayed. I said that by going round and round he could avoid facing the value and importance of his analysis because it would prevent him making any valuable contact with me. By projecting his tramp self into me he created a devalued picture of me, but by having this devalued union with me he also devalued the possibility of using his own gifts. In this way he was bound to feel that he was going round and round and not getting anywhere. In fact he complained during this period that there was nobody helping him to be creative.

He then had a dream where the girlfriend whom he had appreciated very much, and who was in reality a sensitive, sensible, and well adjusted person, was suicidal and went to Rome. He also had a dream that one of our best known psychoanalysts in England was extremely depressed and suicidal. This man actually married very late in life and was now very successful after a successful analysis. Adam himself was afraid that he was too old to get over his illness and he was depressed on beginning to realize what was preventing him from getting better. In the dream about the suicidal analyst he projected his depression into him, again an attempt to devalue me because he could not identify himself with him and me being successful. He did the same thing with his most appreciated girlfriend, namely projecting his depression into her and sending her off to Rome. His phantasy had always been that he would live in Rome if he could not be cured. Here again was his problem that even a woman he appreciated was devalued so that because he felt too bad about continuing his constant envious attacks he was unable to receive love and appreciation from her. In consequence he found it very difficult to believe that he was capable of any affectionate relationship with women without insisting immediately on a sexual relationship. This spoilt his capacity for allowing any loving relationship to develop which could lead to a happy marriage. A striking fact in Adam's analysis, however, was the clarity of his dream communications, combined with his inability to make use of the insight the analysis gave him about them in this period.

The clinical material which appeared in the following week showed Adam's conflicts and difficulties about acquiring a satisfactory identity through identification with me as a satisfactory and important person. Adam had been preoccupied with wanting to buy an overcoat in a Scottish shop in Kensington. He had, however, changed his mind and gone to Harrods, a better known and more important shop, and there in the adolescent department he had found a coat which suited him perfectly. It was not at all expensive because he found it in the adolescent department and not the grown-up section of the shop. However, in coming away from the shop he was very disappointed to find that the Harrods label was not on his coat. He felt cheated and that his coat, which he had appreciated, was now devalued. He believed it would not give him any warmth. He then told me a dream which related to a friend of his childhood who had been very wealthy. The friend's father had made first-class coats and supplied these coats to other firms. In this dream Adam felt excluded by his friend, who had a party in the evening to which he had not been invited. He asked his friend what he was doing in the evening and was determined to go to the party even if he was not invited. Adam associated a party to which he had been invited the night before at a London scientific institute where he listened sometimes to lectures. He was surprised that they had invited him because he went there for only a few lectures. He found these people very nice and interesting. He enjoyed their company and wondered why he never invited them to his own flat.

I think that Adam's attempt to find a coat which fitted him well in the adolescent department at Harrods and his sudden violent disappointment are explained by the dream. In it he feels resentful and excluded from the home and party of his friend, the son of the maker of beautiful coats. The famous department store, Harrods has my initials, 'H.A.', and the beginning of my name, 'Ro'. So it could stand for me as the father who makes beautiful coats which fit well and keep people warm. Adam realized that he could get such a coat from me if he acknowledged that he was really an adolescent who still has to grow up. The terrible disappointment occurs when Adam sees that his coat does not bear my name ('H.A.R.O.(D.S.)', and his complete disillusionment about the coat shows how really he wants to bear my name and to be completely identified with me. The nearest way of doing this is to be my son. The awful exclusion from my home is experienced in the dream when the real son of the coat-maker does not accept him as a brother. In the dream Adam is obviously determined to be my son and he indicates that he will force himself into this position. In his associations to the invitation to a scientific society he feels sorry for his previous superiority and contempt for it and he can admit how much he longs for being part of a family who appreciate and welcome him. This must also relate to a greater admission of being treated well by me, but it seems now that it is mainly his possessiveness of me, wanting to own me and to bear my famous name, H.A.R.O.(D.S.), which makes him still feel so resentful and left out by me. At this time Adam's homosexuality and overwhelming feminine identification had not appeared sufficiently in the analysis.[2]

Narcissistic omnipotent object relations and a negative therapeutic reaction

I shall now describe material from a later stage of the analysis where some aspects of Adam's narcissism related to his psychosis and hypochondriasis could be more clearly understood. A predominant hypochondriacal anxiety at that time related to fears of cancer and of gangrene of the penis, which was stimulated through herpes of his (glans) penis. In addition, there were occasionally hypochondriacal fears of suffering from diabetes, stimulated by a persistent fungus infection of the nails. Adam's anxieties lasted for several months and reached a climax during the period I am about to describe, before gradually disappearing. His fears of cancer were foreshadowed by a dream which he had on the first day of the Christmas holidays. In the dream, he had cancer of the seminal canal, and a girl was exciting him sexually and probably had intercourse with him. He was not able to identify the girl in the dream. From my knowledge of Adam's previous material and from his attitudes during the session, it seemed to me that the girl in the dream represented his feminine self, which was stimulating his masculine self. I interpreted the dream as an expression of his narcissistic bisexuality where he emphasized independence from the analyst as the mother.

In a dream the next day, he was ill, had long hair, and was going to have an operation. He went to bed with a man who was depressed and had left his wife and daughter and who also had a son who suffered from cancer. This dream seemed to have a fairly obvious homosexual meaning, and one could assume that the operation represented castration so that he could be turned into a woman. Adam himself thought that the depressed man stood for me as the father who preferred him to his family. While the homosexual transference and the desire of Adam to seduce me away from his family seemed to be on the surface, I thought that the dream had in addition a more hidden meaning: Adam's narcissistic resistance in the transference. I therefore mainly interpreted his negative attitude as an attempt to depress me by seducing me into being his father. In this way we would forget the importance of myself as the analyst who has to be father and mother at the same time.

A fortnight later, the feelings and anxieties related to his bisexuality came strongly to the surface. In one session, he was full of complaints that his girlfriend neglected him, but his main complaint, which he expressed in a paranoid complaining way for at least twenty-five minutes, referred to his feeling insufficiently valued by his colleagues. He emphasized that he had made important contributions to his science, but these were disregarded, and he felt particularly annoyed that he was not asked to teach. The longer he went on with his complaints, the more resentful he seemed to get. He threatened to leave England and also the analysis if the situation did not change. In listening to him, I felt that he expected me to change this situation and that this complaint related to his feeling neglected by me, because I was treating him as a patient and not as my wife. I was refusing to allow him to have children, or, as he put it, not allowing him to have pupils. This I interpreted, and his paranoid outburst died down. He told me a dream. In it he was looking into the eyes of a girl, and there was something wrong with them. Apparently, they were infected, and he pressed on them like a boil. Suddenly, a great deal of pus popped out of them. He appeared excited about this dream and gave many associations. He talked about masturbation and ejaculation, and mentioned his satisfaction in pressing on pimples and watching their contents coming out. It seemed that he wanted me to take notice of both the dream and the material which he was pressing out of himself. I was able to interpret that the girl in this dream represented himself. *The next day*, he started the session by telling me that he had become aware that the stuff he was pressing out of the eyes of the girl referred to hallucinations, because throughout the night *he was afraid of going mad and was beginning to hallucinate.* He had feared that he might not be able to sleep and dream. However, he had dreamt. I noticed that while he related the dream to me it was curious that there was no sign of the very severe anxiety which must have troubled him during the night.

In the dream, Adam was sitting in a room, and his brother was lying on the couch crying. He was probably psychotic. Adam had become his brother's analyst. He saw a little boat flying in the air, and many things were going on under the surface of the sea. He thought that his state had something to do with his girlfriend not wanting to see him. His associations were connected with his recognition that he used his compulsive sexual relations to evacuate his psychotic anxieties. He talked in some detail about the hallucinations which he had as a child, but very little about the anxiety of the night before. While he talked, he was holding a paper in his hand on which he had made notes of his dreams. I had the distinct impression that he wanted to impress me that the material would teach me about psychotic disturbances. In other words, the attitude of the day before, when he stressed that he wanted to be a teacher, seemed to come right into the transference situation. I concentrated, therefore, mainly on analysing his behaviour. I interpreted that he was acting as if he was the mad girl who wanted to show off to me her important hallucinations for me to admire. He wanted me to recognize them as an important contribution to the science of analysis. There were also other elements. He seemed to express resentment that I would use the material which was coming to the surface in order to be more effective in my analytic role, and this would reveal that he was the psychotic depressed patient on the couch. I interpreted that he was envious of me and resented my insight and capacity to help him. This was the reason why he reversed the roles in the dream – he became the analyst and I the psychotic patient. I thought that this dream implied that I was beginning to arouse increasing envy as in the mother transference I represented the creative mother who could understand his illness and look after him. In other words, he was warding off the dependent object relationship.

Adam reacted to my interpretations with great resentment. At once he complained that I was not satisfied with his important material. He had done a great deal of work to produce this analytic report for me. This complaint confirmed my impression that he was acting out the reversal of the dream. At the same time, there seemed to be some appeal to me, as the father, to recognize him in the creative feminine role. I felt that in this session the overpowering domination and idealization of his feminine psychotic self were coming to the surface. This meant that an infantile feminine part deluded herself that she was not a baby but a grown-up woman who had breasts and babies. Everybody, including the analyst, should recognize these delusions as reality. In spite of all his protests, I tried to repeat my interpretation, explaining that his deluded self was denying his need for me. I was the feeding mother whom he denied out of envy but with the consequence that he could not get any help from me on the level where he needed me most. I also stressed that it seemed that his deluded feminine self had completely overpowered, at the present time, this dependent infantile baby self who needed me and was able to have insight into what was going on. There was apparently no response to this interpretation in this session.

On the next day, Adam first reported a dream in which he was looking through a list of telephone numbers to pick up a girl to have intercourse with. In the second dream, there was an important English book or essay which had been translated into Italian, but when Adam read the Italian translation he realized that most of the value of the English text had been lost in the translation. The Italian translation read quite differently, and he was very angry about it. In another part of the dream, he travelled to Italy with a suitcase, but there was something wrong with it, as it seemed much too light. He suspected that somebody had stolen something from the case. As an afterthought, he thought perhaps he had not taken enough with him from England. In the last part of the dream, he felt that his penis was shrinking.

In his associations, Adam talked about his fear that his penis was getting smaller and that he was trying to find another girlfriend with whom to have intercourse, in order to reassure himself. He gave a long dissertation about symbolic transformations, but this seemed rather intellectual and pseudo-scientific. Adam often idealized Italian thinkers in literature, in philosophy, and also in his own science, and he often insisted that Italian girls were much sexier than the English ones. It was surprising that he himself did not recognize that this dream represented a criticism of his constant idealization of Italy and his desire to travel abroad. I thought that the translation from English into Italian implied an eroticization of the transference by changing the good feeding relationship with the analyst/mother into a sexual one, represented by Italy. I interpreted that he felt that the session the day before had been valuable and important and was represented in the dream by the valuable English essay. But translating it into Italian and eroticizing it implied an envious alteration of the session which took the real value and meaning out of it. By now it had become unrecognizable and insignificant (light). The first dream, looking for a girl to have intercourse with, could also be understood as providing an alternative to the session of the previous day. Travelling with a suitcase which was too light was an acknowledgement that Adam, by acting out, either by going to Italy or by changing the analytic relationship into an erotic one, was losing the value of the analysis. However, he felt persecuted and robbed by the envious part of himself who was the cause of his constant loss. Because he wondered whether he had taken in enough from the analysis the afterthought in the dream brought him more into contact with the real situation.

The anxieties in the dream relating to the changing and diminishing importance of the analytic situation are in the end connected with the shrinking penis. His difficulty in taking in the help from the analysis (representing the good breast in the feeding situation) ultimately interfered with his becoming an adult and developing a potent masculinity. Clinically this interrelationship was particularly important in view of the patient's compulsive need to act out sexually, something which the dream reveals as an emptying-out process which becomes manifest only in a hypochondriacal anxiety: the shrinking penis. I felt that these dreams represented a protest by the saner part of the patient's personality against the destructive and acting-out activities of the psychotic narcissistic parts of him. At the time of these dreams, there were as yet no conscious changes or insight into a need to protect the healther from the psychotic parts of his personality.

During the next weeks, the hypochondriacal anxieties relating to his penis appeared on the surface with great force. About a fortnight after the Italian translation dream, he complained that some herpes which had developed on his penis was getting worse and he was afraid that his penis would become necrotic or gangrenous and would fall off. He wondered how he could live without a penis. He also complained of the fungus, which he asserted was not properly treated in England. He considered going to Italy to consult doctors because nobody in England seemed to care about his physical health. But again, after complaining bitterly that he had not been sufficiently recognized by his colleagues as a teacher, he admitted that the night before he had again had hallucinations and felt that he was being driven into a psychotic state. After this he reported a dream about a friend of his who gave up flying some years ago because he had realized it did not suit him and made him feel sick. Another friend was also a flier and advised this friend either to go on flying or to go on with something else which was not specified in the dream. After telling me the dream, Adam immediately continued worrying about his diseases. He was convinced that he had diabetes and that he did not get proper treatment. He also complained that he could not eat by himself and he wondered whether his girlfriend could feed him.

I interpreted that he made it clear in the dream that a part of him realized years ago that flying away to other countries, which implied turning away from me to other objects, made him ill. At the same time there seemed to be another part of him which had been persuading him to go on acting out by flying off to other objects or simply ignoring the analysis and the realization of the real sense of his sickness. I said that he had been submitting to this part of the personality, which gave him bad advice, for years. This was the part that was preventing him from using my help and interpretations so that he could not experience that he was getting better. I also related this to his complaint that he needed somebody to feed him. Immediately after my interpretations, Adam had a phantasy of consulting a doctor in another country. When I interpreted this in similar terms, he said he was thinking of taking a girlfriend out for a meal. So he quickly changed his role and had become the feeding mother, the analyst. When this was interpreted, he said he was busy thinking of presenting a paper to some learned society. Each time I made an interpretation, he seemed to move in the opposite direction, so I connected this acting out during the session to his constantly flying off and turning to other situations and objects. I interpreted that it was this behaviour that was making him sick. I also related it to the dream a fortnight before in which the acting out was experienced as a shrinking attack on his penis.

Adam replied that he had been reading that schizophrenic patients behaved in this way and proceeded to give me a lecture on the behaviour of schizophrenic patients. When I again interpreted this as not wanting to acknowledge that anything important was being given to him by me, he told me that he had a phantasy of being James Bond. I replied that he idealized himself now as the James Bond who could deal omnipotently with all situations. He could fly or swim anywhere and could seduce all the girls. He had no need for me as the analyst/mother who could give him the interpretations representing the food he needed to get better. With this the session ended.

I have presented the foregoing session in some detail to illustrate to what extent, in spite of very insightful dreams, the omnipotent psychotic attitude can be acted out in an extreme way, and a negative

79

therapeutic reaction continues unabated. The reason for the opposition against the analysis seems to lie in the attempt of the omnipotent psychotic part of the patient to maintain its power by preventing the interpretations from reaching the infantile dependent part of the personality. Adam's hypochondriacal complaints were emerging under the pressure of the psychotic narcissistic aspects of his personality. This managed to remain in control by trying to persuade and probably hypnotize the infantile part of Adam to believe that to fly abroad to Italy was not the cause but the cure of his sickness.

During the next days Adam still complained about his fear of gangrene or cancer of the penis. He often had hallucinations and distorted visions during the night and reported many dreams which illustrated in greater detail some of the aspects I have already reported. But a change in emphasis began to be observed. He insisted that the psychotic part was felt to be like a Nazi, murdering an infantile part of himself which he regarded as a child of mine. He felt this to be a particularly destructive hurting attack directed against me, representing both parents.

In spite of the progress Adam had made there were still further negative therapeutic reactions, although the quality of hypochondriacal thoughts took on a more depressive tone. During this time the patient had a dream. He was in the analyst's house. The analyst was talking in the kitchen. The patient's father was doing acrobatics, pulling himself up on the wardrobe in the bedroom, and was doing very well. The patient knew in the dream that the father was dead (he had, in reality, died some time ago). He remembered his funeral and asked his mother whether she could see his father too. At that moment his father felt very upset, and the patient woke up with a severe pain in his heart and was afraid of dying. The patient added that, in the dream, the analyst knew the father. In his associations he talked with admiration of how strong and acrobatic his father had been.

It seemed to me that the main significance of this dream was the appearance of the analyst in the dream representing the feeding mother who helped him get in contact with the infantile situation which revived his admiration and jealousy of the father in the Oedipal situation. But in the dream the father, not the patient, is made to feel small and left out. This triumph over the father causes the patient to wake up from the dream with a pain in his heart and the fear that he is going to die. This dream seems clearly a move forward from the narcissistic position to dependency, the Oedipal situation, and the depressive position.

Two days later Adam was very disturbed with severe pain in his chest and reported a nightmare. In the nightmare he was living in a flat with his mother. A very paranoid, megalomanic Indian insisted that the flat belonged to him and tried to force his way in and take it over by threatening to shoot Adam in the chest with a bow and arrow. At first Adam wanted to shoot him because he was so dangerous but then he felt afraid of the Indian, who was much younger, and so he gave in. He woke up again with an intense pain in his chest, fearing that he was going to die. He associated his latest girlfriend to the Indian. He explained that, while he had admired her greatly for a long time, recently he had become frightened of her as he realized how narcissistic she was. Adam could think of no other associations to the Indian and he stressed how paranoid and deluded he seemed to be. I had explained previously that his girlfriend had stood for his feminine omnipotent self, which recently had been more clearly revealed in dreams as mad and deluded. This feminine self was now being simply described as a paranoid and deluded dark or anal man, representing his own omnipotent narcissistic self, which was an acknowledgement that the feminine delusion had diminished. In the dream this psychotic, mad part (similar to that part of him represented in the 'Nazi' dreams previously mentioned) is making a take-over bid, claiming possession of the flat which represents both his ego and his relationship to the mother/analyst, but the father is absent. However, the attack is not directed against the mother but against the sane, dependent part of the patient, who when threatened with death gives in to the omnipotent narcissistic part, allowing it to regain charge of his ego and of the analysis. This dream was still followed by a set-back which lasted for several weeks and it illustrates again the struggle involved in the negative therapeutic reaction. It is the narcissistic omnipotent delusional part of the patient which feels threatened by progress and insight. The progress of the analysis in making contact with the infantile part of the patient had mobilized envy on an infantile level, particularly envy of the feeding breast. This threatened to expose the emptiness and delusional quality of the narcissistic structure which was beginning to break down at that time, so that depressive anxieties, particularly relating to the analyst, were experienced more frequently.

In another dream, both Adam's mother and father had mental breakdowns and were in analysis. In another dream the same night, his father was an analyst but had cancer. Adam consulted several doctors for him, but there was no hope, he was much too ill. Adam woke up from these dreams with a terrible biting pain in his heart. I thought that these dreams were expressing the beginning of a change in his attitude. The attack on my mental health, represented by the patients, was clearly admitted in the dreams, and there seemed to be a strong depressive anxiety about both the combined parents and the analyst/father, who seemed to represent to Adam not only the partner of the mother in the Oedipal situation, but the main support of the analyst/mother in the dependent feeding relationship. The beginning of depressive anxiety was also clearly indicated by the hypochondriacal biting pains in his heart which woke him up from the dream. It is a significant and interesting feature in the treatment of hypochondriasis, reported many years ago by Melanie Klein (1935), that progress in treatment shows itself first by changes in the anxiety content of the hypochondriacal symptom. They then increasingly lose their persecutory quality and acquire a more depressive content.

During the following weeks, infantile parts of Adam, represented as babies or young children, often appeared in dreams, showing that his dependent infantile parts, essentially linked with the sane part of his personality, were gradually growing in strength. It is interesting that the hypochondriasis of the penis gradually subsided during this period and was superseded a few months later by a prolonged fear about the heart, which had been foreshadowed by the pain in the heart dream.

Summary

Adam was a patient with a narcissistic omnipotent character structure who frequently tried to improve during the analysis by attempting to have more loving and appreciative object relations. But he was pulled back time and time again by the narcissistic omnipotent part of his personality which would overwhelm his saner healthier part. At such moments the hypochondriacal symptoms flared up. It was particularly striking that symptoms and problems constantly shifted, a process which could be traced clearly to the transference experience. He dealt with his intense envy, which was stimulated in a dependent and good relationship to the analyst, by quick devaluation and by constant moving to different object relations and even different countries. Such patients find it very difficult to bear the pain of normal ambivalence, so they are slow to learn to accept both their love and envy in a holding relationship which helps them to bear depressive anxiety and gradually leads to a diminution of the power of the narcissistic structure and the hypochondriasis. Even in successfully treated patients, as in this case, the improvement is very gradual and slow and is constantly interrupted by negative therapeutic reactions which have to be interpreted carefully.

Notes

1 In dealing with patients who are suffering from severe hypochondriasis, we have to decide whether the hypochondriasis forms part of a mental illness such as senile depression or whether it dominates entirely the symptomatology and has to be regarded as a disease entity. When we have diagnosed that we are dealing with a hypochondriacal disease entity, we have to differentiate again between two forms of this disease: first, the hypochondriasis which is characterized by bizarre delusions relating to the state and function of the body and bodily organs, a disease which belongs to the schizophrenic group and is very difficult to treat by psychoanalysis. In the second form of severe hypochondriasis, bizarre delusions are comparatively rare, but the patient is almost constantly preoccupied with fears of suffering from certain physical illnesses such as cancer, TB, or heart disease. Most of these patients are mainly preoccupied with one illness at any time. However, when the anxiety relating to one disease begins to fade, hypochondriacal fears about an entirely different disease affecting another organ will soon appear. This chronic hypochondriasis has been regarded by most psychiatrists as a psychosis of a non-determining type. Sometimes it is combined with a physical illness which may easily be overlooked, as the hypochondriasis is generally in the foreground.

In my book *Psychotic States* (Rosenfeld 1965), I have described the psychopathology of hypochondriasis in some detail. I argued that severe hypochondriasis was often a defence against a schizophrenic or paranoid condition. In the patient to be described the psychotic state underlying the severe chronic hypochondriacal anxieties was often clearly noticeable. The hypochondriacal anxieties of this patient should not be regarded simply as a conversion of the psychotic state into physical symptoms since, as I shall try to show, whenever the analysis or external experiences made an impact on the narcissistic psychotic state and threatened its rigid control, the hypochondriacal anxieties increased. The hypochondriasis should therefore more correctly be described as an expression of the conflict between the more normal non-psychotic part of the personality and the narcissistic psychotic organization which tried to dominate the whole personality, and it was this that caused the constant negative reaction and with this an increase of the hypochondriasis.

2 The incident of the Harrods coat and the dream of forcing himself into the coat-maker's family, which showed that he wanted to be part of my

family and to have my name, 'H.A.R.O.(D.S.)', seem outwardly identical with the delusion of the hebephrenic patient, Maria, of Dr N., who had the long persisting delusion of being the analyst's daughter and bearing his name (see Chapter 12). But the psychopathology is entirely different. In Maria's case her delusion of bearing the analyst's name seems to be an idealized oneness and closeness with the analyst to deny her confused aggressive feelings with which she fears that neither she nor the analyst could cope. However, in Adam's case the closeness and warmth of the coat, his need for closeness with me, were spoilt for him by having to realize that he was not me, that he could not acquire my name, which meant for him not only quality but fame and importance. So the narcissistic identification, the desire to assume my identity, was still stronger than his need for closeness. However, in the incident of being invited to the scientific society he recognized that he had rejected people who valued him and wanted to be close to him because he was rather superior and had looked down on them and devalued them, which he began to regret.

5

Narcissistic patients with negative therapeutic reactions

Negative reactions to psychoanalytic treatment were first described by Freud (1916) when he mentioned the story of a young, adventurous woman who had rebelled against her parents and run away from home. After many difficulties she became reconciled to her family and found a young artist who wanted to marry her. From that time onward she began to neglect the house, imagined herself persecuted by her lover's family, hindered her lover in his work and social life, and then succumbed to an incurable mental illness. Freud realized that the paradoxical behaviour of this woman was caused by guilt which had set in motion dangerous and forbidden wishes. In other words, he regarded this reaction as being induced by her conscience. Two years later Freud (1918: 69) wrote of 'The Wolf Man' that he had the habit of producing transitory 'negative reactions' every time something had been conclusively cleared up in the analysis. Freud felt this reaction related to the way children respond to prohibitions before they accede to them. Typically they repeat the prohibited act once more and only then stop it. In this way, Freud felt, they create the impression that changing their ways is under their control and so maintain some degree of omnipotence. In 1923 Freud introduced the term 'negative therapeutic reaction'[1] and in subsequent writings linked it with disorders in super-ego development and with his theory of the death instinct (Freud 1923, 1924).

Since Freud, many analysts have described chronic resistance to analysis and have developed their own theories about it – very often following Freud in drawing attention to problems connected with guilt, super-ego formation, and omnipotence. Among them Abraham

(1919) mentioned the importance of the patient's superior attitude and the influence of envy and narcissism[2] – a view echoed by Horney (1936)[3] and by Klein (1957). Abraham also stressed the hidden way in which negative therapeutic reactions seem to occur.

Turning to the technical problems of handling patients with a negative therapeutic reaction Riviere (1936),[4] among others – for example, Klein (1957)[5] – has emphasized the need to pay direct attention to the patient's inner world of phantasized object relations and, especially, to the aggressive wishes therein. She stressed the need to be cautious about both encouraging positive aspects of a patient's narcissism and overdoing the interpretation of aggressive impulses. Both tendencies, she felt, could aggravate or even create negative therapeutic reactions.

Among more recent contributors to the literature on this subject, Olinick (1964, 1970) has emphasized the importance, for the successful psychoanalysis of some patients, of allowing negative therapeutic reactions to develop. His stress is on how some patients need to repeat past experiences in reverse in order to regain control over them. In this situation the danger is that the analyst will be unable to bear the experience of being made a failure in his counter-transference and set up a collusive sado-masochistic relationship with his patient.[6] Asch (1976) takes a rather similar view to Olinick, emphasizing the underlying cause of the phenomenon in faulty super-ego development.[7]

I have always been interested in negative therapeutic reactions and, like the authors I have mentioned, also stress the role of envy, superior attitudes, and destructiveness. In this chapter I want to present some views about the negative therapeutic reaction in relation to my ideas about narcissistic omnipotent object relations.

When I first put forward my ideas about narcissistic object relations, one of the key points I had in mind was that this was a way of being which defended against feelings of aggression caused by dependence, frustration, and envy. It is particularly related to the latter that the narcissistic patient either keeps up his feelings of superiority by devaluing the analyst, or when he benefits by the analysis, gives himself the entire credit for it (Rosenfeld 1964b). It is by omnipotent projective identification that the patient takes over the analyst's capacity and feels very concretely that he is inside the analyst and able to control him, so that all the analyst's creativity and understanding can be attributed to the patient's ego.

Later, as I described in Chapter 1, I formulated the concept of destructive narcissism, related to Freud's concept of the death instinct and also particularly pertinent to the negative therapeutic reaction

(Rosenfeld 1971). I stressed the way destructive omnipotent parts of the self can be idealized but remain disguised or silent and split off so that their existence is obscured. In these cases one is aware only of an apparent lack of any relationship to the outside world. In fact, of course, modes of relating of this kind have a very powerful effect in preventing dependent object relations and keeping external objects permanently devalued, with serious consequences for psychoanalytic therapy.

Since 1971 I have become aware that the structure of the narcissistic omnipotent self varies considerably. Omnipotent phantasies may be stimulated during all phases from infancy to adulthood. None the less we have to remember that the omnipotent phantasies originated in infancy at a time when the individual felt helpless, small, and incapable of coping with the reality of being born and all the problems related to it. From birth onwards he not only built up a phantasy of an omnipotent self but also omnipotently created objects (at first part-objects) which would always be present to fulfil his desires. In this situation separation, overindulgence, or, particularly, the lack of a holding and containing environment increases the development and persistence of narcissistic structures.

As I illustrated in describing Adam's analysis in Chapter 4, once a firm narcissistic way of living has been established beyond infancy, relations to self and object will be controlled in order to try to maintain the delusional omnipotent belief. Any contact with reality or self-observation inevitably threatens this state of affairs and is felt as very dangerous. In my experience careful examination allows one to detect the fact that this omnipotent way of existing is experienced and even personified as a good friend or guru who uses powerful suggestions and propaganda to maintain the status quo, a process which is generally silent and often creates confusion. Any object, particularly the analyst, who helps the patient to face the reality of his need and dependence is experienced as dangerous by this good friend, who is afraid of being exposed as a phantom. Anything which might enable the patient to become aware of how completely dominated and imprisoned by his omnipotence he is, is silently criticized, belittled, devalued, and distorted. When the patient's capacity for self-observation improves and he becomes conscious of this process and tries to free himself from being controlled, the persuasive, seductive nature of the omnipotent structure changes; it becomes sadistic and threatens the patient with death. Only then does one become aware that hidden in the omnipotent structure there exists a very primitive super ego which belittles and attacks the patient's capacities, observations, and particularly his attempt to accept his need for real objects. The most confusing element in this process is the successful disguise of the omnipotent structure of relating and the envious destructive super-ego as benevolent figures; this disguise makes the patient feel guilty and ungrateful towards them when he tries to improve. It is the particular sense of guilt created in this way which is an important factor in producing negative therapeutic reactions.

The process which I have observed clinically resembles Freud's (1923) psychological explanation of the negative therapeutic reaction, when he argued that it was due to an unconscious sense of guilt which was a hidden (dumb) phenomenon related to the death instinct, the force which pulls the patient away from life, from object relations and from recovery. Indeed, in 1971 I wrote: 'Freud must have realized the obvious relation between narcissism, narcissistic withdrawal and the death instinct but he did not work it out in any detail either theoretically or clinically' (Rosenfeld 1971: 170). He believed that the resistance to analysis related to the silent opposition of the death instinct 'could not be analysed unless it emerged as an open negative transference and that interpretations could do nothing to activate it (1971: 170).[8]

Given the nature of narcissistic omnipotent object relating, it is not surprising that it is after a session where the patient quite openly admits that he feels better, and realizes that the analysis has helped him, that negative therapeutic reactions are most likely to occur. In these circumstances the patient may come late, completely forget what happened in the last session, and seem so entirely out of contact as if something has occurred which has completely wiped out the experience of the day before. It is not only the good experience with the analyst which has disappeared. That part of the patient which received help also appears to have been lost. Thus, when the patient is able to talk in such situations he complains of feeling cut off and imprisoned. Sometimes he describes the feeling of being completely overpowered, or he says that something has been killed or lost. Generally he is unable to give any information about the reason for this state, which seems to him to come completely out of the blue. During the analysis the patient only gradually becomes more able to report and observe the detail of his reaction. I shall illustrate this phenomenon with case material from two patients.

Peter

One of my patients, Peter, had a psychotic episode many years ago and in his analysis developed many negative therapeutic reactions which repeatedly left him feeling unable to think and observe what was going on inside him. He would feel paralysed and sleepy for several days. Only gradually was he able to describe how, at these times particularly, a part of his personality was arrogant and superior. It often made speeches to him criticizing the analysis and throwing doubts on my interpretations. When his trust and co-operation in the analysis increased and he allowed himself to be helped by me the omnipotent part criticized him for being weak and inferior and belittled him so violently that he came to the next session feeling shocked, battered, and almost smashed to pieces. He would fear that he would break down completely, as he could not stand up against these attacks. He complained, 'What is the good of making any progress if I am torn to shreds afterwards?' He was particularly aware that his capacity to think came under attack at such periods and that everything he had gained from the analysis was in danger.

Peter's life had been geared to having prostitutes once or twice a day for many years. The analysis had gradually helped him to understand the meaning of this compulsion, which he had used for evacuating any anxiety or concern and had also prevented any loving dependent relationship. During the time that he began to resist going to prostitutes for several weeks the internal attacks became particularly violent, and at the same time a voice seductively told him that it would be good for him to have a prostitute and that everything would be all right again if he followed the suggestion. The relationship to prostitutes related to Peter's phantasies of ruthless power and control over women with whom he felt he could do anything he wanted. He realized he was being blackmailed by a part of himself to believe that if he gave up any progress, particularly any meaningful relationship to the analyst, and would allow his omnipotent narcissistic part to regain control so that it could indulge in uncontrolled masturbatory pleasures without any care for his objects, he would be all right again. However, when the analysis progressed in spite of the negative therapeutic reactions, murderous rages against people in the outside world appeared which led to constant obsessional anxieties about having killed somebody in-advertently. Eventually, when we were able to trace the origin of his murderous feelings, he admitted that they always occurred when he started to compare himself with other people. It was particularly when he felt that somebody was superior to him that these murderous feelings came to the surface – in other words that the murderous, omnipotent envy which was hidden behind his narcissistic omnipotent control had been able to emerge.

Peter's case illustrates the fact that negative therapeutic reactions can at first be silent or dumb, as Freud has described. It was only when Peter recovered his capacity for self-observation that was he able to describe his omnipotent self and its violent attacks and punishments directed against that part of himself which had co-operated with analysis and wanted to be helped by it. He was also able to report the seductive disguise of the omnipotent self which tried to lure him back into his addiction to prostitutes by false promises and blackmail.

In my experience there are several important technical matters if the silent resistance of the negative therapeutic reaction is to be overcome. One has to understand first that the patient feels helpless and completely unaware of what is going on, and therefore that there is *no point* in insisting that *the patient* is resistant or wants to withhold information. On the other hand, interpretations which can make the patient aware that there is *a force* at work inside him, which is powerfully suggestive and prevents him from thinking and observing what is going on, are experienced as helpful and ego-supportive. This approach gradually mobilizes self-observation. But most patients need a great deal of help to understand and overcome this silently undermining process because it is very frightening and confusing. What is particularly confusing is the existence of a split-off self or object inside the patient who by persuasion and suggestion exerts a powerful influence over him and assumes the role of an adviser. Under other circumstances this figure becomes extremely threatening and critical. It can also be guilt-provoking and act *as if* it were the patient's conscience. The point to be observed, of course, is that this adviser or conscience operates under false pretences and has as its main function the aim of keeping the patient's narcissistic delusional way of being in power. Any good dependent relationship the patient is gradually developing, such as that to the analyst, is therefore attacked and belittled. Detailed investigation of this way of relating reveals that it is intensely destructive to the patient and his important object relations. In these circumstances I think it is rather confusing to speak of the internal structures which represent this way of relating as 'super-ego'. Certainly, if one diagnoses this structure as a primitive super-ego, one has to be aware of its violence and omnipotence, but this has little relationship to the super-ego as it is normally conceived. It would be better to call it a narcissistic omnipotent structure. It does indeed often create guilt but this is a false sense of guilt quite different from the emotion which is self-preservative.

Michael

Michael, a man of about forty, came from southern Europe to England for an analysis. He was married and had two children. He had been fairly successful in his professional work in the social field, but almost every day he would have to withdraw from his wife and children for several hours to read poetry and to listen to music. He was so absorbed by his preoccupation that he almost entirely lost contact with his family. He felt very superior going into this withdrawn state and looked down on and belittled his wife, whom he realized was more sociable and normal than he. In some previous therapy in his own country he had gradually come to realize that he was living entirely in a false, isolated world which he had highly idealized and he was beginning to get depressed. He realized that he needed more analysis as he felt bad and worthless and so he came to me.

Michael had very grandiose phantasies about himself which attached themselves to his knowledge and his obsession about being so rich that he could fulfil all his wishes. During his first weeks in London he felt more depressed, because he had to reduce his standard of living, and consequently he felt resentful against me, his analyst, and humiliated that he had been forced by his illness to give up a very comfortable life and professional work which he could not continue in its lucrative form in England. After the initial resentment and difficulty he began to function a little better. He enjoyed analysis and his new understanding. But the state of self-absorption and self-idealization continued, because he started to read voraciously, and his wife and children began to complain about him. He realized he had to overcome this problem because now, more than before, he was aware how much his wife and children needed him and how much he had been depriving them through his behaviour. But he also noted the very strong resistance against bringing about any change in his behaviour.

Whenever Michael succeeded in being a little better and more able to relate to his family and to resist his tendency to withdraw, at first he felt happy and satisfied. But then he would suddenly be overcome by a great anxiety about his ability to stay in England. He had invested money to fulfil his dream of being rich in the future, but would become afraid that by doing so he had spoiled his wish and his need to stay in England. The anxiety about this mistaken and grandiose investment was justified, and he really needed to take corrective action about it. But this he could never do. His anxiety

91

would also appear whenever he made some progress and realize how badly he needed treatment.

During these states of depression or anxiety he would come very late and even miss sessions and had great difficulty in saying anything in the analysis. When he spoke he insisted that he had nothing to say and there was no point in coming. The only thought which seemed to force itself into his mind was an insistence that he had to go back to his own country. This thought was also accompanied by an inner argument which was going on that it was impossible for him to improve and to overcome any of the mistakes he had made. Gradually it became possible to help him to become conscious that all this was the product of an inner figure who insisted that analysis was useless. It would certainly end in failure because his problems could not be overcome. He was a fool to stay here any longer and should go back to his own country as soon as possible. When Michael was able to report his experience to me, I became aware that what he was describing was no mere dialogue with an internal figure. Rather, he seemed to be entirely hypnotized and overpowered by these internal attacks against the analysis which were also made against himself and his capacity to think. This is characteristic of what happens in a negative therapeutic reaction. At such times patients are unable to think about the problems which are most disturbing to them and which brought them for help. Under these circumstances the patient is generally entirely dependent on the analyst.

Whenever I succeeded in helping Michael to express some of the thoughts which were going on inside him, or when I guessed what was going on inside him, he was generally able to agree with what I was saying and to be relieved. At the end of the session he would be more hopeful that this repetitive but frightening situation could be understood.

To illustrate the difficulty in more detail I want to discuss a problem which preoccupied Michael and me during the first three months of the analysis. Michael had heard that his father was very ill and probably dying and that he wanted to see him very urgently. But this desire for his father and his threatening death aroused no concern in Michael. Instead he felt enormous hatred, contempt, and abuse. In this situation he expressed himself very freely and in his hatred felt his father was absolute rubbish and fit only to be thrown away. In spite of the urgency of the situation the patient's resentful, almost incredibly vulgar attitude towards his father continued for some weeks.

His father had been very successful professionally and had been kind to Michael when he was small and supported him in going to the best schools; but his father's favourite had been Michael's sister. Michael felt that she was loved because she was beautiful and kind. He was expected to work hard in school and be active, while his sister was not at all good in school, perhaps not even intelligent. However, this did not seem to worry his father. He loved her just the same. When she was about nineteen years old she suddenly died and his father was heartbroken and became very depressed. He eventually gave up work. Michael remembers that he was briefly concerned about his father after the death of his sister but, when his father did not respond to him immediately, he became very cold and withdrew from him. Michael was intensely bitter and jealous about his father's love for his sister and in his coldness he expressed his revenge. He had evidently never forgiven his father and refused to give him any love after his sister's death.

In listening to Michael's abuse against his father I tried to make him aware that behind this abuse were feelings of affection and love for him: feelings which he tried to destroy because he did not want to realize how painful it was for him to understand that his father was now dying. He also felt guilty that he had neglected him for such a long time. I also showed him that he had always denied his love for his father and his own wish to be his father's favourite daughter. In becoming cold and more and more masculine and competitive he had denied not only his love for his father but his own feminine wishes and feelings. In fact he wanted to be warm and lovable like his sister. Gradually, his coldness broke down and his love for his father appeared. He then went to see his father and stayed with him for a fortnight. While he was there he actually managed to help his father to get over his severe depression by being able to treat him with affection for the first time in many years.

Michael was very happy on returning from his visit to his father and he also recognized that something very important had opened up to him. He then had a dream where he had not only a penis but also a vagina. In the following session he was able to acknowledge that he also had a feminine part in himself which he would express by showing greater affection to his children and his wife. He also managed to find some work. He seemed to be improving. However, a typical negative therapeutic reaction was to follow.

After a particularly fruitful session on a Thursday, when he had been able to express himself better and showed much more appreciation for me, he came forty minutes late on the Friday. He was overcome with shock and disgust with himself. He admitted that he had been drinking heavily on the Thursday evening. He had slept deeply and could not remember anything about Thursday. He had also the greatest difficulty in getting up. He felt blocked and could not think, but felt very guilty that he had spoilt everything. He could not understand what had forced him to behave like this. How could he do something like this both to somebody he loved and to himself? As he could not think, he could not pursue what had been going on in his mind before he started drinking. He only felt bad that drink had affected and spoilt his mind, a mind of which he was very proud.

On the following Monday he was at first also unable to think or to remember anything that had been happening on Thursday. But in the middle of the session he suddenly remembered a dream he had had the previous night. In it he had a therapeutic session with a woman, a social worker he knew. He greatly admired her attitude and the atmosphere which surrounded this woman in the dream. He felt that she was warm and understanding and talked in a very straight and clear way. She said to him in the dream, 'You are the most self-centred, narcissistic person I have ever met in my life.' In the dream Michael felt that this woman was completely right and he reacted inside himself with such severe pain that he felt it was almost unbearable. But he had no wish to excuse himself or defend himself because he felt that the atmosphere which the woman had created was so understanding. He also felt that she was completely devoted to the truth and had transmitted this to him. He felt she cared for him only as a patient and felt she had to be firm in order to help him to get better. He emphasized several times that he had never had such an experience before in his life. He had sometimes agreed with his previous therapist, with me, and his wife that he was terribly selfish and preoccupied with himself but he had never been able to respond to any interpretation, any truth, so strongly. He felt deeply grateful to the woman in the dream for touching him through her way of talking to him. The woman in the dream reminded Michael of a woman he worked with whom he admired.

I thought that the woman in the dream seemed to be a highly idealized version of me, but why was I presented in the dream as a woman? Was this a hidden attack on me as a man? And what was the relationship of the dream to the negative therapeutic reaction, creating this sudden bout and compulsion to drink? It seemed clear both in the dream and in Michael's association that what had impressed him most was not the interpretation, which was in any case simply a confrontation, but the therapeutic atmosphere. This related to Michael's need to become more aware of the feminine part of his personality, which he realized could help him to become less narcissistic. I felt that the dream therapist succeeded in conveying his problem to him without appearing superior and narcissistic, and this was what Michael felt he needed. But he also deeply envied the therapist for behaviour he would have liked to be capable of himself. In the dream Michael could allow himself to feel the pain of the truth although it hurt him. He became aware of the extent of his selfishness and narcissism. In the negative therapeutic reactions he had always attacked his self-awareness, admiration, and grateful response to analysis. I gathered that, simultaneously with his progress in analysis and the breaking through of strongly affectionate, admiring feelings, he must have been overwhelmed by an intensely envious response which, as so often, had been silent. I did not interpret a great deal of the dream but I conveyed to Michael that he felt he was responding to the therapy with me and felt deeply touched. He could express this in the dream. I also noted that there were feelings which came up at the same time which had attacked this good experience.

In the next session Michael told me that soon after the last session he was suddenly overcome by such an intense feeling of envy of me and my helpful attitude to him during the sessions that it frightened him. He wanted to be like me and to be capable of treating his own clients in the way I was treating him. He felt it was almost unbearable to think that he had to wait so long and needed more treatment. He was afraid that he could never become like me and the woman in the dream. It was now clear to me that this last severe negative reaction must have been caused by an overwhelmingly positive response to the Thursday session. He had not been able to cope with it, and it had stirred up in him an almost unbearable feeling of envy. He avoided the painful experience by drinking, which seemed at first to wipe out the whole experience completely, but after a few days the dream relating the 'marvellous' session helped him to remember and express some of the feelings which had been so unbearable.

In Michael's case the negative therapeutic reactions can be regarded as a way of acting out both positive and negative feelings which were too painful for him to bear. The interesting point with him was that the overwhelming negative therapeutic reaction, leading to the drinking bout, did not last very long. In spite of Michael's feeling of despair and fear of having spoilt everything the dream emphasized not the negative reaction but the positive progress which he felt he had made. This is a very important aspect of the negative therapeutic reaction to consider.[9]

After the dream, Michael's wish to be instantly like me became a major issue in the analysis. It was, of course, a wish for a narcissistic identification, and one could see that there would now be many problems about Michael feeling he was advanced and had reached an ideal state. While this did happen, there were thereafter only occasional negative therapeutic reactions.

Discussion

The examples I have given make it clear that the understanding and analysis of envy, in the context of narcissistic omnipotent object relations, are an important element in understanding the negative therapeutic reaction. So is an understanding of guilt and of hidden destructiveness. I mentioned at the beginning of the chapter that both Olinick and Ashe have drawn attention to the similarity between depressive patients and those suffering from frequent negative therapeutic reactions, and to the importance of super-ego formation. I agree with them that the super-ego is an important factor in most negative therapeutic reactions. It is, however, difficult to differentiate the attack by the super-ego on the ego from the violent attacks derived from the narcissistic omnipotent organization which turns against the infantile part of the self. The super-ego in the negative therapeutic reaction is an extremely primitive structure closely related to the patient's narcissistic omnipotence. It is not easily accessible to direct interpretation, as Freud (1923: 50) pointed out. It seems mainly to have a persecutory character and contains many envious components which give it a begrudging, delusional, and spoiling character that tries to destroy any success and progress in the treatment. It is also important to realize that this primitive super-ego is probably always disguised as a very seductive and persuasive ideal figure. It is only through the detailed analysis of the destructiveness and envy in the analytic transference relationship, and of the related persecutory anxieties projected on to the analyst, that the primitive super-ego and the negative therapeutic reaction become more accessible to analysis.

Notes

1 Freud (1923: SE 19:49) explains the phenomenon that patients get worse during treatment in the following way:

'In the end we come to see that we are dealing with what may be called

96

a "moral" factor, a sense of guilt, which is finding its satisfaction in the illness and refuses to give up the punishment or suffering. We shall be right in regarding this disheartening explanation as final. But as far as the patient is concerned his sense of guilt is dumb: it does not tell him he is guilty; he does not feel guilty, he feels ill. This sense of guilt expresses itself only as a resistance to recovery which it is extremely difficult to overcome.'

In his paper on 'The Economic Problem of Masochism' (1924) Freud returned to the discussion of the negative therapeutic reaction. He speaks here of the difficulty in making patients aware of the unconscious sense of guilt and wonders whether it would not be better to speak instead of the need for punishment. He also pointed out that the sadism of the super-ego and the masochism of the ego complement one another, resulting in a severe sense of guilt or conscience, both the sadism and masochism being derived from the destructive or death instinct. In his paper 'Analysis Terminable and Interminable' (1937) he confirms that he regarded the negative therapeutic reaction as related to the death instinct.

In describing the negative therapeutic reaction Freud apparently wanted to provide evidence for the usefulness of the concept of the super-ego (Spillius 1980). But as he described the dumb unconscious structure which resisted analysis and could not be made conscious it is understandable that Freud attempted to link this phenomenon with his clinical experience of silent responses which he believed could not be activated and which he related to the silent influence of the death instinct (1937).

It seems to me important to try to understand those hidden factors described by Freud in more detail because our therapeutic results in dealing with negative therapeutic reactions may depend on the successful activation of the elusive destructive factors, and this in turn would make the super-ego more accessible to investigation.

2 As early as 1919 Abraham described chronic resistances to analysis which were hidden. He found that these patients begrudge the analyst any remark that refers to the progress of the analysis; Freud mentioned identical observations in describing in 1923 the behaviour of patients who developed negative therapeutic reactions. Abraham also stressed that he finds the need to be superior in these patients, a point which Freud briefly referred to but regarded as too superficial. Abraham emphasized that these patients do not want to free-associate or to allow the analyst to be the cleverer one. In fact they want to do the analysis by themselves and do it better. Abraham did not actually describe a clear negative therapeutic reaction in his patients, because when they made any progress in the analysis they became able to verbalize their resentment and envy of the analyst. He did not make it clear whether they relapsed. He related the

patient's attitude to envy and anal eroticism and stressed that the patient feels the 'analysis is an attack on his narcissism, that is on that instinctual force upon which our therapeutic endeavours are most easily wrecked' (1919: 310). Abraham gives a number of clinical examples in this paper, and I think it should be regarded as an important contribution to the negative therapeutic reaction; his observations are still relevant today. For example, he clearly links narcissism and envy to explain this negative therapeutic reaction. His description of the outwardly eager attitude of his patient to analysis would suggest that much of the envy remained hidden (silent) and was defended against. It was actually Abraham's analytic work which brought the hidden envy to the surface. Abraham regards envy in this paper mainly as an anal character trait but in the later paper 'The Influence of Oral Erotism on Character Formation' (1924a) he stressed the origin of envy in the oral sadistic phase.

3 Horney in her paper on 'The Problem of the Negative Therapeutic Reaction' (1936) made a number of important clinical observations and offered technical suggestions on how to handle this difficult problem. She observed that the negative therapeutic reaction occurs most frequently after a particularly good interpretation, which is experienced by the patient as a sign of the analyst's superiority and high intelligence, to which the patient reacts with resentment, disparagement, and belittlement, leading to attempts to assert his own superiority over the analyst. As a second point she stresses the narcissism of the patient, his need to be perfect, flawless, and beyond reproach. As a good interpretation exposes some weakness in the patient, he experiences it as a severe narcissistic blow and feels humiliated. Horney thinks that it is the analyst's effectiveness which endangers the patient's belief in his absolute supremacy, and he retaliates by trying to humiliate the analyst and make him feel insignificant and ineffectual. Thirdly, she stresses the patient's fear of improvement through the analyst's help since such success is always related in his mind to 'crushing others and maliciously triumphing over the crushed adversaries' (1936: 37), an attitude necessarily leading to a fear of retaliation and failure. The fear of success may be phrased in the following way. 'If I attain success I shall incur the same sort of rage and envy that I feel towards the success of other people.' Horney sees similarities between Freud's view and her own. Freud, however, stresses the guilt feelings in this type of patient, while Horney emphasizes fear of envious retaliation, a persecutory anxiety situation, which would link up with Melanie Klein's observations on an envious super-ego. Horney deliberately refrains from relating the problems connected with the negative therapeutic reaction to infancy but emphasizes that 'I select out of the material offered by the patient those parts which I can relate to his reaction to the analyst, and interpret those only' (1936: 43).

4 Riviere (1936) is concerned with investigating the question as to why the negative therapeutic reaction should be regarded as more unanalysable than any other obstacle to treatment. She argues that Freud regarded psychotic and narcissistic patients as equally inaccessible to treatment. She implies that the negative therapeutic reaction may be a reaction not to a good interpretation but to an incorrect one which should lead the analyst to look for deeper causes of this problem.

Riviere proposes that, in especially refractory cases of the narcissistic type, we should pay more attention to the analysis of the patient's inner world of object relations, which is an integral part of his narcissism, and that we should not be deceived by the positive aspects of narcissism but should look deeper for the depression which will be found to underlie it. She gives a detailed description of the manic defence against depression, the patient's omnipotent denial of psychic reality, and the denial of affects, particularly regarding the ego's object relations and its dependency on them. She also stresses manic contempt and depreciation of objects and the control and mastery over them which, in her view, explain the narcissistic patient's denial of the value of everything the analyst says. Riviere emphasizes the narcissistic patient's need to maintain the status quo by his omnipotent control, because the lessening of the manic omnipotent defence brings him face to face with his hopeless despair related to his depressive anxiety which he fears will become reality to him. She believes that what makes the negative therapeutic reaction so stubborn is the unconscious love and anxiety for the destroyed or dying internal objects, producing an unbearable sense of guilt and pain. The patient needs to sacrifice his own life for others who represent these internal objects, and therefore faces death or suicide. She states that this situation is not identical with Freud's unconscious sense of guilt. She relates the negative therapeutic reaction to the patient's feeling that he deserves no help from the analyst and is unworthy of it until he has helped to restore and cure his internal objects. She also suggests that omnipotent control is specifically related to the negative therapeutic reaction; if the patient's state begins to change he loses control and so he quickly has to reinstate the former situation which has proved bearable. Her paper is full of technical and clinical details as to how to deal with this difficult clinical problem.

Riviere specifically warns the analyst *not to overdo the analysis of aggressive impulses*, because she feels that nothing will more surely lead to a negative therapeutic reaction than the analyst's failure to recognize anything but aggression. She says, for example, that *not all negative reactions to treatment should be regarded as attempts of the patient to defeat the analysis*. The patient's feeling of prior obligation to rescue damaged internal objects may take precedence over his freedom to accept help for himself.

5 In her book *Envy and Gratitude* (1957: 13, 11) Klein discusses how 'envy and the defences against it play an important part in the negative therapeutic reaction in addition to the factors discovered by Freud and further developed by Joan Riviere'. She states that 'with some patients . . . this helpful interpretation may soon become the object of destructive criticism. It is then no longer felt to be something good [they have] received and [have] experienced as an enrichment.' She explains that the envious patient grudges the analyst the success of his work, and the interpretation which she has given is spoilt and devalued by the patient's envious criticism. This interefers with the acceptance of interpretations. The envious patient may also, out of guilt about devaluing the analyst's help, feel that he is unworthy of benefit by psychoanalysis. (This sense of guilt is clearly related to Freud's view on the importance of the sense of guilt in the negative therapeutic reaction.) Melanie Klein's observations of envy being aroused by good interpretations is almost identical to Horney's (1936) description of the competitive patient who devalues the analyst and the interpretation. Horney relates it to the negative therapeutic reaction, however, only in terms of the patient's fear of envy of other people which prevents him from attaining success.

Klein stresses the danger of success when envy is stimulated. The patient manically triumphs over the analyst, representing the good object, and devalues him. This leads to severe guilt feelings and depression. In this situation it is clear that the negative therapeutic reaction does not occur as a result of the breakdown of the manic defence, as Riviere (1936) observed, but is itself caused by the destructive element in mania represented by envy. The depression following an envious attack contains not only guilt feelings but severe persecutory anxieties. The persecutory fear relates to fear of being enviously attacked both by external objects as well as by internal objects, represented by an envious super-ego, which is experienced as devaluing and disparaging and which grudges the ego any goodness and success. When envy is located in the super-ego it becomes an important part of the negative therapeutic reaction. As the envious super-ego is particularly difficult to bear, it leads to denial and splitting (this would link up with Freud's comments on the sadistic super-ego and the difficulty in making it conscious). Horney gives the impression in her paper that competition, rivalry, or envy appears in the analysis of patients showing negative therapeutic reactions in a quite undisguised way. It is, however, apparent from the study of Klein's work that the most powerful negative therapeutic reactions occur when the envy remains hidden or silent, due to the creation of powerful defences against envy. Defences against envy include splitting, idealization, confusion, flight from the original object leading to dispersal of feelings, devaluation of objects and self, violent possessiveness, and reversal of the envious situation by stirring up envy in others through success and possessions. Some of these defences, particularly idealization and splitting, are identical with those which Klein and previously described as the very earliest defences of the ego belonging to the paranoid schizoid position, which are directed mainly against the destructive or death instinct.

This is in line with her view regarding early oral envy as a derivative or expression of the death instinct and stressing its existence from the beginning of life. Klein gave a detailed description of the importance of split–off envy, which she frequently observed clinically as an incapacity to accept with gratitude interpretations that in some part of the patient's mind were recognized as helpful. The splitting off and projection of envy into the analyst are an important hindrance in the analytic situation because the analyst is constantly mistrusted since he is unconsciously again and again turned into a dangerous and retaliating figure. When through the analysis of the split–off aspects of envy the ego is strengthened, and when the feeling of responsibility becomes stronger and guilt and depression are more fully experienced, 'the projection onto the analyst diminishes so that the analyst in turn finds it easier to help the patient toward further integration. That is to say, the negative therapeutic reaction is losing its strength (Klein 1957: 75–6). It is clear from this description that envy and the defences against it prevent the integration of the ego which is necessary for reaching the depressive position. It is therefore often noticeable that patients showing long–drawn–out negative therapeutic reactions tend to be rather more schizoid than depressive, and it is only when the envy has become conscious and has been worked through in the analysis that the depressive anxieties can be fully experienced and worked through. The negative therapeutic reactions which Riviere described – namely, the manic defence against depressions – are generally less severe and intractable, but there are exceptions to this as when, for example, excessive envy has become part of the patient's manic system.

6 Olinick (1964, 1970) examines the negative therapeutic reaction (NTR) as a special kind of negativism. He stresses that this syndrome itself represents the nucleus of the patient's defences. These defences are highly cathected narcissistic devices originally evoked in the phase of necessity during infancy and childhood, which become reinvoked in the genetic and dynamic regression of childhood. This would imply that some patients inevitably would experience negative therapeutic reactions in a successful analysis. He also has the impression that those people who display the negative therapeutic reaction are endowed from birth with greater than average aggressive orality and anality, which in turn make the mothering relationship more stressful; the mothers have to cope with

these masterful children, a situation being repeated in the analysis. From his description, however, it is clear that he regards the NTR mostly as a normal phase of transference resistance in some patients. He sees negativism as part of the negative therapeutic reaction, a defence against a loss of self inherent in the ambivalent relationship with a depressed pre-Oedipal maternal love object, with which the patient tends to fuse.

Olinick regards the negative therapeutic reaction as a transference resistance which occurs in certain patients with anal–sadistic tendencies as a repetition of their behaviour to their mothers. He stresses that the long-drawn-out negative reaction in analysis occurs only when the analyst colludes in being pulled into a constant sado-masochistic relation with the patient, which implies counter-transference problems in the analyst. I would agree with Olinick that it is very important to avoid a masochistic collusion with the patient and that this causes an impasse in analysis, but this is an artefact created by the analyst's problem rather than by the patient.

7 Stuart Asch (1976) considers that whereas Freud's concept of the negative therapeutic reaction limits its aetiology to the sense of guilt or need for punishment, he himself has found it clinically useful to add the following aetiologies to the theory of the NTR: (1) a masochistic ego responding to a special psychopathology of the ego-ideal; (2) a defence against the regressive pull-back to symbiosis with the depressed Oedipal object; and (3) an extension to Freud's category of the unconscious guilt to include early pre-Oedipal anxieties and phantasies such as having castrated the mother. These three roots of the NTR are elucidated in analysis in terms of structural deformities of both the ego and the super-ego due to pathological introjections related to early experiences with the mothering object. Asch agrees with Olinick in the necessity of understanding and analysing the transference projection in the NTR; the core of the transference is the projection of the sadistic super-ego on to the representation of the analyst, followed by an attempt to provoke the analyst into a punitive sadistic response. Counter-transference problems are the response to the covert sadistic component in the patient's masochism, which constantly belittles the analytic work. Sadism is also revealed through the disguised omnipotence, the arrogant narcissism.

It is interesting that while Olinick (1964) and Asch (1976) refer to narcissistic problems in the NTR only in passing, Olinick (1970: 671–72) in summing up the Symposium on the Negative Therapeutic Reaction in New York, throws up the question: 'If it is agreed that the negative therapeutic reaction is to be found among the narcissistic neurosis or disorders, how is this relevant to superego development and to the classification of the negative therapeutic reaction as a superego resistance?' In the Symposium there was general agreement that the super-ego of which all the participants spoke was archaic or primitive, consisting in forerunners that were not structured in what is generally called the mature super-ego. I regard Stuart Asch's observation that a negative therapeutic reaction may be a defence against a regressive pull-back to symbiosis with the depressed Oedipal object as important but I have found this only on rare occasions, while the negative therapeutic reaction in narcissistic patients is exceedingly common.

8 It seems appropriate here also to quote details of Loewald's important contribution to the theory of the negative therapeutic reaction (1970, 1972). He bases his formulation of the psychopathology of the NTR on Freud's definition as discussed in 1923 but developed more in detail in 1937; and he comes to the conclusion that Freud ultimately thought that the NTR was based on the prevalence of the death instinct in the economy of psychic life. The sense of guilt represents the workings of that portion of the death instinct which is psychically bound by the super-ego. The person with an intractable unconscious sense of guilt in Freud's sense resists improvement. Improvement to him is a sign of a lessening of self-punishment which he requires. In the last analysis according to Freud improvement represents to him abandoning the life–death struggle within him in which the death instinct always has to maintain the upper hand. Often the accent seems to be on self-punishment, an indication of the importance of narcissistic omnipotence including the omnipotence of bisexuality and its relation to the death instinct. The Oedipal early disturbances in infancy where destructive forces got out of hand and affected the very fibre of the person are an important factor in negative therapeutic reactions. In discussing the early mother–child relationship Loewald says that the intensity of destructive tendencies and of their narcissistic entrenchment in the NTR would depend predominantly on early interactions (between mother and infant) which favour a distorted organization of both destructive and libidinal and destructive and creative drives. In this primitive situation interpreting in terms of guilt, conscience, and need for punishment could hardly be effective. Loewald feels that when it comes to early psychic exchanges Freud underplays the crucial importance of the individual psychic development and in his view does not stress the importance of often invidious and primitively structured counter-transference problems for some therapeutic failures. Loewald is one of the few analysts who have tried to apply Freud's death instinct theory and recognized the clinical importance of Freud stressing the working of the death instinct as an important factor in the negative therapeutic reaction. It is unfortunate that Loewald in his interesting paper offers no detailed clinical material which would make his contribution much more alive and useful to colleagues who want to use his experience. Asch and Olinick describe the mechanisms which they

regard as clinically important in cases of negative therapeutic reaction in some detail but they do not give any case material, which would be very helpful to those who want to study their experiences in more detail. In the work of both Asch and Olinick one does not feel that in their discussion they are focusing on the actual negative therapeutic reaction as it occurs in the clinical situation; they seem instead entirely preoccupied with therapeutic impasse and not with a temporary negative therapeutic reaction. They seem to concentrate on the transference/counter-transference problems which may occur during the negative therapeutic reaction and make the working through of it in certain cases rather difficult. I would agree with Asch and Olinick that if there is a transference/counter-transference confusion and collusion occurring between patient and analyst negative therapeutic reactions would cause an impasse. I would, however, agree with Robert Langs (1976) that the transference resistances leading to collusion between patient and analyst should not be called negative therapeutic reactions. A great deal of confusion could be created if our understanding of the pathology of the negative therapeutic reaction were to become confused with transference/counter-transference reactions, which have obviously more to do with the pathology of the therapist than with the patient.

9 Limentani (1981) came to similar conclusions in his cases. However, in my experience these negative therapeutic reactions, which act as a kind of shock and help the patient to make positive progress, are comparatively rare.

6

Destructive narcissism and the death instinct

The experience of analysing the transference relationships of patients whose psychopathology is dominated by narcissistic omnipotent object relationships and consequent negative therapeutic reactions (such as those of the patients discussed in the last two chapters) has drawn my attention to the important role of recognizing and analysing aggression and destructiveness and the special ways in which these are incorporated in the life of the narcissistic individual. In studying narcissism in some detail it seemed to me essential to differentiate between its libidinal and destructive aspects.

In considering the libidinal aspect of narcissism one can see that the over-valuation of the self plays a central role, based mainly on the idealization of the self. Self-idealization is maintained by omnipotent introjective and projective identifications with ideal objects and their qualities. In this way the narcissist feels that everything that is valuable relating to external objects and the outside world is part of him or is omnipotently controlled by him. The negative consequences of such processes are obvious, and narcissism was generally discussed by Freud (1914) in relation to the distribution of the libido into the ego and its pathological consequences. In Freud's belief there was in narcissistic conditions a loss of all object cathexis and the absence of a transference (indifference to objects). But Freud also described narcissism in relation to the narcissist's love of his self and in relation to self-regard. He stressed, for example, that 'everything a person possesses or achieves, every remnant of the primitive feeling of omnipotence, which is experienced as confirmed helps to increase the self-regard' (1914: SE 14: 98). In my view this type of narcissism often acts as an essential protector of the self, and some patients become exceedingly vulnerable when through frustrations and humiliations the narcissistic protection is fractured and develops holes. This makes it so essential to differentiate the positive side of self-idealization from its negative side. I want to emphasize, therefore, alongside my focus on the negative consequences of narcissistic processes, that I am also careful to examine positive effects. The analysis of all narcissistic phenomena in the same way can be disastrous therapeutically.

When considering narcissism from the destructive aspect, we find that self-idealization again plays a central role, but now it is the omnipotent destructive parts of the self that are idealized. They are directed against both any positive libidinal object relationship and any libidinal part of the self which experiences the need for an object and the desire to depend on it.[1] The destructive omnipotent parts of the self often remain disguised or they may be silent and split off, which obscures their existence and gives the impression that they have no relationship to the external world. In fact they have a very powerful effect in preventing dependent object relations and in keeping external objects permanently devalued, which accounts for the apparent indifference of the narcissistic individual towards external objects and the world.

Experience suggests that, in those narcissistic states in which the libidinal aspects predominate, open destructiveness becomes apparent in the analytic relationship as soon as the patient's omnipotent self-idealization is threatened by contact with an object which is perceived as separate from the self (as in Adam's case, discussed in Chapter 4). Such patients feel humiliated and defeated by the revelation that it is the external object which, in reality, contains the valuable qualities that they had attributed to their own creative powers. A primary function of the narcissistic state has been to hide any awareness of envy and destructiveness and to spare the patient these feelings. However, as the analysis brings the existence of such wishes to the patient's notice, his feelings of resentment and revenge at being robbed of his omnipotent narcissism diminish. Envy can then be consciously experienced, and the analyst can gradually be recognized as a valuable external person who can help.

By contrast, when the destructive aspects of narcissism predominate the difficulty is that this destructiveness is much more difficult to bring into the open. Envy is usually more violent and more difficult to face. There is an overwhelming wish to destroy the analyst, who becomes via the transference *the* object and *the* source of life and goodness. The patient can become extremely frightened of the destructiveness that is revealed to him by the analytic work. This development is therefore often accompanied by the appearance of violent self-destructive impulses. In terms of the infantile situation, such narcissistic patients are determined to believe that they have given life to themselves and are able to feed and look after themselves without help. Thus when they are faced with the reality of being dependent on the analyst (standing for the parents, particularly the mother), they seem to prefer to die, to become non-existent, to deny the fact of their birth, and to destroy any analytic and personal progress and insight (representing the child in themselves which they feel the analyst, representing the parents, has created). At this point such patients frequently want to give up the analysis but more often they act out in other self-destructive ways by spoiling their professional success and personal relations. Some of these patients become very depressed and suicidal, and the desire to die, to disappear into oblivion, is expressed openly. Death is idealized as a solution to all problems. To understand more about the way such destructive narcissism operates and how to prevent and deal with the negative therapeutic reactions that result when trying to treat them is the main purpose of this chapter.

The death instinct

In the last ten years I have made further detailed observations and have changed my views in so far as I believe that some deadly force inside the patient, resembling Freud's description of the death instinct, exists and can be clinically observed. In some patients this destructive force manifests itself as a chronic paralysing resistance which can hold up analysis for many years. In others it takes the form of a deadly but hidden force which keeps the patient away from living and occasionally causes severe anxieties about being over-whelmed and killed. It is this deadly force which resembles most closely Freud's description of a death instinct that remains mute and hidden but opposes the patient's desire to live and to get better. Freud himself did not think it would be possible to activate the destructive impulses hidden in the mute death drives. But our modern technique of analysis can often help the patient to become more aware of something deadly inside himself. His dreams and phantasies can reveal the existence of a murderous force inside him. The force tends to become more threatening when the patient tries to turn more towards life and to rely more on the help of the analysis. Sometimes the deadly force inside threatens both the patient and his external objects with murder, particularly when patients feel overwhelmed by a deadly destructive 'explosion'.

When Freud (1920) introduced his dualistic theory of the life and death instincts he instigated a new era in the psychoanalytic understanding of destructive phenomena in mental life. He emphasized that there was a death instinct which was silently driving the individual towards death and that it was only through the activity of the life instinct that this death-like force was projected outwards in the form of destructive impulses directed against objects in the outside world. In 1920 (SE 18: 258) Freud wrote that the 'erotic (life) instincts and the death instinct would be present in living beings in regular mixtures or fusions, but "defusions" would also be liable to occur'.

In 1933 (SE 22: 105) Freud returned to the discussion of the fusion of the erotic and the death instincts. He added that 'fusions may also come apart and we may expect that functioning will be most gravely affected by defusions of such a kind. But these conceptions are still too new; no one has yet tried to apply them in our work.' He argued that generally the life and death instincts were mixed or fused to varying degrees, and that neither instinct was likely to be observable in a 'pure form'. Many analysts objected to the theory of the death instinct and were tempted to discard it as purely speculative and theoretical. However, Freud himself, along with others including Melanie Klein,[2] soon argued that it was of enormous clinical importance – employing it to understand masochism, the unconscious sense of guilt, negative therapeutic reactions, and resistance to treatment.[3]

In discussing this psychoanalytic approach to narcissistic neurosis Freud (1916) emphasized the impenetrable stone wall he encountered. However, when in 1937 he described the deep-seated resistances to analytic treatment, he did not explicitly relate the resistances in narcissistic conditions to the resistances in states of inertia and in negative therapeutic reactions, both of which he attributed to the death instinct. None the less there is an obvious relation between narcissism, narcissistic withdrawal, and the death instinct in his work.[4] The infant must develop a self or ego, the means for dealing with the impulses and anxieties deriving from the life and death instincts, and find a way of relating to objects and of expressing love and hate. In this context Freud's theory of the fusion and defusion of the life and death instincts seems crucial. He argued that the development of inner psychic structure involves 'binding' derivatives of the life and death instincts so that they do not overwhelm the individual. Whereas in normal development instinctual impulses experienced within object relations are gradually recognized and directed towards appropriate external objects (such as aggression, love, hate, destructiveness, etc.), in pathological situations, where there is severe defusion, a destructive narcissistic organization tends to develop. These generally omnipotent forms of organization exert in a sometimes open but more often hidden way a powerful destructive influence; they are directed against life and destroy the links between objects and the self by attacking or killing parts of the self, but they are also destructive to any good objects by trying to devalue and eliminate them as important.

I consider that the development and perpetuation into adulthood of narcissistic omnipotent object relations are commonly found in patients who are very resistant to analytic treatment. They often respond to analysis by profound and persistent self-destruction. In these patients the destructive impulses have become defused (unbound) so that they actively dominate the entire personality and all the relationships a patient has. In analysis such patients express their feelings in an only slightly disguised way by devaluing the analyst's work through persistent indifference, tricky repetitive behaviour, and sometimes open belittlement. In this way they assert their superiority over the analyst (representing life and creativity) by wasting or destroying his work, understanding, and satisfaction. They feel superior in being able to control and withhold those parts of themselves which want to depend on the analyst as a helpful person. They behave as if the loss of any love object including the analyst would leave them cold and even stimulate a feeling of triumph. Such patients occasionally experience shame and some persecutory anxiety but only minimal guilt, because very little of their libidinal self is kept alive to feel concern. It appears that these patients have dealt with the struggle between their destructive and libidinal impulses by trying to get rid of their concern and love for their objects by killing their loving dependent self and identifying themselves almost entirely with the destructive narcissistic part of the self which provides them with a sense of superiority and self-admiration. When analysing clinical symptoms, such as the wish to die or to withdraw into a state of nothingness or deadness, which at first sight might be thought of as manifestations of the death instinct, described by Freud as a primary drive towards death, I have generally, on more detailed investigation, discovered that some active destructiveness is involved which was directed by the self not only against objects but against parts of the self. In 1971 I called this 'destructive narcissism', by which I meant that destructive aspects of the self are idealized and submitted to; they capture and trap the positive dependent aspects of the self (Rosenfeld 1971). They oppose any libidinal relations between the patient and the analyst.

One narcissistic patient I encountered, Simon, illustrates this phenomenon. For a long time he managed to keep all his relations to external objects and the analyst dead and empty by constantly deadening any part of his self that attempted object relations. On one occasion he illustrated this through a dream. In it a small boy was in a comatose condition, dying from some kind of poisoning. He was lying on a bed in a courtyard and was endangered by the hot midday sun which was beginning to shine on him. Simon was standing near to the boy but did nothing to move or protect him. He only felt critical and superior to the doctor treating the child, since it was he who should have seen that the child was moved into the shade. Simon's previous behaviour and associations made it clear that the dying boy stood for his dependent libidinal self which he kept in a dying condition by preventing it from getting help and nourishment from me, the analyst. I showed him that, even when he came close to realizing the seriousness of his mental state, experienced as a dying condition, he did not lift a finger to help himself or to help me to make a move towards saving him, because he was using the killing of his infantile dependent self to triumph over me and to show me up as a failure. The dream illustrates that the destructive narcissistic state is maintained in power by keeping the libidinal infantile self in a constant dead or dying condition. However, after much work it was sometimes possible to find that part of Simon which did not feel self-sufficient and dead, and to communicate with him in such a way that he felt more alive. He would then admit that he would like to improve but soon he would feel his mind drifting away from the consulting room. He would become so detached and sleepy that he could scarcely keep awake. This was an enormous resistance, almost like a stone wall, which prevented any examination of the situation. Only gradually did it emerge that Simon felt pulled away from any closer contact with me, because as soon as he felt helped there was not only the danger that he might experience a greater need for me but also the fear that he would attack me with sneering and belittling thoughts.[5]

Simon's case illustrates my argument that contact with help is experienced as weakening the patient's narcissistic omnipotent superiority and exposing him to conscious feelings of overwhelming envy which were strictly avoided by his previous detachment. It also illustrates the view I have developed in recent years: namely, the need to recognize clearly and to distinguish between the operation of a highly organized chronic and active narcissistic defensive organization and a more surreptitious and hidden deadly force which can be a chronic paralysing resistance holding up the analysis for many years. The latter, which operates in a manner very much akin to the way Freud described the functioning of the death instinct as a mute and hidden force opposing all progress, and which (like the death instinct) involves a deep preoccupation with death and destructiveness, often lies behind the narcissistic defensive organization and supports it. It is characterized by overwhelming murderousness and a feeling of being dead or deadly, hidden in which there is often concern for the consequences. The patient feels he is dead or the analyst is dead or that they will become so if the deadly force is admitted. This frightens the patient, as in Simon's case, to such an extent that it has to be kept hidden. The patient often secretly believes that he has destroyed his caring self, his love, for ever and that there is nothing anybody can do to change the situation. Our modern technique of analysis, however, involving the careful observation of the patient's dreams and behaviour in the transference, allows us to help the patient to be aware of this belief and the force which gave rise to it and to become aware of the support the belief gives to the destructive omnipotent way of living for which he has settled. Frequent interpretation and firm confrontation of Simon's destructive narcissistic thoughts and behaviour, to my complete surprise, brought about a considerable change in the patient's personality and attitude to other people. He seemed helped by my understanding and interpretation that a part of himself, particularly his infantile self, had masochistically colluded and accepted this paralysing deadly state by submitting to torture rather than admit a need and hunger for life. When he stopped treatment he was better although he could admit how improved he was only after some time when his symptoms had disappeared. Later, he had a very successful career in which he had to deal with many people and was greatly appreciated.

The destructive omnipotent way of living of patients like Simon often appears highly organized, as if one were dealing with a powerful gang dominated by a leader, who controls all the members of the gang to see that they support one another in making the criminal destructive work more effective and powerful. However, the narcissistic organization not only increases the strength of the destructive narcissism and the deadly force related to it, but it has a defensive purpose to keep itself in power and so maintain the status quo. The main aim seems to be to prevent the weakening of the organization and to control the members of the gang so that they will not desert the destructive organization and join the positive parts of the self or betray the secrets of the gang to the police, the protecting super-ego, standing for the helpful analyst, who might be able to save the patient. Frequently when a patient of this kind makes progress in the analysis and wants to change, he dreams of being attacked by members of the Mafia or adolescent delinquents, and a negative therapeutic reaction sets in. This narcissistic organization is in my experience not primarily directed against guilt and anxiety, but seems to have the purpose of maintaining the idealization and superior power of the destructive narcissism. To change, to receive help, implies weakness and is experienced as wrong or as failure by the destructive narcissistic organization which provides the patient with his sense of superiority. In cases of this kind there is a most determined chronic resistance to analysis, and only the very detailed exposure of the system enables analysis to make some progress.[6]

In some narcissistic patients the destructive narcissistic parts of the self are linked to a psychotic structure or organization which is split off from the rest of the personality. This psychotic structure is like a delusional world or object, into which parts of the self tend to withdraw (Meltzer 1963, personal communication). It appears to be dominated by an omnipotent or omniscient, extremely ruthless part of the self, which creates the notion that within the delusional object there is complete painlessness and also the freedom to indulge in any sadistic activity. The whole structure is committed to narcissistic self-sufficiency and is strictly directed against any object relatedness. The destructive impulses within this delusional world sometimes appear openly in a patient's unconscious material as overpoweringly cruel, threatening the rest of the self with death to assert their power, but more frequently they appear disguised as omnipotently benevolent or life-saving, promising to providing the patient with quick, ideal solutions to all his problems. These false promises have the effect of making the normal self of the patient dependent on or addicted to his omnipotent self, and to lure the normal sane parts into this delusional structure in order to imprison them. When narcissistic patients of this type begin to make some progress and to form some dependent relationship to the analysis, severe negative therapeutic reactions occur as the narcissistic psychotic part of the self exerts its power and superiority over life and the analyst, standing for reality, by trying to lure the dependent self into a psychotic omnipotent dream state which results in the patient losing his sense of reality and his capacity for thinking. In fact there is a danger of an acute psychotic state if the dependent part of the patient, which is the sanest part of his personality, is persuaded to turn away from the external world and give itself up entirely to the domination of the psychotic delusional structure.[7]

Clinically, in these situations, it is essential to help the patient to find and rescue the dependent sane part of the self from its trapped position inside the psychotic narcissistic structure, as it is this part which is the essential link with the positive object relationship to the analyst and the world. Secondly, it is important gradually to assist the patient to become fully conscious of the split-off destructive omnipotent parts of the self which control the psychotic organization, because this can remain all-powerful only in isolation. When this process is fully revealed it becomes clear that it contains the destructive envious impulses of the self which have become isolated, and then the omnipotence which has such a hypnotic effect on the whole of the self gets deflated, and the infantile nature of the omnipotence can be exposed. In other words, the patient becomes gradually aware that he is dominated by an omnipotent infantile part of himself which not only pulls him away towards death but infantilizes him and prevents him from growing up, by keeping him away from objects who could help him to achieve growth and development.

Robert

The first case I want to report, involving Robert, who had a chronic resistance to analysis, is intended to illustrate how a split-off omnipotent destructive aspect of a patient's functioning can be made visible in the analysis, with good results. The patient had had many years of analysis in another country, but his analyst eventually concluded that his masochistic character structure was not analysable.

Robert was a married man with three children. He was a scientist and very keen to have more analysis and to overcome his problems. From his history it is significant that he heard from his mother that when he developed teeth as a baby he started to bite her breasts regularly and so viciously that they always bled after feeding and her breasts became scarred. His mother did not withdraw her breast when she was bitten and seemed to be resigned to suffer. He thought he was breast-fed for more than a year and a half. Robert also remembered having very painful enemas from very early childhood onwards. It was also important to understand that his mother ruled the household and treated her husband as a very inferior being who had to live in a cellar-like basement. Robert co-operated at first in the analysis quite well and made good progress. But in the fourth year of analysis his progress slowed down. He was very elusive and repeatedly undermined the therapeutic effort. Robert had to leave

London occasionally for short professional trips and he often returned too late on Mondays and so missed either part or the whole of his session. He frequently met women during these trips and brought to analysis many of the problems which arose with them. It was clear from the beginning that some acting out was taking place but only when he regularly reported murderous activities in his dreams after such weekends did it become apparent that violently destructive attacks against the analysis and the analyst were hidden in the acting-out behaviour. Robert was at first reluctant to accept that the acting out of the weekend was killing, and blocking the progress of the analysis, but gradually he changed his behaviour, the analysis became more effective, and he reported considerable improvement in some of his personal relationships and his professional activities. At the same time he began to complain that his sleep was frequently disturbed and that he woke up during the night with violent palpitations and itching of his anus which kept him awake for several hours. During these anxiety attacks he felt that his hands did not belong to him: they seemed violently destructive as if they wanted to destroy something. He scratched at his anus violently until it bled profusely; his hands were too powerful for him to control, so that he had to give in to them.

He then dreamt of a very powerful arrogant man who was nine feet tall and who insisted that he had to be obeyed absolutely. His associations made it clear that this man stood for a part of himself and related to the destructive overpowering feelings in his hands which he could not resist. I interpreted that he regarded the omnipotent destructive part of himself as a superman who was nine feet tall and much too powerful for him to disobey. He had disowned this omnipotent self, related to anal masturbation, which explained the estrangement of his hands during the nightly attacks. I further explained this split-off self as an infantile omnipotent part of himself which claimed that it was not an infant but stronger and more powerful than all the adults, particularly his mother and father and now the analyst. His adult self was so completely taken in and therefore weakened by this omnipotent assertion that he felt powerless to fight the destructive impulses at night.

Robert reacted to the interpretation with surprise and relief and reported after some days that he felt more able to control his hands at night. He became gradually more aware that the destructive impulses at night had some connection with analysis because they increased after any success which could be attributed to it. This he saw as a wish to tear out and destroy a part of himself which depended on the analyst and valued him. Simultaneously the aggressive narcissistic impulses which had been split off became more conscious during analytic sessions, and he sneered, saying, 'Here you have to sit all day wasting your time.' He felt that he was the important person and he should be free to do anything he wanted to do, however cruel and hurting this might be to others and himself. He was particularly enraged by the insight and understanding which the analysis gave him. He hinted that his rage was related to wanting to reproach me for helping him, because this interfered with his omnipotent acting-out behaviour.

He then reported a dream, in which he was running a long-distance race and was working very hard at it. However, there was a young woman who did not believe in anything that he was doing. She was unprincipled and nasty and did everything to interfere and mislead him. There was a reference to the woman's brother, who was called 'Mundy'. He was much more aggressive than his sister and he appeared in the dream snarling like a wild beast, even at her. It was reported in the dream that this brother had had the task of misleading everybody during the previous year. Robert thought that the name 'Mundy' referred to his frequent missing of the Monday sessions a year before. He realized that the violent uncontrolled aggressiveness related to himself but he felt that the young woman was also himself. During the last year he had often insisted in his analytic sessions that he felt he was a woman, and was very contemptuous of and superior to the analyst. Lately, however, he occasionally dreamt of a little girl who was receptive and appreciative of her teachers, which I had interpreted as a part of him which wanted to show more appreciation of the analyst, but was prevented from coming into the open by his omnipotence. In the dream the patient admits that the aggressive omnipotent part of himself, represented as male, which had dominated the acting out until a year ago, has now become quite conscious. His identification with the analyst is expressed in the dream as a determination to work hard at his analysis. The dream, however, was also a warning that he would continue his aggressive acting out in analysis by asserting in a misleading way that he could present himself omnipotently as a grown-up woman instead of allowing himself to respond to the work of the analysis with receptive feelings relating to a more positive infantile part of himself. In fact Robert was moving in the analysis towards a strengthening of his positive dependence, which enabled him to expose openly the opposition of the aggressive narcissistic omnipotent parts of his personality; in other words, the patient's severe instinctual defusion was gradually developing into normal fusion.

Jill

My second case, Jill, illustrates the difficulties that arise when the deadly force I have mentioned earlier combines with and supports a destructive narcissistic way of living.

When a patient's destructive narcissism is fused with his omnipotent psychotic structure he cannot believe that there is anybody who can oppose his destructive overpowering attacks. This increases his excitement and the splitting off of any positive feelings. The detailed exposure of the destructive narcissistic structure during the analysis diminishes the strength of the omnipotent feelings, and so gradually the split between the destructive and positive impulses lessens. The positive impulses which have been previously completely dominated and controlled by the destructiveness can then start to come to life again so that the patient's self-observation and co-operation in the analysis can improve.

It is of course always essential to study the case history of our patients in detail in order to recognize the specific interpersonal relationships and traumatic experiences which existed in the past and contributed to building up the narcissistic structures. Even patients who appear to be completely identified with the narcissistic structure are from time to time aware that they are caught up and trapped but they do not know how to escape from this prison. With Jill, I would like to illustrate how difficult it is to assess the nature of the hidden secret opposition to life and progress. Gradually in analysis a destructive narcissistic structure was exposed. It was possible to help Jill to recognize how overwhelming she found the pull to turn away from life because she confused this with her wish to achieve an infantile state of fusion with her mother. When Jill gradually began to turn more to living it was interesting to see how very soon she was threatened with murder in her dreams. This marked the emergence into awareness of a destructive narcissistic organization, long referred to as 'they', which was fused with a confusing deadly force.

Jill had received psychoanalytic psychotherapy in another country for many years. At the beginning of this treatment she had a violent impulse to cut her wrists and when she succeeded in doing so she was hospitalized by her therapist for more than three years. Here the staff attempted sympathetically to understand her psychotic behaviour and thinking. She felt glad to be in the hospital because for the first time in her life her sickness, as she called it, was being taken seriously. She felt that her parents could not stand her being ill and would therefore not believe how ill she was. Her manifest psychotic

116

state was an attempt to be more open about her feelings. Previously she had felt so encased by her psychotic rigidity that to make her blood flow out was felt not so much as a wish to die but as an attempt to become more alive. Moreover, in the private hospital she felt it was wonderful to belong to a gang of patients who smashed windows and destroyed furniture and broke all the rules of the hospital. Any softness or need was ridiculed by her and regarded as being 'goody-goody'.

Even more than ten years later, during the treatment with me, she often longed for the days at the hospital where she could do what she wanted and felt alive. But in fact whenever she was a little more successful in her life she became overwhelmed by an unknown force which she called 'they' against which she could do nothing and which compelled her to retire to bed. She put on all the heaters in her bedroom to create a stifling hot atmosphere, drank alcohol, and read detective stories, which helped her to empty her mind of all meaningful thought. She felt this behaviour was necessary to appease 'them' (meaning the destructive forces), which threatened her when she tried to come alive.

At the time when she was beginning to develop insight into her problems she had a dream that she had been kidnapped from herself, but the kidnappers allowed her to walk about freely on parole bound by a promise that she would not escape. It really seemed at first as if she was caught up in her illness for ever. Only very gradually did she understand that the idealization of her destructiveness did not give her freedom, and that this was a trap into which she had fallen through the hypnotic power of the destructive self which posed as a saviour and friend who pretended to take care of her and give her whatever warmth and food she wanted so that she would not have to feel lonely. It was this situation that was acted out during the withdrawal state. In fact, however, this so-called friend attempted to spoil any contact she was trying to make in relation to work and to people. During analysis she gradually became aware that this exceedingly tyrannical and possessive friend was an omnipotent very destructive part of her self, posing as a friend, that became very threatening if she attempted to continue co-operation in analysis or any progress in her life. For a long time she felt too frightened to challenge this aggressive force and whenever she came up against this barrier she identified herself with the aggressive narcissistic self and became aggressive and abusive towards me. Sometimes I seemed to represent her mother and at other times her infantile self, which she projected into me. However, the main reason for her violent attacks related to my challenging the domination of her aggressive narcissistic state, my impudence in wanting to help her or even cure her, and she demonstrated that she was determined to do everything to defeat me. But after a few days of these attacks I also felt that there was a secret hope that I, and I included here also the self which was directed towards life, might win in the end. I also began to realize that the only alternative to her violent attack on me was her admission that she really wanted to get well, and this exposed her to the danger of being killed by the omnipotent destructive part of herself. After we had worked on this situation for many months the patient had a dream which confirmed and illustrated this problem.

In the dream the patient found herself in an underground hall, or passage. She decided she wanted to leave but she had to go through a turnstile to get out. The turnstile was obstructed by two people who were standing there, but when the patient investigated she found they were both dead and in the dream she decided they had recently been murdered. She realized that the murderer was still about and she had to act quickly to save herself. Near by there was an office of a detective, and she rushed in unannounced, but had to wait in the waiting-room for a moment. Even while she was waiting the murderer appeared and threatened to kill her because he didn't want anybody to know what he was doing, and what he had done, and there was a danger that she, the patient, would give him away. She was terrified and burst into the detective's room and so was saved. The murderer escaped, and she feared that while temporarily she was saved the whole situation would be repeated. However, the detective seemed able to follow the trail of the murderer, and he was caught, to her almost unbelievable relief.

Jill realized immediately that the detective represented myself, but the rest of the dream was quite a surprise. She had never allowed herself to think how frightened she was of being murdered if she were to trust me and come for help and give me all the information and co-operation she was capable of, particularly the information about the nature of her own murderous self. In fact the two dead people in the dream reminded her of previous unsuccessful attempts to get better. In the dream the analyst as a detective was, of course, highly idealized as the person who would not only protect her from her madness and murderous self and her destructive impulses but also free her from these fears for ever. I took the dream to mean that a part of her had decided to get well and leave the psychotic narcissistic state which was equated by her with death. But then the deadly power became actively murderous because of this decision. It is interesting that since this dream the patient has in fact turned more to life, and her fear of death has gradually lessened. Theoretically and clinically the work with this patient seemed to confirm the importance of the destructive aspects of narcissism, which in the psychotic states completely dominate and overwhelm the libidinal, object-directed, sane part of the self and try to imprison it.

The way Jill was again and again pulled away from life into a paranoid withdrawn state illustrates the way the deadly force I mentioned earlier works silently to support a destructive narcissistic way of being. Murderous violence lay hidden behind this silent death drive for a long time before it was revealed by the dream. After the murderer had appeared in the dream the analysis could make better progress, and the negative therapeutic reactions definitely lessened. This was possible partly because of Jill's gradual improvement and the surfacing of a much more loving and warm part of her personality.

Claude

Patients like Jill are never certain whether it is they who are murderers or whether they have a deadly force inside themselves. They often feel they need very strongly to keep their fear of death and of being a murderer a secret. Claude, a patient reported by Dr W. in one of my seminars, illustrates this very graphically. He had a severe fear of death between the ages of four and seven as well as later. This terror occurred when his parents were close by, but he stressed that they never knew anything about it, even when he felt at death's door. Complete independence from his parents seemed to him the only way to protect himself from his fear. He also remembered that occasionally he had secret murderous feelings against his mother, particularly when she was reassuring. He once missed an analytic session because he found the windscreen of his car smashed up. He believed he had done it himself in a dreamy state to prevent himself from coming to his session. He felt a strong need to keep the destructive feelings against the analysis secret even from himself. He once went on a skiing holiday with a girlfriend during the analysis. He mentioned this holiday to Dr W. only the day before. He hoped to feel better by being away from analysis but in fact he felt so disturbed with this girlfriend that he had to withdraw from her in order to protect her from himself, and he had also to give up skiing, which he loved. He spent most of the time reading a book of the mystical writer Carlos Castaneda. When he returned to analysis he only gradually revealed that he was quite paralysed and enormously exhausted during the holidays and he realized that there was something in him which was threatening to overwhelm him and could probably pull him to death. He felt that Castaneda's book brought some help to him. That is why he clung to it. Castaneda explains in his book his own terror of death but he advises everyone to make death their only friend in order to appease it, because death is terrifyingly possessive. It seemed clear to me that Claude feared that if he made the analyst and the analysis important, death changed from being a friend into a jealous murderous enemy. In Claude the murderous feelings related to death were directed more towards himself than others. The death drive seemed to appear in an almost undisguised form after a long period of having to hide his fear of death, a secrecy which is typical for all problems related to the death drive. Claude attempted to see death as a very good figure and he avoided all the dangers by allowing himself to be completely dominated by death. With the help of Castaneda's book he tried to do this, but the slightly tricky attempt to make death his friend failed, and he believed he was nearly killed during this so-called holiday.

Richard

My fourth case, Richard, illustrates the existence of a hidden destructive narcissistic way of being which was idealized so that the patient depended very much on functioning in this way and submitted to it as the most desirable way of living imaginable. Richard's psychopathology exemplifies the way narcissistic object relations invade all aspects of a patient's personality and how pathological fusion can be created. Above all he was intensely confused about what was good and bad for him, and this often led to profound disappointment. He often misjudged situations and would then be carried away by his apparent enthusiasm so that he could not recognize his mistake. Then he would become dogmatic, superior, and arrogant, with occasionally serious consequences for his life situation.

The patient was the youngest child in his family; he seemed to have always been treated with a great deal of indulgence by his brothers and sisters. He had an early trauma because when he was three months old he was suddenly separated from his mother, who had to go into hospital for several months because of a broken thigh. He had memories from a later period of her being sometimes seductive and indulgent but that often she was extremely strict and reproachful, which he found confusing. The father was reliable and supportive, but the mother tended to look down on him, and in earlier life he was apparently deeply influenced by her. In childhood Richard was very much attached to a dog whom he treated as an object with which he could do whatever he wanted, which implied that the dog was not only loved but also often grossly neglected by him. Early on in the analysis he dreamt of an otter which was living under his house and was very tame and followed him everywhere. In his associations he thought of his dog and also of a cow's udder. The dream suggested that Richard had formed early on in his life a very possessive part-object relationship to his mother's breast, a situation which was continued with his dog and other objects. He remembered a little girl with whom he played sexual games when he was about four to six years old. She tried to stop the games when they grew older. But he was so infuriated by her decision to abandon the sexual partnership that he killed her most beloved object, her cat. So his possessive love turned easily to murderous cruelty when he was thwarted.

The difficulty in Richard's analysis, as in his life, was the ease with which he turned away from objects internally and externally and seemed to follow impulses which presented themselves to him in a very seductive way, which generally misled him. He seemed keen to come for analysis but he often idealized his own contribution to the analysis. In the third year of treatment he had the following dream which gave us a clue to a better understanding of some of the problems with which he was struggling.

In the dream there was a weekend, and he suddenly realized that he had no milk in his house; he thought that there might be a shop open where he would get some milk but he remained undecided and did not know what to do to get some milk quickly. He then thought of his neighbour, to whom he had often turned for help, which he did also on this occasion. The neighbour told him that he could give him some milk but he confirmed that in fact a certain dairy shop was open on Sundays and he would accompany him to the shop. When Richard arrived at the shop there was a long queue but he accepted that he would have to wait. Two dairy maids dressed in white were looking after the customers. Before entering the shop the neighbour had shown the patient a cornered fivepence coin. The neighbour had not joined the queue and now he suddenly appeared, quickly approached the cash-register, and exchanged the small coin for a large bundle of £10 notes. He disappeared as quickly as he had come without being seen by the milkmaids. Richard was dumbfounded. He thought at first of informing the two women about this ruthless arrogant theft but then he remembered that his responsibility was

121

primarily to protect himself and not to interfere or intrude upon the milkmaids' business, which was their responsibility; but the real reason was that he was afraid for his life. He thought that the women in the shop would not be able to protect him against the ruthless man, who, once Richard was outside the shop, would doubtlessly retaliate. Why should he endanger his life because of such a theft and because of the fact that the women did not care for their money by leaving the till open? When the neighbour rushed out with the money the patient began to feel extremely guilty about the fact that he had not said anything and in that way had colluded with the neighbour. He then left the shop before his turn had arrived, feeling very guilty and selfish, knowing that it was wrong to keep quiet; he felt morally very weak. The dream continued. In the next moment the patient was in a dark back-yard alleyway dressed in old dirty rags, all alone. He was a 'down-and-out', the lowest of society, all apathetic, totally paralysed by hopelessness and helplessness due to guilt. He felt that there was nothing good in him and that he was a ruthless thief himself. He was a pitiful merciless coward who was unable even to inform about the theft, not to mention stopping it. It served him right to be wretched and forgotten by everybody. He felt he would die and that would be right. Then his first girlfriend came by and stroked his cheek gently with warmth and sympathy. He was surprised and glad and filled with some warmth inside. Then he began to think she must be ill and blind herself in some way to show him, who was such a hopeless, spineless wretch of a man, some warmth. Was she unconsciously colluding with him? Then his present wife came by and showed him some warmth as well. He felt that they both were in a danger of having their lives destroyed by associating themselves with him.

The manifest content of the first part of the dream is the more striking because Richard reveals here so clearly his dependence on the idealized neighbour and the complete denial of the neighbour's ruthlessness, greed, and cruelty. In the dream the neighbour is not only ruthless but also murderous, for if he found out that Richard knew what a ruthless criminal he was he would kill him. This is again the typical personality structure of patients who are controlled by a destructive narcissistic aspect of themselves which poses as an ideal friend and helper. In the dream the idealization breaks down, and the patient becomes aware of his collusion with the destructive part of himself which the neighbour represents. He realizes he has been completely unprotective and passive towards the caring milkmaids, who primarily stand for the good relationship to his mother in the feeding situation, and for his dependence on the

122

analyst. This problem had played a very important role in the analysis. Frequently when the patient acted out through thoughtlessness and ruthlessness he blamed me for it and asserted that I should have known beforehand and warned him of the problem. In the dream Richard corrects this attitude because he admits that it is his collusion with the destructive part of himself, the neighbour, which makes him such a tricky patient in analysis because he kept important information about himself from me.

In the second part of the dream Richard now takes full responsibility for the destructive delinquent part of himself, which in his waking state he found practically impossible to do because he feared, as the dream shows, not only that he himself was threatened and murdered by a destructive part of himself, but that he would actually become wholly bad. He was afraid that no goodness could exist in him because he had been false. In the dream he admits that he needs to be loved, but he cannot accept love because he feels he does not deserve it; he deserves only to die. Thus in the first part of the dream Richard is afraid of being murdered by a bad destructive part of himself, but in the second part he becomes afraid of being killed by his conscience, his super-ego, which would condemn him to death. This problem centres particularly on the false nature of his idealization of his neighbour, because Richard seems now to doubt the basis of any admiration and love, and fears that all love is phoney and that he obviously must be all bad. This is also the reason why he distrusts anybody who loves him; he fears that everyone who loves him must be colluding with his badness, and therefore everyone is false.

It is because he recognized his false admiration of the neighbour that Richard now felt it very difficult to trust anybody, including myself in the analysis whenever I made any sort of positive interpretation. However, if one interpreted only destructive intentions to a patient like this, the analyst would of course be identified with the very destructive super-ego which sees only destructiveness in him and does not give him any credit for wishing to recover from his bad state. Clinically it is extremely important to distinguish the false idealization of the destructive narcissistic self (which plays such an important role in the addictions to drugs and alcohol, chain-smoking, etc.) from the idealization of a basically good experience with good objects in the past or present. There is both a clinical and a theoretical danger if all the 'narcissistic' aspects of the personality, including those which have been described by many authors as healthy or normal components of the personality, are regarded as destructive.

Richard's dreams were very useful because they made it evident that his false idealization of a destructive self, posing as a good and ideal object, had contributed considerably to a confusion of good and bad aspects of his personality, with the danger that all the good aspects of the self could become equated with or overwhelmed by the bad ones. It is essential to distinguish between the forces of life and the forces of death. They are basically opposed to one another; when the good and bad parts of the self come together there is a danger that good and bad parts of the self and also good and bad objects will become so confused that the good self is overwhelmed and temporarily lost in the confusion. This tends to occur when the destructive parts of the self predominate. It is this process which I call pathological fusion. In normal fusions the aggressive forces of the self are mitigated by the libidinal parts of the self. This synthetic function is absolutely necessary for life – both for the survival of the self, which implies the development of the ego, and for the strength and constancy of object relations, for normal narcissism, and the capacity to fight for the protection of objects and for oneself. I also want to stress here the pathological fusions or fixation of the patient in the early paranoid schizoid level of development. Normal fusions are necessary for working through the depressive position, a process which Melanie Klein regarded as essential for any normal development. However, to establish normal fusions it is clinically and theoretically necessary to uncover firmly and distinctly the confusions of good and bad objects and good and bad aspects of the self, because nothing positive or sound can develop from the confusions, and there is a danger that a permanently weak and fragile self will result.

The dream of the neighbour explained much of the patient's repetitive behaviour in the analysis. For many years the patient had been unable to report to me any self-observation or conflict which had led up to his omnipotent behaviour, which always seemed to come out of the blue. I could show him through the dream of the neighbour that whenever he was in difficulties or felt thwarted he did not remember that I could help him and look after him because then he would have to wait for me and acknowledge his dependence on me. In his frustration and impatience he bypassed his memory of me and turned to an omnipotent and delinquent part of himself who acted ruthlessly on impulse, devalued the analysis, which was described as a mere fivepenny piece, and quickly grabbed whatever he wanted. He had not even been aware to what extent his destructive and delinquent narcissistic self, which he unconsciously had been proud of because it could get its way so quickly without being seen, had kept his dependent self completely under control by murderous threats so that he felt unable to co-operate in the analysis. In the dream it was made clear that he also felt that there was a collusion between his dependent self and his omnipotent greedy narcissistic self, as he disowned any responsibility for having to report his observations about the neighbour to the milkmaids. On the other hand, as I have mentioned, I had often found that when he did report a dream or gave associations he gave all the credit for progress to himself. This is of course a typical problem in the analysis of narcissistic patients who insist that the analyst, like the breast of the mother, is owned by them. Therapeutically it was essential to expose in this patient the domination of his whole self by his omnipotent destructive narcissistic self: because this enabled Richard gradually to use his analysis better, so that a satisfactory therapeutic result could be achieved.

Notes

1 André Green (1984) (see Chapter 1, note 6) has also made this point in a rather different way.
2 Abraham went much further than Freud in studying the hidden negative transference and in clarifying the nature of the destructive impulses which he encountered in his clinical work with narcissistic patients. In psychotic narcissistic patients he stressed the haughty superiority and aloofness of the narcissist and interpreted the negative aggressive attitude in the transference. As early as 1919 he had contributed to the analysis of the hidden negative transference by describing a particular form of neurotic resistance against the analytic method. He found in these patients a most pronounced narcissism, and he emphasized the hostility and defiance hidden behind an apparent eagerness to co-operate. He described how the narcissistic attitude attached itself to the transference and how these patients depreciate and devalue the analyst and grudge him the analytic role representing the father. They reverse the position of patient and analyst to show their superiority over him. He emphasized that the element of envy was unmistakable in these patients' behaviour and in this way clinically and theoretically he connected narcissism and aggression. It is interesting, however, that Abraham never attempted to link his findings with Freud's theory of the life and death instincts.

Reich (1933) was opposed to Freud's theory of the death instinct. He did, however, make fundamental contributions to the analysis of narcissism and the latent negative transference. He also emphasized, contrary to Freud, that the patient's narcissistic attitudes and latent conflicts, which include negative feelings, could be activated and brought to the surface in analysis and then worked through. He thought that 'every case without exception begins analysis with a more or less explicit attitude of distrust and criticism which, as a rule, remains hidden' (1933: 30).

Reich considered that the analyst has constantly to point to what is hidden and he should not be misled by an apparent positive transference towards the analyst. He studied in detail the character armour where the narcissistic defence finds its concrete chronic expression. In describing the narcissistic patient he stressed their superior, derisive, and envious attitude, as well as their contemptuous behaviour. One patient who was constantly preoccupied with thoughts of death complained in every session that the analysis did not touch him and was completely useless. The patient also admitted his boundless envy, not of the analyst, but of other men, towards whom he felt inferior. Gradually Reich realized and was able to show the patient his triumph over the analyst and his attempts to make him feel useless, inferior, and impotent so that he could achieve nothing. The patient was then able to admit that he could not tolerate the superiority of anyone and always tried to tear people down. Reich states (1933: 58): 'There then was the patient's suppressed aggression, the most extreme manifestation of which had thus far been his death wishes.'

Reich's findings in connection with latent aggression, envy, and narcissism have many similarities to Abraham's description of the narcissistic resistance in 1919.

There are a number of serious analysts apart from Freud who stress the importance of the death instinct and have related it in detail to their clinical work and experience. Federn (1932: 148), in a paper called 'The Reality of the Death Instinct' – in German 'Die Wirklichkeit des Todestriebs' – stresses that the drive towards death can be observed in its purest form in the melancholias where the destructive impulses are quite defused from any libidinal feelings:

> 'It is an awful sight to see how the melancholic in whom the death-instinct is at work without any connection with Eros constantly utters hatred and perpetually tries to destroy all possibilities of good fortune in the outer world in a most cruel way. Death-instinct within him fights Eros without.'

Federn also related the death instinct in great detail to the guilt feelings of the melancholic.

Eduardo Weiss in a paper published in 1935 in *Imago* on 'Todestrieb und Masochismus' described how secondary narcissism was related not only to libido turning towards the self, but also to aggression, which he called 'Destrudo', which behaved in an identical way. Unfortunately this paper, which contains many interesting ideas, is written in a rather obscure German.

Of all analysts probably Melanie Klein, who accepted the importance of Freud's theory of the interaction between the life and death instinct and used it theoretically and clinically, made the most notable contributions to the analysis of the negative transference. She found that envy, particularly in its split-off form, was an important factor in producing chronic negative attitudes in analysis, including negative therapeutic reactions. She described the early infantile mechanisms of splitting the objects and the ego, which enable the infantile ego to keep love and hate apart. In her contributions to narcissism she stressed more the libidinal aspects and suggested that narcissism is in fact a secondary phenomenon which is based on a relationship with an internal good or ideal object, which in phantasy forms part of the loved body and self. She thought that in narcissistic states a withdrawal from external relationships to an identification with an idealized internal object takes place.

Melanie Klein wrote in 1958 that she observed in her analytical work with young children a constant struggle between an irrepressible urge to destroy their objects and a desire to preserve them. She felt that Freud's discovery of the life and death instincts was a tremendous advance in understanding this struggle. She believed that anxiety arises from the 'operation of the death instinct within the organism, which is experienced as a fear of annihilation' (1958: 84). We see therefore that she conceived of the death instinct as a primary anxiety in the infant related to the fear of death, while Freud generally denied that a primary fear of death was in existence. The only clinical situation where he sees the death instinct terrorizing the self or the ego of the patient is described by him in 1923. He discusses here the extraordinary intensity of the sense of guilt in melancholia and suggests that the destructive component, a pure culture of the death instinct, has entrenched itself in the super-ego and turned against the ego. He explains here the fear of death in melancholia by saying that the ego gives itself up and dies because it feels itself hated and persecuted by the super-ego instead of being loved. This situation Freud relates to both the primary anxiety state at birth and the later anxiety of separation from the protecting mother.

In Melanie Klein's view, in order to defend itself against this anxiety the primitive ego uses two processes: 'Part of the death instinct is projected into the object, the object thereby becoming a persecutor; while that part of the death instinct which is retained in the ego causes aggression to be turned against that persecutory object' (Klein 1958: 85).

The life instinct is also projected into external objects, which are then felt to be loving or idealized. Melanie Klein emphasizes that it is characteristic for early development that the idealized and the bad persecuting objects are split and kept wide apart, which would imply that the life and death instincts are kept in a state of defusion. Simultaneously with the splitting of the objects the splitting of the self into good and bad parts takes place. These processes of ego splitting also keep the instincts in a state of defusion. Almost simultaneously with the projective processes another primary process, introjection, starts, 'largely in the service of the life instinct; it combats the death instinct because it leads to the ego taking in something life-giving (first of all food) and thus binding the death instinct working within' (1958: 85). This process is essential in initiating the fusion of the life and death instincts.

As the processes of splitting of the object and the self and therefore the states of defusion of the instincts originate in early infancy at a phase which Melanie Klein described as the paranoid schizoid position, one may expect the most complete states of defusion of instincts in those clinical conditions where paranoid schizoid mechanisms predominate. We may encounter these states in patients who have never completely outgrown this early phase of development or have regressed to it. Melanie Klein emphasized that early infantile mechanisms and object relations attach themselves to the transference, and in this way the processes of splitting the self and objects, which promote the defusion of the instincts, can be investigated and modified in analysis. She also stressed that through investigating these early processes in the transference she became convinced that the analysis of the negative transference was a pre-condition for analysing the deeper layers of the mind. It was particularly through investigating the negative aspects of the early infantile transference that Melanie Klein came up against primitive envy, which she regarded as a direct derivative of the death instinct. She thought that envy appears as a hostile, life-destroying force in the relation of the infant to its mother and is particularly directed against the good feeding mother because she is not only needed by the infant but envied for containing everything which the infant wants to possess himself. In the transference this manifests itself in the patient's need to devalue analytic work which he has found helpful. It appears that envy representing almost completely defused destructive energy is particularly unbearable to the infantile ego and early on in life becomes split off from the rest of the ego. Melanie Klein stressed that split-off, unconscious envy often remained unexpressed in analysis, but nevertheless exerted a troublesome and powerful influence in preventing progress in the analysis, which ultimately can be effective only if it achieves integration and deals with the whole of the personality. In other words the defusion of the instincts has gradually to change to fusion in any successful analysis.

3 In Freud's writings following his more speculative approach in *Beyond the Pleasure Principle* (1920), it became clear that he used the theory of the life

and death instincts to explain clinical phenomena. For example, in 'The Economic Problem of Masochism' (1924: SE 19: 170) he said: 'Thus moral masochism becomes a classical piece of evidence for the existence of fusion of instinct. Its danger lies in the fact that it originates from the death instinct and corresponds to the part of that instinct which has escaped being turned outwards as an instinct of destruction.' In *Civilization and its Discontents* (1930: SE 21: 122), Freud concentrates more on the aggressive instinct. He says: 'Man's natural aggressive instinct, the hostility of each against all and of all against each, opposes this programme of civilization. This aggressive instinct is the derivative and the main representative of the death instinct which we have found alongside of Eros.' Later he adds (p. 122): 'This problem must present the struggle between Eros and Death between the instinct of life and the instinct of destruction, as it works itself out in the human species.'

Here Freud does not clearly differentiate in the discussion between the death instinct and the instinct of destruction, as he wants to explain that there is a force which he calls the death instinct or the instinct of destruction that is in constant struggle with the life instinct, the wish to live.

In the *New Introductory Lectures* (1933: SE 22: 105) he discussed the fusion of Eros and aggressiveness and attempted to encourage analysts to use this theory clinically, arguing:

'This hypothesis opens a prospect to us of investigations which may some day be of great importance for the understanding of pathological processes. For fusions may also come apart, and we may expect that functioning will be most gravely affected by defusions of such a kind. But these conceptions are still too new; no one has yet tried to apply them in our work.'

He also said there:

'At some remote time . . . an instinct must have arisen which saw to do away with life. . . . If we recognize in this instinct the self-destructiveness of our hypothesis, we may regard the self-destructiveness as an expression of a "death instinct" which cannot fail to be present in every vital process.

'The death instinct turns into the destructive instinct when, with the help of special organs, it is directed outwards on to objects. The organism preserves its own life, so to say, by destroying an extraneous one. Some portion of the death instinct, however, remains operative *within* the organism and we have sought to trace quite a number of normal and pathological phenomena to this internalization of the destructive instinct.' (1933: SE 22: 107, 211)

129

In this paper Freud emphasizes particularly the self-destructive feelings as a direct expression of the death instinct and he stresses that there are special organs through which the death instinct turns into destructiveness and is directed outwards on to objects. In this description Freud's views are to some extent similar to Melanie Klein's ideas expressed at a later date. She argues that it is the primitive ego that projects some aspects of the death instinct into external objects, which in this way become persecutors while the rest of the death instinct is turned into direct aggression which attacks the persecutors.

Only four years later, in 'Analysis Terminable and Interminable (1937: SE 23: 242), Freud returned to the clinical application of his theory of the death instinct for the understanding of deep-seated resistances against analytic treatment, saying:

> 'Here we are dealing with the ultimate things which psychological research can learn about: the behaviour of the two primal instincts, their distribution, mingling and defusion. No stronger impression arises from the resistances during the work of analysis than of there being a force which is defending itself by every possible means against recovery and which is absolutely resolved to hold on to illness and suffering.'

He linked this with his previous theory of the negative therapeutic reaction, which he had related to an unconscious sense of guilt and the need for punishment, now (1937: SE 23: 243) adding:

> 'These phenomena are unmistakable impressions of the power in mental life which we call the instinct of aggression or of destruction according to its aims and which we trace back to the original death instinct of living matter. . . . Only by the concurrent or mutually opposing action of the two primal instincts – Eros and death instinct – never by one or the other alone, can we explain the rich multiplicity of the phenomena of life.'

Later on in the same paper he suggested that we may have to examine all instances of mental conflict from the point of view of a struggle between libidinal and destructive impulses.

4 One of the main reasons for this omission may be that Freud's theory of narcissism had originally been based on the idea of a primary narcissism, in which an individual directs his libido towards the self, and a secondary narcissism, in which he withdraws libido from objects back to the self (Freud 1914: 74). It was only after he had clarified his ideas on the pleasure principle and the reality principle in 1911, and brought these ideas into relation to love and hate in 'Instincts and their Vicissitudes' (1915), that he began to write about an important connection between a pleasurable

narcissistic stage and hatred or destructiveness towards the external object, when the object begins to impinge on the individual. For example, in 1915 (SE 14: 136) states: 'When during the stage of primary narcissism the object makes its appearance, the second opposite to loving, namely hating, also attains its development.' In the same paper he emphasizes the primary importance of aggression: 'Hate, as a relation to objects, is older than love. It derives from the narcissistic ego's primordial repudiation of the external world with its outpouring of stimuli' (p. 139).

Something of the same line of thought can be seen in Freud's view of the nirvana principle, which he sees as a withdrawal or regression to primary narcissism under the dominance of the death instinct – where peace, an inanimate state, and giving in to death are equated.

Hartmann, Kris, and Loewenstein (1949: 22) seem to have had a similar impression of Freud's ideas on the relation of aggression to narcissism when they wrote: 'Freud was used to comparing the relation between narcissism and object love to that between self-destruction and destruction of the object. This analogy might have contributed to his assumption of self-destruction as the primary form of aggression to be compared with primary narcissism.'

5 The history of this patient was significant. Simon told me that he had heard from his mother that he was an exceptionally difficult child to feed from the first three months onwards. When he was a year and a half he seemed to be an expert in throwing away all the food that was given to him by spoon or which he was allowed to eat himself from his plate; he would make a proper mess on the floor and look triumphantly at his mother, who would be rather anxious. These scenes occurred time and time again. His father criticized his mother as ineffective in looking after him but did nothing himself to support her or to deal with him. Eventually an expert nurse was employed. After a year the nurse told his mother she had to admit that her work with the child was a complete failure. She had never had a child before who so persistently and clearly, but with obvious satisfaction, refused all her attempts to feed and look after him. She resigned, leaving the mother to struggle on herself.

The striking symptoms of this patient were impotence and a rather obscure perversion. He was very schizoid and detached and had difficulties relating to other people. I was the patient's second analyst.

6 In many of these patients the destructive impulses are linked with perversions. In this situation the apparent fusion of the instincts does not lead to a lessening of the power of the destructive instincts; on the contrary, the power and violence are greatly increased through the eroticization of the aggressive instinct. I feel it is confusing to follow Freud in discussing perversions as fusions between the life and death instincts because in these instances the destructive part of the self has

taken control over the whole of the libidinal aspects of the patient's personality and is therefore able to misuse them. These cases are in reality instances of pathological fusion similar to the confusional states where the destructive impluses overpower the libidinal ones.

7 This process has similarities to Freud's (1914) description of the way in which in the narcissistic object cathexes are given up and libido is withdrawn into the ego. The state I am describing indeed implies the withdrawal of the self away from libidinal object cathexis into a narcissistic state which resembles primary narcissism. The patient appears to be withdrawn from the world, is unable to think, and often feels drugged. He may lose his interest in the outside world and want to stay in bed and forget what has been discussed in previous sessions. If he manages to come to the session, he may complain that something incomprehensible has happened to him and that he feels trapped, claustrophobic, and unable to get out of this state. He is often aware that he has lost something important but is not sure what it is. The loss may be felt in concrete terms as a loss of his keys or his wallet, but sometimes he realizes that his anxiety and feeling of loss refer to having lost an important part of himself, namely the sane dependent self which is related to the capacity for thinking. Sometimes the patient develops an acute and overwhelming hypochondriacal fear of death. One has here the impression of being able to observe the death instinct in its purest form, as a power which manages to pull the whole of the self away from life into a death-like condition by false promises of a nirvana-like state, which would imply a complete defusion of the basic instincts. However, detailed investigation of the process suggests that we are dealing not with a state of defusion but with a pathological fusion similar to the process I described in the perversions. In this narcissistic withdrawal state the sane dependent part of the patient enters the delusional object, and a projective identification takes place in which the sane self loses its identity and becomes completely dominated by the omnipotent destructive process; it has no power to oppose or mitigate the latter while this pathological fusion lasts; on the contrary, the power of the destructive process is greatly increased in this situation.

7

The problem of impasse in
psychoanalytic treatment

I have always been interested in patients who were difficult to treat and in finding out why some analyses ended in an impasse or failure. In Chapter 6 I illustrated how sometimes a mute deadly force constantly caused negative therapeutic reactions in my patient, Jill. Only after a very long time, as she seemed to feel more able to turn towards life, did a murderer appear in her dreams who was trying to murder her. In other cases the open appearance of murderousness, whether it is directed against the analyst or against people in outside life, is a serious problem, particularly if the patient tries to put this murderousness or criminality into action. Such patients seem to feel no regard for life and have no concern about their murderousness, making analysis very difficult.

I remember one such patient, Sheila, who was seen apparently successfully for about four years before a severe impasse developed. She had improved during the analysis but had not succeeded in reaching the perfect state of health and achievement to which she felt entitled. As a result she began to feel so disappointed and cheated by the analysis that she decided to take revenge on her analyst. He was blamed for withholding the perfect treatment from her. She therefore started planning how to murder him in such a perfect way that he could not possibly defend himself against her intention. The problem of analysing such a patient was related to the fact that she put all her pride and sense of achievement into her planning of this perfect crime, preventing her analyst from mobilizing in her any positive feelings or awareness which might weaken her resolve. In such situations there is a real danger that the analyst will have to stop working with a patient, so that the analysis will have to end in an impasse. Sheila is therefore one of the clearest examples of what can happen if destructive narcissistic omnipotence is determinedly and unrelentingly idealized.

Caroline

One of my patients, a doctor in general practice with a part-time psychiatric appointment, whom I shall call Caroline, illustrates another impasse caused by the difficulties of treating someone in whom a destructive narcissistic mode of relating is dominant but split off. Caroline, whom I treated more than twenty years ago, had a destructive, murderous, and criminal part in her personality which was both so completely split off and, eventually, so powerful and so serious that I came to know about it (along with her husband and indeed, in some ways, Caroline herself) only through a newspaper story and the intervention of the police.

Caroline approached me for analysis because she wanted to learn more about herself. She was slightly manic and diagnosed herself as a schizoid personality but was apparently happily married with one child. She reported nothing disturbing or unusual about her childhood experiences and she seemed to have a very good relationship to both parents, towards whom she felt very supportive.

During the analysis there was only one incident which worried me greatly. After about one and a half years of analytic work she reported that she had suddenly been dismised from her part-time job in the psychiatric clinic. She said that no reason was given to her about this dismissal. She felt that it must have involved some misunderstanding or misrepresentation about her, and she wanted to protest. I pointed out to Caroline several times how important it would be in these circumstances to contact her chief in the clinic and ask him what had happened; unless she did this the whole situation would be left as something very mysterious as well as detrimental. She reported later that she had written to her chief but received no reply. The only other incident she ever mentioned to me that was possibly related to this incident concerned one occasion when she had been disconcerted because, when she was in the lavatory of the clinic, some of the nurses sometimes looked over the partition walls at her in a way which she felt was quite extraordinary. She thought they must have suspected her of drug addiction, which was ridiculous as she never used drugs herself although she had looked after some drug addicts in the clinic. Caroline was so distressed and outraged about her dismissal that I felt a mistake must have been made but continued to be very puzzled.

After this incident Caroline reported an increase in her interest in treating drug addicts and trying to help them and eventually that she had been appointed by the National Health Service as a director to a special clinic for addicts. This was exactly what she had wanted to achieve, and she was thrilled. At the clinic she also had an assistant. During the following months Caroline became more and more interested in her clinic and she felt she was very successful in dealing with the drug addicts. Only occasionally did she report some problem with a drug addict whom she was trying to wean off the drugs.

At the time I was aware that she seemed to be becoming more and more preoccupied with this clinic and so pointed out to her to what extent all her interest seemed to be drawn in this direction, while, in contrast, all other aspects of our analytic work took second place. She defended what was happening by saying that there were a number of anxieties that were stirred up in her by working so intensely with drug addicts. She needed the analysis more than ever to cope with their problems.

Direct evidence that something unusual was going on came to my attention only when Caroline told me that the police had questioned her about criminal drug-prescribing following a newspaper article which she described to me as very poisonous. She reported this to me immediately it occurred and was very upset. She believed that some very envious person was trying to defame her and asserted that she was completely innocent. However, the police insisted on taking her into custody and would not allow bail, so she could not attend her sessions. After some time I was visited by Caroline's solicitor, who told me that he had investigated all the police allegations and had unfortunately found they were true. Caroline had sold prescriptions to drug addicts for large sums of money. Her solicitor thought she was probably schizophrenic and wanted me to co-operate with him by telling the courts that I had been treating her for schizophrenia. This put me in a difficult position because at the same time Caroline was writing many letters to me from prison protesting her innocence. She insisted that I should tell the solicitor and the courts that she was both sane and innocent.

Caroline was sent for observation to a major London mental hospital for more than a week, but the professor there diagnosed only a hypomanic state, finding no sign of a severe mental illness such as schizophrenia. The split in Caroline's personality was so severe that neither her husband, her friends, nor I had the slightest notion about her criminal activities. Yet these were so extreme that while she was in prison awaiting her court case she tried with a large amount of money to hire someone to murder her assistant. He was the one Caroline accused of having got her into this terrible situation. The courts took a very serious view and brought an additional charge against her for attempted murder. Caroline was found guilty but soon afterwards became so persecuted and disturbed that the authorities realized that schizophrenia had developed. She was detained at Her Majesty's Pleasure, which implied that she was found to be unsound and had to be detained for her own protection as a dangerous criminal.

The outcome of Caroline's treatment was a severe shock for me, although I could not see that there was anything I could have done to prevent it. What seems so incredible even now is the extent of the split between the destructive criminal part of the patient and the part with which she related to me. The first represented the complete opposite to the second. Consciously her ambition was to be a specially caring and successful healer who wanted to devote a great deal of her time to the welfare of her patients and make them better. Drug addicts are notoriously difficult to treat, and it is clear that during the last six months of her treatment with me, when she was so preoccupied with curing and helping her drug addict patients, she was pulled more and more into collusion with them and probably identified with their destructive narcissism. However, she never expressed any disillusionment or sense of failure in connection with the treatment of these patients. On the contrary, she claimed, as far as my contact with her was concerned, that she was very successful. It was because of her success with her patients that she had become the director of this clinic. One might wonder whether pathological lying played a role in Caroline's case, because patients suffering from *pseudologia fantastica* behave similarly in psychoanalytical treatment, in so far as they manage to persuade the analyst to believe that they are making a great deal of progress and doing good work when in fact they do absolutely nothing and remain complete failures in their achievement. The lying in these cases is so complete that the analyst is generally taken in and does not know that he is being lied to. With Caroline one never had the feeling that she was lying. She seemed to have split off her criminal and murderous ruthless self utterly, so that when this was acted out disastrously in real life it was uncontrollable.

Caroline has a great deal in common with the patient just mentioned, Sheila, who suddenly developed murderous intentions against her analyst. They both had uncontrollable impulses on which they intended to act. When the murderous intentions appeared,

136

Caroline seems to have split off entirely her positive self, who had previously co-operated with the analyst and had apparently made a great deal of progress. Such a split is so violent that the analyst has the impression that the patient seems no longer aware that a positive, co-operative part of himself ever existed. Fortunately the split between the murderous destructive narcissistic self and the positive part of the patient is not always so deep and persistent as in these cases.

Pauline

A second impasse I want to describe was with a patient of mine, Pauline, whom I treated thirty years ago. She suddenly developed delusions about me after six years of analysis. At the time I feared that a latent schizophrenic state had been activated by the analysis, because I was unable to help her reach any insight whatsoever about it. The analysis broke down in an impasse.

During the six years of her analysis Pauline had very gradually become more and more hesitant in speaking and often gave the impression that she had come up against some block, but I could not find out what it was. It often created in me a feeling that she and I could never bring the analysis to a successful end. In the first years of the analysis I had felt hopeful about the patient's progress. She was well qualified and very interested in becoming an analyst herself. But when the patient's difficulties in speaking became worse and worse I seriously doubted that I had been right in my hope that she might be able to become an analyst. Clearly, then, my feelings towards the patient had been changing.

One day Pauline suddenly told me that she understood what was holding her back. I was at first happy and relieved that she had apparently decided to let herself go but I must confess that I was rather shocked when she told me that she was dissatisfied with the colour in all the rooms in her house. She had decided to paint them all dark brown, including the kitchen and bathroom. Dark brown in one or two rooms can, of course, be rather attractive, but I felt apprehensive and a short time after I was horrified as a complete delusional system appeared. She had been having difficulty conceiving a child but was eventually successful. She had a fairly normal pregnancy and had delivered a child without too many problems. However, when this child was nearly a year old, Pauline told me that she knew that I had always been rather critical about her having a child and had all the time been trying to produce an abortion. She also said that it was obvious that I was sexually interested in her and that she was disturbed about my constantly wanting to seduce her. I want to stress here that consciously I was not physically attracted to the patient but, as I explained, I had had hopes that one day she might become an analyst herself.

When this delusion appeared, Pauline lost all insight and became angry that I did not agree with her that the analysis was now successfully concluded. She insisted that what had now appeared in the analysis was her true self, and I should be pleased about it. She said her only reservation was some disagreement with me about analytical theory and she wrote a paper which she gave me to read to prove her health and sanity. The paper was terribly confused and pretentious. She wanted to publish it, but I persuaded her to show it first to someone whose opinion she trusted. She sent the paper to Ernest Jones, who asked her to come and see him. He was very tactful with her but said the paper was neither good nor clear enough to be published.

Jones wrote to me to say that he was sorry that I had such an alarming and disappointing experience with the patient and added that such sudden psychotic eruptions occurred sometimes. Looking back I realize that I made several mistakes. Instead of trying to help Pauline to gain some 'real' insight into her delusional state, which was not possible, I should have taken some responsibility for what I was doing in her analysis. I should, perhaps, have explained to her that it was obvious that she had been feeling critical about me for some time and wondered whether there was an occasion when something I had said or done might have hurt her. That might have enabled Pauline to tell me more of what had been going on inside her and what she really felt about me. I do remember that once, when she wanted to apply for a very important research grant, for which she wanted a recommendation from me, I had said something to put her off that she did experience as a 'put-down'. Anyhow I had not felt that I could recommend her.

Pauline stopped the analysis three months later, remaining convinced she was well. She wrote me a very friendly letter several years later, explaining that she had by then had some more analysis and realized that she had been confused when she broke off the analysis with me. We would nowadays classify a patient like Pauline as a borderline state and be on the look-out for transference/counter-transference problems as a possible cause of confusion and transference psychosis. In these cases the treatment generally consists of stopping interpretations for a while so as to be able to think through and explore what transference collusion might be operative.

Diagnosing impasse

Counter-transference problems in a long analysis frequently occur when the analysis is not making progress and an impasse is threatening. Impasses, however, are of different kinds, and it is important to try to differentiate them. One type occurs during the final stages of an analysis when some of the patient's symptoms which have often been analysed before appear again in an exaggerated form. They have to be worked through at least once more. Such impasses are a very positive development in the sense that they provide the opportunity to reinforce the understanding of the disturbing processes which have dominated the analysis.

A second type of impasse occurs when a patient has made particularly good progress but suddenly exhibits a negative reaction. He comes late, or forgets to come to the analysis, or cannot remember what work has gone on in the earlier sessions. In these circumstances, as I have discussed at length in earlier chapters, it is likely that hidden envy has been mobilized and is being acted out through destructive behaviour aimed against the analytic progress. To deal with this situation one has to be very careful to scrutinize the patient's dreams and associations for the kind of material I have presented in Chapters 4 and 5.

I believe it is important to distinguish the kinds of impasse mentioned so far, and particularly to differentiate the true negative therapeutic reaction just mentioned, from a different kind of impasse in which severe negative reactions to analysis do not follow real progress and where it would not, therefore, be appropriate to speak of negative feelings being due to envy of therapeutic progress. If an analyst misdiagnoses such chronic negative reactions as a negative therapeutic reaction and interprets envy and triumph over the analyst in the transference situation, the impasse will only become worse. If the patient holds a grudge against the analyst or has criticisms of what he has been doing, like Sylvia (Chapters 2 and 3) or the patient just mentioned, Pauline, the repeated interpretation of envy (or a preoccupation with 'real' problems) will imply to the patient that the analyst is out of touch with what is going on in him. He feels rejected and still more frightened to express his criticism, because he feels that the analyst will not listen. In these cases a severe deterioration of the relationship between analyst and patient and a gradual worsening of the patient's mental and physical state are an invariable consequence. In fact these situations produce the most severe form of impasse. Equally invariably an important source of such impasse is some difficulty in the counter-transference.

I shall now present material from the analysis of one of my patients, Eric, whose previous analysis had reached an impasse and whose analysis with me was also very difficult.

Eric

Eric was about forty when he approached me for analysis. He was very hesitant and frightened to do so because he felt almost sure that he would be rejected by me. After about fifteen years of psychoanalysis with a very experienced woman analyst, Dr U., he found himself in a shocking mental condition. He experienced anxiety all day long and at night and he was also frightened to eat, particularly in the morning, because he frequently vomited. He explained to me that after he had been in analysis for about eight years there was a session in which Dr U. mentioned the ending of the analysis. Shortly after, he was suddenly overcome by strong feelings of contempt for the audience to whom he was at that moment lecturing. These feelings were so strong that he was scarcely able to finish the lecture. Eric not only felt that it was unpleasant to experience such contempt for his audience; he was also deeply ashamed of his complete inability to control these feelings. He was very shocked by the incident because lecturing had been an activity he always enjoyed and he had always felt this was one thing he did well. Suddenly his life's achievement seemed to be threatened.

Eric described to me how his experience at the lecture had an enormous impact on him and made him feel a very much increased need for help and understanding through his analysis. He said, however, that he felt in a great dilemma because Dr U. seemed to be as shocked and at a loss as he was about what had happened; this may have been true. He knew that he very badly needed sympathetic understanding of and help with his problem but said he had not felt able to detect any such feeling in her. This impression may perhaps have been influenced by the fact that it appeared Dr U. had concentrated her interpretations after the lecture incident almost entirely on the triumph and contempt which she thought Eric was expressing towards her. He reported, for example, that she said that he wanted enviously to destroy the success of the analysis and make her look entirely incompetent. Interpretations of this kind were felt by Eric as critical angry remarks which increased his hopelessness and isolation and made him feel unable to put anything in order.[1]

When I first saw Eric, he told me that he had felt very critical of

Dr U. at that time. He felt she seemed to be unconcerned about the pain, depression, and hopelessness he was feeling. He had wanted to have a second opinion, particularly after his condition deteriorated over the following years. However, this was apparently discouraged by Dr U., and he was too frightened to carry on regardless. He described how he felt threatened by her hostile power if he did not completely obey her. Eventually, as Eric did not respond to treatment and deteriorated further (in other words, when an impasse had been reached), Dr U. reduced his sessions to once a week. Eric experienced this reduction both as a further threat and as an illustration of Dr U.'s cruelty. He managed to consult another analyst, myself, only when Dr U. eventually stopped the treatment altogether.[2]

When I first spoke to Eric he was terrified that I, also, would reject him and agree with the way he had been treated previously. He expected me to regard him as a hopeless case not deserving any further analysis. In such a situation it is important to try to assess the patient's character structure and some of the transference/counter-transference reactions from the last therapy which dominate the patient. I also thought it would be important to examine whether Eric had really been so much better when the negative reaction occurred, and whether there were good grounds for Dr U. to interpret the fact that his envious feelings had gone out of control as a result of his improvement. I wondered if there were other factors which had not been sufficiently analysed. In fact, as I shall shortly describe, Eric had accumulated an enormous amount of criticism against the way he had been treated in childhood as well as by Dr U., and much of this, repeating his history, was fully justified. I was to find out that during his analysis with Dr U. a great deal of criticism had accumulated which had remained unexpressed and had not been analysed. There was evidence that Eric felt constantly hurt, injured, and belittled by Dr U., which created a dangerous accumulation of narcissistic rage and revenge against her with which Eric did not know how to cope. In fact during this long negative reaction to the treatment Eric experienced that he was being pulled entirely away from life, success, and people towards death and isolation. In particular the satisfaction and joy he had learned to get from his work success disappeared, and he was in a constant state of terror. This created very unpleasant symptoms. The further he travelled from his home, the more terrified he became, so that eventually he could not travel at all. He was frightened of meeting people. He admitted that he had been very arrogant and superior at one time and was constantly preoccupied with narcissistic phantasies. He would watch himself and try to imagine himself as an important person engaged in many occupations. However, such attempts to regain his self-confidence seemed to make matters worse. By the time he saw me he was near collapse. He felt a complete failure and devalued.

Eric had to wait for some time until I could find a place for him but at first he responded very well to the treatment with me. It is of course very easy for any analyst taking over a patient of that kind to understand the need to be careful and to allow him to recover from the previous experience. It is therefore easy to avoid the old pattern from a previous analysis and to beware of repeating some of the interpretations he had become used to and which he was almost in the habit of making to himself. I think it took only a month or so for Eric to feel more relaxed so that he could say things without feeling that he was immediately being criticized.

Eric soon informed me that his mother had often told him that, as a baby, he was always crying. She insisted that he cried before, during, and after breast-feeding and that she had become desperate about this and didn't know what to do. In a case like this it is also essential to examine details of the patient's early history in order to understand how much of earlier events in his life had repeated themselves during the analysis and got entangled with the analytic situation. I soon noticed such an entanglement. Eric told me that during the years of impasse his analyst had often interpreted that he behaved in analysis exactly as his mother described his behaviour to her as the baby. However, as Eric's feelings of being very unhappy and not comfortable in his relationship to Dr U. were not analysed sufficiently, he understood Dr U.'s remarks simply as meaning that she felt he was a difficult and ungrateful baby and patient, or that she felt desperate and did not know what to do with him. He therefore felt deeply rejected.

Eric's mother had herself worked with small children and must have felt very hurt that her own baby seemed to reject her. His mother was apparently depressed when he was born. Generally, she had great difficulty in getting pleasure from being alive, and Eric seems to have been deeply affected by this, particularly as she tended to pull him into her own way of thinking. He reported, for example, how when he wanted to enjoy himself she often said, 'This is not for us.' To add to the strong background of feeling rejected by his parents, his father, who was a schoolteacher, regarded him as stupid when he was ten or eleven. However, in spite of his background he seemed to have been ambitious and very keen to be successful, and to gain recognition. He was therefore very disappointed when, later, when he did become successful, going to university and starting to write papers and even books, that his father was apparently never willing to say that he was pleased with him.

When I started analysis with Eric he told me that he constantly felt that there was something inside him which belittled him and ran him down. There was no doubt that he was very narcissistic, but he was no longer able to use his narcissistic defences successfully or to feel confident and superior. It seemed that his narcissism had been smashed but, apparently, without anything positive being created in its place. Moreover, the previous analysis seemed to have created or mobilized an enormous amount of guilt about his narcissism without confronting his tendency to be superior and triumphant – which clearly still existed, as illustrated by the outbreak of contempt during the lecture. I have mentioned that when Eric came to me he was afraid that his criticism of Dr U. might be wrong and for this reason had suppressed it for such a long time. Given the context of a great deal of hurt and suppressed narcissistic rage not expressed towards Dr U. (not least as the transference representative of the parents), I came to the view that the lecture incident was not really a negative therapeutic reaction. It seemed to be more of an attempt to draw Dr U.'s attention to the fact that Eric felt far from well, depressed, and in need of help. If this is so, a considerable misunderstanding existed between patient and analyst at the time when he got worse, and this misunderstanding persisted as an impasse right to the end of the analysis.

After several months of analysis with me Eric felt very much better but could still become very easily upset and discouraged when he had a slight set-back. He had felt quite hopeful that he could cope with the first long holiday and he had also allowed his wife to leave him for a while at the same time. He decided during the holiday that he would buy himself a new leather coat. He had always wanted one and suddenly felt he had the courage to buy one. When he bought the coat he was at first very pleased with it. However, he became almost immediately very anxious and depressed. For some days he felt overwhelmed by the depression but he eventually managed to understand for himself that by buying the coat he felt he had rejected both his wife and me. While the leather coat was a good permanent protective skin it was not a substitute. In fact when he realized what had gone on inside him he began to feel gradually better, and he came through the holidays well enough.

Eric occasionally had negative reactions. After about a year in analysis he told me how very well he felt I understood him and compared and contrasted me with both his mother and his previous analyst. However, soon after this, when he started to be able to leave his house and went with his wife to the theatre, he felt absolutely dreadful and had such a shock that he started to sweat and felt that life wasn't worth living. He completely lost both any desire and appetite and feared that he had relapsed more than ever before. None the less, such set-backs did not last very long.

The way Eric used feelings to triumph over me and his previous analysis became clear only after a session in which he had felt particularly well understood. He suddenly experienced a violent rage against his parents and an even more murderous rage against Dr U. These feelings were welling up in him and getting out of control, and he had the phantasy that he was meeting one of Dr U.'s patients and told him, or her, what a rotten person she was. He had never had any experience before as bad as with her. Eric realized that in this violent phantasy he felt very triumphant, resentful, and revengeful. He was also aware that he believed that when he was treated well he could not feel that it would make him better. Rather, he felt secretly indulged by me in this violent destructive attack. The next day he felt dreadful and very guilty. He tried to make things up to his wife because he felt he didn't give anything to anybody. He realized that in the previous breakdown he felt he could not do anything better than want to kill himself. However, at the same time, he began to remember that in fact he hadn't always felt so badly treated by his mother. His mother had sometimes been happy. It was only when she was sad that she could not enjoy anything. He now remembered that one day she had been crying and had said to him. 'I can't spend money. I can't enjoy it.' She had given him £5 and said, 'Use the money because I can't use it myself.'

After this memory Eric began to feel sorry for his mother, whereas in the past he had felt only resentment. He realized that feelings of sympathy for her had been missing all this time. By now there had been a gradual improvement; however, Eric's anxiety about not being able to go on holiday persisted, and he felt rather depressed and incurable about it. At the same time he reported to me some things about himself and his life which were very striking but about which he had only recently become more aware. He said it was very peculiar because, although his wife had been rather aggressive towards him for some time and had not been helpful, she was now trying to help and had tried to make him aware of certain factors which he had never observed in himself before. For example, she had noticed that when his anxiety was quite strong it was accompanied by such a strong smell that it was almost unbearable for her to be near him while it lasted. On the other hand, he also reported that he did not understand why, when he wrote something for publication,

144

his wife was never interested in it. She saw only the ugly side of him and never his good points. I reminded him that he had told me something similar about his previous analyst. After eight years in analysis she had got so fed up with him that it seemed to him that she was interpreting only the destructive and bad parts of him and no longer saw anything good. He replied that he would have to consider whether, perhaps, he had the power to make people lose their good image of him as somebody who could be attractive and valuable. He then described to me, in detail, his anxiety when I went on holiday. Normally one might have thought of what he was saying as expressing a fear of separation and of being left alone. However, from his description it seemed to me that he was envious that I was free to go, while he could not. Moreover, while he continued talking to me he said his anxiety intensified and he felt a particularly great anxiety growing in his stomach. He said he thought this could be related to his conviction that he could create in me a bad picture of himself. At the end of the session he said he didn't feel any better.

At the beginning of the next session Eric told me immediately that as soon as he had arrived home after the last session and was alone by himself he had felt relaxed. He was surprised that he felt so well. He had thought I would still be worrying about him and perhaps not be able to get him out of my mind. So I could see that I was left with the anxiety and he could enjoy himself alone in his room feeling very good. It had become apparent that there was a strong sadistic relationship being enacted in the analysis, which was related to his feeling envious of my well-being. He obviously felt satisfied about having spoilt my enjoyment in trying to help him, so that I would have to worry about him while he was sitting comfortably at home with no worry. As an afterthought he added that he did still feel some envy towards some aspects of my activities but this he left rather vague. Eric continued by telling me that he felt there was a woman inside him who was very ugly, and he had to keep her very ugly because there was a danger that if she was beautiful she would be violently attacked by others, particularly by other women. This was her way of keeping herself comfortable. He added, 'Of course, if she was ugly and unpleasant nobody would want to be with her.' He then became aware that there was a feeling in him that he actually liked to remain cruel and bad and that it was a situation he enjoyed. He continued telling me another story in which there was a man who had a mistress who was very tricky and had a nasty character. So he had killed her. Afterwards he was lying in bed with his wife, who was very kind and to whom he was outwardly friendly. But he then found that he actually hated her. He missed the nasty and deceitful mistress and realized that he had been very much in love with her.

I then tried to show him that the mistress, who was so nasty, seemed also to be the ugly woman – that is, his own destructive narcissistic self with which he was so much in love. I added that he seemed to be afraid that I would cure him because he feared that in this event he would be bored. In fact, he actually wanted to go on as he was. It was now possible to see why it had been so difficult to get at the real cause of Eric's troubles. These were mainly caused by a secret and hidden determination to hold on to the status quo, a preference for nasty and sadistic behaviour over and above everything else and a belief that nothing else could be better. He was terrified that I would take away this inner destructiveness with which he was so much in love. Until it suddenly emerged, the cause of this problem had been very carefully disguised. But now Eric confessed to me that a few weeks before, after he had left a session feeling very much better, he had been hoping to try enjoying the good relationship with his wife. But then he suddenly felt an impulse to start a violent quarrel with her. In fact, however, he had been able to stop this quarrel and was glad about it. He was glad too that he had become more aware what was going on inside him.

I was surprised about the extent of Eric's destructiveness, which had been hidden from me for most of the time. Usually, the destructive narcissistic aspect of a patient's personality shows itself after a patient has made progress and some positive aspects of him have come more to the foreground – as in Jill's case, described in Chapter 6. It is the destructive part of a patient which appears in the negative therapeutic reaction. However, Eric's attachment to an ugly, nasty, narcissistic self remained much more hidden and created a very powerful chronic negative reaction to analysis. He was afraid, even convinced, that he might be incurable, and his deadly fear pervaded his being. In Eric's case the destructive narcissistic self had paralysed his capacity to relate to men or women, and it was essential to show him this. He could never allow himself to be attractive and affectionate, despite consciously hoping he would learn to do so, and always failed to make friends.

After Eric presented this material to me there were many ups and downs in the analysis. I gradually formed the impression that he had used destructive narcissism to hold himself together and to give himself strength, even if it was a false strength. He felt that his capacity to love was weak, sometimes even absent, but he could not believe that love could ever give his personality any strength. Eric had had a number of experiences in his life where his confidence in his own strength and capacity had been severely shaken. In these situations he had felt deeply humiliated, hurt, and most disappointed about close colleagues. In the analysis he felt strongly suicidal when these problems were being touched upon. His destructive narcissistic phantasies seemed to be organized in a defensive system of strength and superiority on which his survival depended. When Dr U. had made very forceful attacks on his narcissism Eric had felt smashed and defeated and after that he felt increasingly unprotected. But, in this treatment with me, there was gradually distinct progress which helped him to gain more confidence in certain aspects of his work. However, an inner paralysis and emptiness seemed to remain which worried both him and me. He felt very vulnerable and thought this should be covered up rather than more exposed. In particular, he felt that other people had desirable objects inside them, like a good breast, which gave them basically good feelings. He thought he lacked this basic experience and felt there was an emptiness, a black hole, inside him. He felt that this problem had interfered in his relationship with his mother from the beginning. He had seemed unable to find any calmness and satisfaction at the breast and so had cried before, during, and after the feed, as his mother had told him. He had actually had two women therapists before me. He felt the first therapist, whom he had consulted during his first breakdown, was at first very hopeful and friendly; but when he did not recover, after taking the exams he had been frightened about, as she expected, and when he was getting worse and worse, she seemed to become disappointed and anxious. She was also cruel to him and handed him over to another therapist. Something similar occurred, he felt, with his second woman therapist, Dr U. She had also seemed to be more hopeful about his capacity to develop at first, but then, at the moment when she hoped he was getting much better, he became worse and worse in the negative reaction I have described. Dr U. also became cooler and more withdrawn from him. In both cases he felt terribly vulnerable, unable to deal with the situation, completely hopeless and abandoned.

As far as one can judge Eric's very complicated pathology, I considered that during the first year of analysis with me he did have a good experience and that some good introjections had taken place. He could then recover through his own insight from the depression which overwhelmed him when he bought the leather coat. For that reason I did not think that his bad early experience, even if he had not been able to introject a good experience with the breast/mother, would entirely prevent any later good introjections. However, we noticed in the analysis that, after the good experiences with me, there was an enormous eruption of suppressed chronic narcissistic rage and revenge. It seemed to be related to earlier humiliating and traumatic experiences. I then became aware that he had developed a pleasurable identification with the ugly rejecting object and seemed to feel caught up in a masochistic and sadistic object relation. He held on to this as if he derived his main strength from it. This investment in a destructive object relation gave him greater security than good object relations, which seemed to him rather uncertain and made him feel constantly afraid of feeling utterly rejected.

Some time after this phase in the analysis Eric began to feel that he was not getting better with me either. In fact, he was getting worse. He noticed this particularly when he left his sessions. He described this feeling as very painful, so painful that he felt suicidal, thinking of death as the only way of finding relief for this pain. He did not wish to kill himself but he had to struggle against a strong feeling of being pulled towards death. He then explained that he hated himself more and more. What was revealed in the analysis increased his self-hatred because he wanted to feel love and confidence in himself. However, when a more hopeful, better picture of himself appeared, he was not able to retain it. He constantly felt disappointed with himself, so his self-hatred increased.

Eric's disappointment in himself was, I think, created not only by the breakdown of a very idealized self-image but also by the growth of a conscious awareness of the masochistic and sadistic narcissistic way of relating he had developed, which had given him a false feeling of protection. At this stage Eric insisted that he did not feel aggressive towards me. Rather he feared he would disappoint me by being unable to use his energies more constructively to write or publish. However, he remained very co-operative in the analysis and attempted to work with me to unearth past experiences which illustrated how he had never been able to stay enthusiastic about anything for very long. For example, he remembered that at one time when he was seventeen he became greatly enthusiastic about wanting to own a clarinet and to play it. He explained to his father about his longing to possess this instrument; his father readily offered to buy him one, and they selected a very nice one. Eric tried to play it but he didn't want to have any lessons. After a short time he felt exceedingly disappointed in the clarinet. He didn't like the tone of it; he looked at the clarinet and felt disgusted by its shape; he felt so disturbed about it that he had to give it back. He had to lie to his father because he felt so ashamed. He made up a story about it causing him asthma. In one session he remembered why the clarinet had been so disappointing. He had often listened to jazz and to a famous clarinet player, Benny Goodman. He had imagined that by having a clarinet he would change into Benny Goodman and play as beautifully as he did.

In this incident one could see how Eric's enthusiasm for the clarinet was related to a delusional possession of an exciting and admired object. So, when he could not play as well as he wanted he felt not only disappointment but also disgusted and persecuted, as if he believed he had changed the clarinet into something horrible which he had to run away from.

There was another very similar incident in his past involving a pair of wonderful binoculars. He was excited at the prospect of owning them because they were the best on the market. But, when he spent all his available money to buy them, after a short time, he again became terribly disturbed and disgusted by them so that he could no longer look through them. In discussing his excited pleasure about the binoculars it emerged that he expected, when he looked through them, to see whatever he wanted, particularly to see what was going on inside other people. They would then be unable to keep any secrets from him. However, he became afraid that his eyesight would be distorted and his eyes damaged so he had to put the binoculars away. This and other experiences made it clear that, when Eric approached such experiences in life with strong pleasurable expectation, there was a danger that powerful omnipotent and omniscient phantasies would appear to overwhelm him. This, then, was one of the reasons why he withdrew so much from life and particularly from other people.

After this work Eric began to wonder whether as a baby at his mother's breast he had experienced similar feelings to those with the clarinet and binoculars. Perhaps he had excitedly wanted to take over and become her nipple but then felt immediately that it had changed into a frightening and terrifying object, causing him to be over-whelmed by crying. He also remembered that when he successfully passed an important university examination he had bought a bottle of champagne to celebrate it with some members of his family and friends but, at the last minute, had dropped it. Again it had been dangerous to desire anything. I now wondered whether this did not also relate to the analysis. Perhaps the help he expected from me was thought of as exceedingly exciting and so very dangerous. He must expect that all good things eventually become disgusting and horrible. Eric did not improve suddenly after this revelation, but I had the feeling that from then on he was not quite as stuck as I had feared.

Some time later Eric confirmed my observation that he had always relied on some positive feeling of omnipotence to be professionally successful and confident. He now remembered more about the early years of his life. He had felt constantly belittled and ridiculed by an older sister while being simultaneously regarded as stupid and a failure by his father – because when he first went to school he had problems learning. In fact, Eric was bright and soon got on very well at the primary school and was also very popular. At ten he passed the entrance examination for a secondary school very well. But when he told his mother she seemed disappointed and almost disgusted with him, shouting, 'He has taken the easy one! He has taken the easy one!' After that she denounced him as lazy. The problem arose because Eric had taken the examination for boys of his own age, while his mother insisted he should take the examination for boys older than he was. Reluctantly he also sat for this more difficult examination and passed it without trouble. But from that time everything went wrong. He hated being the youngest in his class of boys aged eleven to twelve. He felt uncomfortable with them, was not popular, and then he developed learning difficulties. After failing in the school examinations he was put back into a lower class, which he found humiliating. He became withdrawn and started his intense omnipotent day-dreams to compensate for his failures. The day-dreams still persisted when he came to see me.

It became clear that Eric believed that his mother had made a very violent sadistic and envious attack on him after his first successful examination. None the less, he felt forced, masochistically, to submit to her just as he did with Dr U. It seems that this very disturbing school experience damaged Eric's self-confidence severely and increased his narcissistic defensive structure. He was also physically very clumsy and had difficulties with the ball games at school. With enormous effort and concentration he became successful at school and he also overcame his physical clumsiness through joining a very tough army regiment. In this way he began to be sufficiently self-confident to apply for a place at one of the most prestigious universities in England and was accepted. Through these experiences his strong feeling of inferiority had changed to great confidence and determination. On the whole his feelings of superiority as an academic lecturer were benevolent and under his control, and so he could enjoy his job.

It appears that the precarious balance Eric achieved in his university career was jolted by a number of severe disagreements and then by his experience with Dr U. His destructive omnipotent feelings increased during the analysis with Dr U. and became more uncontrollable. Eric confirmed that, about one and a half years before these destructive feelings appeared, he had experienced a number of severe disappointments in his work and career which he found to be deeply disturbing and humiliating. He had prepared himself for many years for a higher examination. He had studied his subject very thoroughly and had a great deal of advice from his colleagues on his thesis. They thoroughly approved of it, but in the event he was nevertheless failed. If he had been lazy and careless he would have understood this failure, but to fail after an incredible amount of work and preparation seemed to him unjust and made him feel helpless, diminished, and enraged. It was, apparently, his accumulated narcissistic rage, which he had tried to put aside but which gradually increased his destructive omnipotent feelings, that suddenly broke through to the surface in the lecture. He wished to take revenge and to humiliate other people as he had felt humiliated, although when this overwhelming feeling of contempt overcame him during the lecture he was completely unaware of what was happening. He was shocked by the experience, which destroyed his self-confidence and made him feel very anxious and dependent. Dr U.'s interpretation that he wanted enviously to humiliate her and triumph over her made matters worse. He felt attacked and criticized by her, and not understood. Under these circumstances his mental state deteriorated increasingly.

The recovery from such deeply disturbing experiences is not easy. The narcissistic patient depends so much on external life, as Eric did on his work success. A patient like Eric is so embittered against life that often he has not got the capacity and charm to create enough positive response in others. This produces a vicious circle. In his analysis with me Eric became very appreciative of the analytic work, and a great deal of his accumulated resentment seemed to lessen, but not in all aspects of his experience in life.

In trying to assess the cause of Eric's strong and long-lasting negative reaction to analysis, which led to impasse and to a severe deterioration in his mental state, I think it is likely that his former analyst, Dr U., had not correctly assessed the type or structure of the patient's narcissism. She was, apparently, not fully aware of his basic over-sensitivity, his feeling of inferiority, and his fear of being ridiculed and humiliated, all of which were defended against by a rather weak narcissistic cover. His defences could not stand up to attacks, particularly humiliating ones. Eric had a bad start in life. He felt weak, inferior, and not supported by his parents and sister. None the less he managed to find some positive narcissistic strength and so to change his severe early failure into success. He had a breakdown at university, after he experienced severe anxiety and temporarily lost confidence in himself, but he managed to get over it in a year or so.

His analysis at a much later date seemed to help him at first, but Dr U., in analysing his narcissism, too often seemed to interpret in a way he found humiliating, belittling, and infantilizing. He also found that Dr U. never examined his criticisms about her. Such doubts as he expressed about her were immediately interpreted as an attack, never as a valid criticism from his point of view. He began to conclude that it was useless to tell her what he was feeling. After the humiliating failure in his higher degree examination matters got worse. He felt utterly unsupported and had to erect an even stronger barrier against the experience of being belittled in analysis.

When his own contemptuous feelings emerged later, in the lecture, making him feel vulnerable and depressed, Dr U. seemed to become even more entrenched in a negative counter-transference. The reality of her humiliating form of interpretation became still more evident. A traumatic repetition of all the earlier traumas of his life took place. He felt the situation to be most damaging but also felt helpless and unable to escape from her because he had become terrified of her power, if he left her.

With narcissistic patients with early traumas, as in this patient, one has to study the traumatic situations very carefully. Frequently, there is an intense interaction between infant and mother in which for some reason the mother feels an intense failure. This often produces not only anxiety in the mother but hostility, and increases any insensitivity which may have existed originally. It is clear from the report of his mother that Eric's early feeding relationship must have been a torture for both the baby and the mother. Something which should have been pleasurable and satisfying, and could have been the basis of security and love, created terror and misery. It seems that the mother was not only depressed but also narcissistic and hurt by this failure and that this whole situation was almost completely repeated in the analysis with Dr U. It seemed that Dr U. identified herself with this Eric-mother and became very angry and accusing against Eric, who was experienced by her not only as frightened and miserable but as aggressive and spoiling Dr U.'s good analysis, the good feeding situation which she believed she had provided. Experiences like this in analysis are very unfortunate and are extremely difficult to overcome and remedy. I want therefore to emphasize my observation that a wrong assessment of a patient in analysis not only leads to wrong interpretations – in this case to a destructive negative form of interpretation – but distorts the helpful counter-transference of the analyst into a more angry and resentful attitude, which can produce disastrous reactions on the part of a patient and must lead to a complete impasse.

Notes

1 We are reminded of Mrs Riviere's remark in her paper on the negative therapeutic reaction (1936) that the analyst should be careful not to concentrate too much in negative therapeutic reactions on negative and hostile feelings of the patient because of the underlying depression, a factor which seems certainly to apply to this patient on first sight.

2 Dr U. once spoke to me very briefly about Eric but only from the point of view of regretting that she had reduced this analysis to once a week. It was clear to me that she must have been influenced by Meltzer (1967b), who recommended reducing a patient's sessions to once a week when he diagnosed that there was an impasse in the analysis. This was a measure that was unacceptable to most analysts because it was considered to be damaging to the patient, as he was bound to experience it as punishment. I noticed that Dr U. felt very regretful about having reduced Eric's sessions to once a week. However, she could not bring herself to explain to Eric that she had realized she had made a mistake, an act of regretful understanding that Eric certainly would have greatly welcomed.

PART FOUR

The influence of projective identification on the analyst's task

8

Projective identification in clinical practice

I mentioned in Chapter 1 that I found Melanie Klein's (1946) concept of projective identification to be seminal for understanding the transference relationship in the treatment of very disturbed patients. The concept of projective identification has been much in vogue since 1946 and is often used very differently.[1] In this chapter I want to set out my ideas about projective identification and the way a precise understanding of it can help clinical practice. In particular I want to explore the way a detailed understanding of the various projective processes (particularly in psychotic states) is essential if the analyst is to maintain his therapeutic functioning and avoid complex transference/counter-transference difficulties and therapeutic impasse. However, before discussing the role of projective identification in daily practice, some consideration of the concept itself and the processes it seeks to describe will be necessary.

As the term 'projective identification' has been used for a variety of similar, but not identical, processes, I shall attempt to differentiate and clarify some of the problems related to this term. Projective identification relates, first of all, to a splitting process of the early ego, where either good or bad parts of the self are expelled from the ego and, as a further step, are projected in the form of love or hatred into external objects. This process leads to a fusion of the projected parts of the self with the external objects; the individual is identical with the relevant aspect of the external object to the extent that he is it. A major consequence of such projective identification is that it gives rise to paranoid anxieties. Objects felt to possess the aggressive parts of the self become persecuting and are experienced by the patient as threatening retaliation. He feels they will try to force

157

themselves and the bad parts of the self which they contain back inside him. Patients using extensive projective identificatory processes are, therefore, constantly threatened by such paranoid anxieties. One technical implication, therefore, is that it is essential to avoid mobilizing these anxieties too quickly in the analysis. The analyst or parts of his activity can very easily become mixed up with the return of the projected parts of the self and so become a dangerous persecutor.[2]

Projective identification as described by Melanie Klein is mainly a defensive mechanism of the primitive self. None the less it implies that some separateness between self and object has to exist. Some patients, however, live in such a permanent state of projective identification that I think one has to consider that in these cases we may be dealing with a different and more primitive, albeit related, process. Primitive primordial forms of projective identification might then be considered a forerunner of the more usual type relating to the very earliest primary states of fusion between mother and baby. First, I have in mind the possibility that some processes of projective identification start even *in utero*. What I mean is that the foetus may be sensitive to certain disturbing mental processes within the mother which are somehow communicated to it in a manner analogous to the underlying process in psychosomatic states. Second, I am thinking of those states of very early fusion between mother and baby which are observed in the paranoid–schizoid position and then later during the depressive position. Some analysts – for example, Steiner (1975, 1982), Tustin (1972), Bion (1980), Felton (1985) – make use of such more primitive forms of projective identification; others do not. I myself feel that significant early processes, probably starting *in utero*, exist, although I am uncertain how to understand these processes better without a great deal more careful clinical observation. None the less there is no doubt in my mind that the children of some parents, suffering from very early disturbances, need a particularly open and perceptive state of mind on the part of the analyst or therapist if he is to understand their communications at this early level. Those who have studied these early forms of communication stress the uncontrollable experiences the baby has with its mother. Her mental processes are somehow transmitted to the baby in a manner akin to osmosis (Steiner 1975, 1982; Felton 1985). They are absorbed by the child without it being able to do anything about it, so that the experience is quite overwhelming.[3]

In many of the borderline and psychotic states, patients seem to be desperately struggling with contradictory, confused, and confusing

158

feelings and thoughts. They seem to find it very difficult to think about their feelings or to know them but none the less communicate or anti-communicate them powerfully in many different ways. I feel sure that this kind of patient is suffering from very early and disturbing experiences of the kind envisaged by ideas about primitive projective identification and osmotic communication. For months rather than days such patients need to communicate non-verbally and are often silent or speak in a very confused, monotonous, or symbolic way. The experience often has a strong physical effect on the analyst and produces sleepiness or physical discomfort. It can cause major difficulties for the analyst's capacity to think or to concentrate. It is as if something has been projected into the analyst in a real and concrete way.

Projective identification and containment

With the considerations just mentioned in mind, I find it useful to think of projective identification in two simultaneous ways. On the one hand, in all projective processes of this kind there is an expulsive quality. The individual, sometimes very violently indeed, is trying to rid himself of unbearable thoughts and feelings and to do so forcibly by imaginatively taking over and controlling others. On the other hand, the process of projective identification can also be considered as an attempt to communicate. If the unbearable and often chaotic thoughts and feelings which are expelled can be contained (Bion 1962b), it is possible that what is happening can be understood and considered, paving the way for the thoughts and feelings to be tolerated and to become less unbearable.

The psychotic patient who projects impulses and parts of himself into the analyst is expelling them. But in doing so he makes it possible for the analyst to feel and understand his experiences and to contain them. In that way the unbearable experiences can lose their frightening or unbearable quality and become meaningful. Through the analyst's capacity to use interpretations to put feelings into words, the patient can learn to tolerate his own impulses and obtain access to a more sane self, which can begin to think about experiences that were previously meaningless and frightening.

From a technical point of view, the fact that the process of projective identification can open a way to dialogue, leading to understanding, depends crucially on the analyst's capacity to exist as a container for the patient's projections. However, in my view, it is essential that we recognize what it means to contain the patient's projections. The word 'contain' can imply a rather passive attitude which might mean that an analyst should remain silent or inactive. While this is occasionally a necessary function of the analyst (as of the mother in normal development), I want to stress that the containing function in fact requires a great deal more than passivity. Essentially, the analyst has to be prepared to enter into an intense relationship and to retain his function of putting experiences into words. Indeed, Grotstein (1981: 205) calls the relationship a form of 'Siamese bonding' which progresses through 'autistic, symbiotic and even separated and in the end individuated relationships'. The analyst has empathically to follow the patient's description of both real and phantasized events, which are often re-enacted by being projected into him. Most patients, particularly psychotic and borderline patients, usually require a great deal of active thinking on the part of the analyst because they themselves lack the capacity for thinking. The analyst has to bring together the diffuse, confused, or split-up aspects of the patient's pre-thought processes in his own mind so that they gradually make sense and have meaning. This implies the need for an integrated and organizing activity on the analyst's part. He must gradually play back to the patient his 'inchoate' communication so that it becomes understandable to the patient – an activity which is almost an art.

Bion has called the analyst's capacity to function in the way I have described 'Alpha function' and he has labelled the psychotic patient's diffused state of mind and his way of communicating as 'Beta' elements, which remain incomprehensible until the analyst, through his containing function, converts these Beta elements into Alpha elements. It is important that the analyst is able to hold his patient's material very clearly and logically in his own mind. He can then play it back to the patient so that he or she can follow the logic of their own way of thinking and feeling. This activity diminishes the anxiety which prevents the patient from holding on to a logical, natural state of mind.

It is important to realize that in so far as projective identification is communicative it is a benign process, which means that the object into which projection has taken place is not changed by the projective process. The emphasis is on the need for the object to function as a container for the not-understandable aspects of the self so that the mental content can be taken back into the self in understandable form with the added experience of feeling understood and accepted by someone. There are other ways in which projective identification can be thought of as a benign and essential part of normal object-relating. I am thinking here of the specific instance of

160

psychoanalytic treatment in which free associations can be considered as projective identificatory externalizations which allow the patient to grow by externalizing his inner mental content for interpretation, leading to self-assessment (Grotstein 1981: 125). I also believe that some projective identification is involved in the process of object cathexis, a term used by many analysts. There is also the projection and externalization of aspects of the self in order to recognize objects by identifying with them, which is the basis of empathy. All such instances of projective identification are necessary for developing object relations.

Recognizing projective identification

If projective identification makes it possible for the analyst to feel and understand the patient's experiences, and so to try to help him face them and make better sense of them, by the same token it makes the analyst's task very difficult. The powerful and overwhelming nature of some forms of projective identification has already been mentioned. I now want to describe some of the specific ways in which projective identification can confuse the analyst's task.

First, as several authors have noted, the essence of projective identification is that it often takes the place of ordinary, more logical, verbal communication. Consequently, whenever projective identi- fication is excessive (as with most psychotic patients) there is a danger that the verbal communication between patient and analyst may break down. At such times the analyst's interpretations are misunderstood and misinterpreted by the patient, while the patient's communications increasingly assume a concrete quality, suggesting that the capacity for abstract thinking has vanished. In investigating such situations, I have found that omnipotent projective identification interferes with the capacity of verbal and abstract thinking to produce a concreteness of the mental processes, which leads to confusion between reality and phantasy. As Segal (1957) has argued, the patient who uses excessive projective identification is dominated by concrete thought processes which cause misunderstanding of verbal interpretations. Words and their content are experienced by the patient as concrete, non-symbolic objects. The basis of a psychotic patient's concrete thinking is the non–differentation between the thing symbolized and the symbol, which is part of a disturbance in the relation between self and object. In excessive projective identification the differentation between the self and the object is obscured. Since a part of the self is confused with the object,

161

the symbol which is a creation and a function of the self or ego becomes in turn confused with the object which is symbolized (Segal 1956, 1957).[4] As a result, it is very difficult to use verbal interpretations with a psychotic patient. Because they are often misunderstood and misinterpreted, the patient can become very frightened and may even cover his ears or try to rush out of the consulting room. An analysis can be in danger of breaking down. At such times the technical imperative is to uncover the projective processes being used for the purpose of communication between patient and analyst. This makes it possible to make simple verbal interpretations once again and to explain to the patient to help him to understand the terrifying situation his concrete mode of experience has created for him.

A second way in which projective identification complicates the analyst's task arises from the way patients use it to deal with primitive aggressive and envious wishes. I have described in several earlier chapters the way in which narcissistic omnipotent object relations allow a patient to avoid intense feelings such as those of envy or separateness. This form of relating is of course maintained by projective identification through which some psychotic patients manage to feel they live inside the analyst's mind and body and possess his help and understanding as part of themselves. They are able to attribute everything they experience as valuable in the analysis to themselves. However, as I have described in earlier chapters, as soon as such a patient begins to feel separate from the analyst an aggressive reaction appears, particularly clearly after a valuable interpretation demonstrating the analyst's therapeutic capacity. Such patients react with feelings of humiliation and complain that they are made to feel small; why should the analyst be able to remind them of something which they need but cannot provide for themselves? In their envious anger such patients try to destroy and spoil the analyst's interpretations by ridiculing or making them meaningless.

From the point of view of this chapter, what matters is that as a result of powerful projective processes the analyst in this situation may have the distinct experience in his counter-transference that he is no good and has nothing of value to give to the patient. Even physical symptoms can be experienced by the analyst with such patients because the patient's expulsions may be so concrete; he may feel sick just as the patient may actually vomit. Such concrete rejection of the analyst's help can often be clearly understood as a re-enactment of some earlier rejection of the mother's food and care, now repeated in the analytic situation. On the other hand, care must be taken to differentiate between a patient's rejection of the analyst's bad handling or misunderstanding (when the analyst does actually repeat a bad feeling situation, as in Eric's case, discussed in Chapter 7) and any envious aggression. Not only is the latter difficult for the primitive ego of the child to tolerate, it also creates a particularly difficult problem for any loving and caring mother or analyst. This is the trouble when a patient who has previously made good progress in the treatment has a negative therapeutic reaction. It is often violent, as if he wants to spoil and devalue everything he has previously received, regardless of the often suicidal danger of such a reaction.

Many patients (and in their counter-transference analysts as well) experience their violent envy directed against the good qualities of the analyst as quite insane and illogical. The sane part of the patient (and perhaps of the analyst) experiences these envious reactions as unbearable and unacceptable. Many defences against this primitive envy are, therefore, created. One such relates to the splitting off and projection of the envious part of the self into an external object, which then becomes the envious part of the patient. This kind of defensive projective identification follows the model of Melanie Klein's description of the splitting off and projection of bad parts of the self, quoted at the beginning of this chapter. Another defence against envy involving projective identification occurs when the patient has omnipotent phantasies about entering the admired and envied object. He takes over his role (for example, doing all the analysis) and in this way insists that he is the object. In such cases of almost total projective identification with an envied object, more direct expressions of envy are entirely absent, until they reappear as the analytic work allows for some separation between self and object.[5] One particular type of object relation I observed is particularly influential in this respect. In this way of relating, the parasitical one, the psychotic patient in analysis, maintains a belief that he is living entirely inside an object – the analyst – and behaves like a parasite living on the capacities of the analyst, who is expected to function as his ego. Severe parasitism may be regarded as a state of total projective identification. It is, however, not just a defensive state to deny envy or separation but also an expression of aggression, particularly envy. This is the combination of defence and acting out the aggression which makes the parasitic state a particularly difficult therapeutic problem.

A patient maintaining parasitic object relations relies entirely on the analyst, often making him responsible for his entire life. He thus behaves in an extremely passive, silent, and sluggish manner, demanding everything and giving nothing in return. This state can be extremely chronic, and the analytic work with such patients is often minimal. For example, one of my depressed patients described himself as a baby, which was like a stone heavily pressing into my couch and into me. He felt he was making it impossible for me either to carry him or to look after him and he feared that the only thing that I could do was to expel him, if I could not stand him any longer. However, he was terrified that he could not survive being left. He felt not only that he had a very paralysing effect on the analysis but that he was paralysed and inert himself. Only rarely was it possible to get in touch with the intense feeling of either hostility or overwhelming pain and depression bound up with this process. There was no joy when the analyst was felt to be helpful and alive, as it only increased the patient's awareness of the contrast between himself and the analyst and at times produced a desire to frustrate him. With this he returned to the status quo of inertia, which was felt to be unpleasant but preferred to any of the intense feelings of pain, anger, envy, or jealousy which might fleetingly be experienced. As I suggested before, extreme parasitism is partly a defence against separation anxiety, envy, or jealousy, but it often seems to be a defence against *any emotion which might be experienced as painful*. I often have the impression that patients, like the one just described, who experience themselves as dead, and are often experienced by the analyst as so inactive that they might as well be dead, use their analyst's aliveness as a means of survival. The latent hostility prevents the patients from getting more than minimal help or satisfaction from the analysis and is very difficult for the analyst to experience.[6]

A third point about the difficulties caused by projective identification is that it can be used to defend not only against experiences of primitive envy and aggression but also against psychic reality in general. In this situation the patient splits off parts of his self in addition to impulses and anxieties and projects them into the analyst for the purpose of evacuating and emptying out the disturbing mental content, which leads to the denial of psychic reality. As this type of patient primarily wants the analyst to condone the evacuation processes and the denial of his problems, he often reacts to interpretations with violent resentment, as they are experienced as critical and frightening. The patient believes that unwanted, unbearable, and meaningless mental content is being pushed back into him by the analyst. The process can be illustrated by some material of a schizophrenic patient. In a particular period of the analysis the patient had a very bad relapse. She had to be hospitalized and developed delusions. When she was able to start analysis again she explained to the analyst that when she felt the analyst did not understand her she had turned away from him to her mother. But her mother had told her that she should evacuate her thoughts. She concretely asked her daughter to take a laxative. This occurred at a time when the patient was already a little anxious about having forgotten about the analysis and about having developed doubts. Suddenly she realized what had happened to her as the result of defecating out her mind – namely, that it left her incapable of understanding words, so that she felt completely stupid.

The fact that projective identification can be used to evacuate and to deny psychic reality has to be recognized alongside the fact that when a patient is trying to push unbearable mental content into the analyst he is also compelling him to share the unpleasant experiences. An attack on an analyst who is believed to be aloof and not caring may be a form of communication, with a faint hope that the analyst, through being forced to share the patient's experience, may find a better solution to the problems than the patient. Such behaviour by a patient is frequently misunderstood and interpreted by some therapists as being entirely aggressive. The result is that the patient feels even more rejected, misunderstood, and alone. He can also feel severely guilty and depressed because he fears that his repeated projections have damaged the analyst and been the cause of his failures, producing a vicious circle of defensiveness. The patient may then not only identify with the damaged analyst but also torture himself with severe masochistic self-punishment. This can often go on for a long time unless the details of the projected experience have been clarified in the analysis. While the projective processes are being acted out, the patient cannot generally observe what is going on in certain sessions, or sometimes in the whole analysis.

The different ways in which patients try both to evacuate and to share feelings and experiences have to be conceptualized very carefully by the therapist lest he be overwhelmed by the process and lose contact with the patient. An example of the difficulties can be illustrated from a case treated by a very experienced analyst whom I supervised between 1966 and 1967. The patient was in an acute psychotic state and had lost her capacity for verbal understanding and communication. She was a severely manic depressive who was cared for in a mental hospital but managed to come from the hospital to the analyst's consulting room for psychoanalytic treatment. At a certain period of the analysis the patient, who had previously improved a great deal, became more and more persecuted by the analyst and tried to invade all the rooms of the analyst's house instead of using the waiting-room. This created a great deal of disorder and noise. At the same time she generally refused to enter the analyst's consulting room, so that the analysis, if it was to be carried on, had to be carried on in the hall or on the staircase. Only occasionally did the analyst succeed in getting the patient into the consulting room, and then she constantly threw accusations at him. When the analyst interpreted that she felt very guilty about her behaviour so that she could not cope with it and that she was pushing her own guilt feelings into him, she rapidly got worse. She accused him of making her worse and worse and said that she could not and would not come any more. It was at this point that I was consulted urgently. The analyst feared that the patient would refuse to be treated by him both in his home and at the hospital and he thought there was a complete impasse.

Listening carefully to the material, I became aware that the patient, who had previously been able to have a relationship with the analyst in which she understood interpretations, had completely lost her capacity to take anything in. So I suggested that the analyst should tell her that he had been treating her now for several years and had understood that she had been able to use the analysis well and had been very much better. But at the present time she seemed to have lost that part of herself that could understand, think, and listen to him. In other words, I suggested he remind her that she had a sane part although it had been lost for the moment and their job was to try to find it. After the analyst tried something along these lines, the patient hesitated for a few minutes. Then she suddenly lay right down on the floor on her front and looked underneath the couch for a few minutes before getting up again. The analyst interpreted that she seemed to have understood this interpretation very well and had been looking for this part of herself which had been temporarily lost and was now hidden somewhere in the analyst's consulting room. Perhaps they could get it out from under the couch so that she could use it again. Almost immediately after this experience the patient was able to communicate and listen much better, and the complete deadlock was over. It seemed miraculous to the analyst. The experience showed me how important it is to remember that even the acute psychotic patient still has the capacity to find somewhere in himself or in the analyst the hidden sane part again so that the treatment can be revived.

Perhaps the most important point to understand about projective identification is the way it can be used by a patient to get into a confused, merged, or fused state of relating to the analyst. This can take several forms and needs to be understood very carefully. On the one hand, there is a basic wish for symbiotic symmetry in which the patient wants the analyst to experience identical complementary feelings and experiences in order to create a mirror-like twin relationship with the patient in which there is perfect communication and understanding.

A patient of mine, whose mother had died when she was ten months old, was overwhelmed with anxiety early on in the analysis during my first long summer holidays. She felt it was unbearable that she could not be near me in spite of being with her very devoted husband. She was convinced that she could feel better only if she could hear or see me. Her husband encouraged her to ring me up, but she could not bring herself to do this because she thought I wanted and needed my holiday; she was also convinced that I did not want to know anything about her during the holidays. In fact she could not even write to me during the holidays but she felt immediately better when she saw me when treatment started again. It took several months for her to realize that it seemed necessary for her to have a picture in her mind of me wanting to see her and look after her. She applied this realization also to her mother. She thought it must have been exceedingly painful for her mother not to be in a position to look after her and feed her when she was ill. Her mother had obviously been torn away from her own feelings for her little daughter when she suddenly died. The patient felt very comforted by these thoughts and felt also much better about her mother's death when I could show her the symbiotic phantasies towards me and her mother. The patient had also feared that she had been projecting forcibly this symbiotic phantasy into me and so she had spent her holidays trying to protect me from any intrusions.

The fact that the patient felt better when I interpreted her wish to intrude into me underlines the difficulties projective identification can cause. Normal symbiotic processes are similar to, but not identical with, projective identification. They relate to very early attempts to ward off acute feelings of helplessness by becoming part of the mother, and to memories of infancy. They are probably connected to a strong symbiotic tie in the mother towards the child, in which the mother could not experience her child as a separate being. However, when such situations are touched on in the analysis the patient's symbiotic longing turns very quickly into a dangerous feeling of being sucked or pulled into a relationship where the patient feels passive, immobilized, and trapped and is unable to find his own self again. He then becomes intensely persecuted and tantalized by the symbiotic object who he feels has seduced him, sucked him in, and now makes no attempt to release him from this trap. The most disturbing aspect of this state is that the patient feels entirely in the power of the symbiotic object and has no possibility of doing anything active. This situation of entanglement generally produces violent rage in which the patient feels that he wants to destroy himself and the object because he cannot get out of the entanglement. When this problem appears in the analysis in a delusional form the analysis is slowed down considerably because the patient actually feels trapped by the analyst and believes that the analyst knows all about this problem, but is determined not to do anything about it. What has often happened is that symbiotic phantasies have combined with projective identification so that a symbiotic phantasy has been projected into the analytic situation. It seems then that the projective process has become part of the symbiotic process rather than an ordinary process of projective identification where one can concentrate on individual elements which have been projected from time to time into the analyst. To treat the symbiotic entanglement simply as an element of projective identification is contra-indicated because the symbiotic phantasy needs to be understood in its whole dimension. In the analysis this most powerful feeling and experience is projected into the analyst, who has to become aware of the symbiotic process which is felt in the counter-transference to be paralysing both to the analysis and to the analyst.

I want now to mention the use of the term 'projective identification' for a very common aspect of the transference relationship of the psychotic patient, an aspect which is aimed at controlling the analyst's body and mind and seems to be based on an early infantile type of object relationship. In analysis, one observes that the patient believes that he has forced himself omnipotently into the analyst, which leads to fusion or to confusion with the analyst and to anxieties relating to the loss of the self. In this form of projective identification the projection of the mad parts of the self into the analyst often predominates; the analyst is then perceived as having become mad, which arouses extreme anxiety as the patient is afraid that the analyst will retaliate and force the madness back into the patient and as a punishment deprive him entirely of his sanity. At such times the patient is in danger of disintegration, but detailed interpretation of the relationship between patient and analyst may break through this omnipotent delusional situation and prevent a breakdown of the treatment.

Another way of living entirely inside an object occurs in severely deluded schizophrenic patients who seem to experience themselves as living in an unreal world that is highly delusional but nevertheless has qualities of a structure suggesting that this hallucinatory world is a representation of the inside of an object, probably the mother (Meltzer: personal communication (1963)). The patient may be withdrawn, preoccupied with hallucinations, in the analysis occasionally projecting the hallucinatory experience on to the analyst, which leads to mis-identifying him and others with his delusional experience. Sometimes the patient may describe himself as living in a world, or object, which separates him entirely from the outside world; the analyst is experienced as a contraption, an actor, or a machine, and the world becomes extremely unreal. The living inside the delusional object seems to be in strong opposition to relating to the outside world, which would imply depending on a real object. This delusional world or object seems to be dominated by an omnipotent and sometimes omniscient part of the self, which creates the notion that within the delusional object there is complete painlessness and freedom to indulge in any whim. It also appears that the self within the delusional object exerts a powerful suggestive and seductive influence on saner parts of the personality in order to persuade or force them to withdraw from reality and to join the delusional omnipotent world. Clinically, the patient may hear a voice making propaganda for living inside the mad world by idealizing it and praising its virtue by offering complete satisfaction and instant cure to the patient. This persuasion or propaganda to get inside the delusional world means that there is a constant stimulus to all parts of the self to use omnipotent projective identification (forcing the self inside the object) as the only possible method to solve all problems. This situation leads to constant acting out with external objects which are used for projective identification. When, however, projective identification becomes directed towards the delusional object, the saner parts of the self may become trapped or imprisoned within this object, and physical and mental paralysis amounting to catatonia may result.

Technical considerations

In so far as a patient is caught up in living predominantly by projective identification there will always be enormous limitations in his capacity to differentiate what he is feeling and what others are feeling about him. Part of the patient, when he is in touch with his sanity, if you like, will be aware of his separate existence and of the analyst as a separate person trying to help. At other times, however, he will be caught up in a delusional system of thinking in which his own feelings and thoughts and his experience with the analyst are constantly split and projected. Such situations are associated with and complicated further by the presence of narcissistic omnipotent object relations and, therefore, underlying aggression and envy. Often the patient will feel that part of himself and the analyst are so violently at war that he will retreat into all kinds of delusions to escape the awful consequences. The patient's own capacities for self-observation in this situation are often very limited, and so he is especially dependent on the analyst and in particular on his capacity for remembering, organizing, and differentiating. What matters in this situation above all, as far as remaining therapeutic is concerned, is that the analyst observe very carefully how the patient is describing him and what he feels him to be communicating about this at any moment; in other words, the analyst must observe the psychotic transference relationship and be particularly alert for its delusional variety. To do this the analyst will need to keep a very careful watch on his own feelings and reactions, because in situations of powerful projective identification this may be the main clue he has about the psychotic transference relationship.

Projective identification operated in infancy mainly on an omnipotent basis, and even in adulthood, as we can observe in our psychotic patients, it is a very powerful mental process. Not only does it affect the aspects of the self which are moved about, but the object under the influence of projective identification is strongly affected by it. It can have a very powerful good influence but can be dangerous and even disastrous if it is abused. So object relations under the influence of projective identification are often strongly manipulative, forceful, and controlling. Seduction also plays a very important part and it often has even hypnotic and telepathic influences.

Projective identification can include transformation of the self and the object, leading to confusion, depersonalization, emptiness, weakness, and vulnerability to influence which goes so far as being hypnotized or even put to sleep. Some analysts I have supervised complain that in treating certain psychotic or borderline patients they get so sleepy that they can scarcely keep awake and they feel that their capacity to think is severely interfered with. However, when the analyst becomes experienced in understanding the psychotic patient's way of communicating it is clear that the overpowering influence of projective identification lessens. It is therefore extremely important in observing the interpersonal processes involved in projective identification to understand that when the person or object has been *transformed by the projection* he is incapable of functioning helpfully as mother to the infant or as the analyst to the patient.

However, if the analyst or mother has effectively and understandingly *transformed the projection* and so has remained unchanged by it, the infant or patient begins gradually to feel safer and better in the relationship. The three cases I shall present illustrate this proposition.

John

The first case I want to describe illustrates the difficulties which projective identification can cause. In some situations powerful projective identification can mean that unless he is very observant an analyst can be unaware of a patient's problems before being suddenly overwhelmed by them.

Dr B., a psychotherapist, reported a case of a 44–year–old man, John, married with two children, who presented himself as depressed and anxious and who had developed acute depression and anxiety after a car accident, which was caused while John was under the influence of drink. After this accident he had attempted suicide and was admitted to the local hospital but discharged very soon afterwards. His general practitioner referred him to Dr B. for twice-a-week psychotherapy. Dr B. reported that John had a very understanding but weak father and a very critical and accusatory mother who often tended to blame John from an early age. There was an incident which threw a deep shadow on the patient's further development. When he was about nine years of age he played with his eight-year-old sister in a derelict house of the town; but this house had not been at all safe, and the girl fell down from the third floor and was killed. How exactly this accident happened is not known, but the mother always accused John of being responsible for his sister's death and of not having taken enough care of her to prevent this accident. John was, of course, deeply affected by this. It is very likely that the recent car accident had stirred up his anxieties about endangering people and being careless, because in the car accident it was he who had been drunk and it was through his not being careful in driving that people had been injured, although not killed.

In the treatment John was depressed and self-accusatory: 'I can't do anything. I am an absolute mediocrity. I can't even kill myself.' In addition, Dr B. felt that John presented a classic paranoid defensive system against feelings of guilt so that a particularly harsh and cold super-ego was projected into other people, who were then felt to be against him for the many offences he had committed. Such hard judgement increased his fear and anger. Often this process was most apparent at the beginning of the session, when he found it difficult to

171

speak due to some guilty act for which he thought he would be condemned and excommunicated by Dr B. For instance, in one session, after a period of silence in which he was furious with the therapist for not talking, he told the following story. In the morning, he had been sitting in a non-smokers' carriage in the underground train but had decided to smoke a cigarette. A man who was sitting opposite told him to stop smoking and thirty seconds later he disembarked. John was furious at being treated in this way, accusing the man of being cold and heartless. Dr B. interpreted that there was some wrongdoing he was holding back from him because he feared that he would also judge him in a cold and heartless way. John then said he had been drinking at lunchtime; he felt that Dr B. would kill him for this. John was a surveyor for a large company and he had a drinking problem. On this occasion he had gone to the toilet when he arrived back at the office and sprayed his mouth with breath-freshener in order to get rid of any evidence of having consumed alcohol. Dr B. was quite sensitive in spotting here John's hidden guilty action in the transference situation, but one would think that this level of interpretation was perhaps too superficial for a patient of this kind and one might wonder how John would present himself after having made some deeper contact with Dr B. In fact, very soon after this session John's feelings of worthlessness increased. He started to avoid going to work and during the weekends stayed in bed, failing to honour family commitments such as going to watch his little boy play football for his school. John admitted that he found it increasingly difficult to work and he was very much afraid of being neglectful of his family and of being a failure.

In one session during the second month, John spoke of giving up and committing suicide. Interestingly enough, Dr B. was not affected by John's depression and suicidal threat in his counter-transference. He apparently felt that he had the therapy quite in control and interpreted that John was being driven into a state of despair and hopelessness by a harsh judge and how this state of mind neutralized the help that the therapist offered him. By withdrawing more from life, expressing his inability to cope, and being overwhelmed by suicidal thoughts, John had projected his over-whelming guilt and fear of suicide into the therapist. The therapist's inability to experience the projection and his not responding to it would be experienced by John as harshness, punishment, and abandonment by the therapist, who thus becomes identified with John's cold super-ego, which would not only fail to help John but make him feel worse. In fact, John did not come for therapy any more. At this moment the therapist became exceedingly anxious and

172

depressed. He had vivid phantasies of John having committed suicide; he reproached himself for having neglected John and having failed him and he also felt deeply that he had let down the other doctors who worked with him, which increased his sense of failure. Fortunately the colleague with whom Dr B. discussed this case was not at all accusatory to him, but he still could not accept any comfort from him and remained exceedingly disturbed and upset for quite a time.

After some weeks Dr B. was told that John had not committed suicide but did not feel that there was any point in coming for therapy after the last session with Dr B., during which he had felt rejected and misunderstood. On examining Dr B.'s mental state after John did not appear any more, one is impressed by the therapist's intense feeling of guilt and responsibility for John's life, believing that he had caused his patient's death through neglecting him. This feeling was so strong that he could not shake himself out of it. If we examine John's deep-seated anxiety and guilt we are aware that this state of mind was related to his feelings after the death of his sister, when he felt himself guilty and neglectful. This was enormously increased by the accusations of his mother, who had accused him of being neglectful and responsible for his sister's death. These accusations and guilt feelings John seems to have projected into Dr B. with such intensity that Dr B.'s depression after John stopped treatment reflects exactly John's own state of mind after his sister's death. At the same time there is in John an intense feeling of failure related to his fear of continually failing and never being able to put right what he believed he had done in the past. This sense of failure, and the feeling of being regarded by his mother and others as a failure, is also mirrored clearly in Dr B.'s feeling of being a failure and of being so guilty and disturbed about what his colleagues might now think about him. I think this is one of the cases where one can be amazed to what extent the projection into the analyst completely mirrors the patient's feelings. In this case of course it was particularly interesting that at first the therapist had no reaction at all, and this response could come to the surface only after John did not return to him. I think Dr B. had too strongly defended himself against any feelings of anxiety and guilt in relationship to this patient and had created a theoretical structure with which he falsely believed he could approach John and also protect himself from him. He hoped to get hold of John's overwhelming guilt without having to make deeper contact with the patient's feelings of depression and guilt. This is not possible. One cannot treat depressed patients, particularly not severely depressed patients, without allowing them access to one's own deeper feelings and showing oneself willing to experience this with them, however depressing and disturbing this might be.

We should realize that in all the severe cases of anxiety and depression the analyst's emotional participation is absolutely necessary in order to be able to create a containing environment, and a purely intellectual approach is equal to a complete failure to contain. This therapist must have learnt a great deal from the disturbing experience, and it will be much easier for him next time to put himself into a frame of mind where he will become open to his patient's projections. Even if the therapist is not able to interpret the patient's projections and state of mind in detail, the emotional participation is generally experienced by the patient and leads to a feeling of being not criticized but accepted. The way John communicated with the therapist, particularly through his suicidal feeling, was an intense appeal for the therapist to realize how disturbing and how unbearable the situation was. He was asking him to feel and sympathize with him about how bad he felt. He hoped that the therapist would not accuse him but gradually help him to feel less guilty.

To understand the patient's inability to cope with his feeling of failure it would be helpful to go into details of the specific feelings that are experienced by him to be so unbearable: his feelings of guilt, responsibility, and failure. All these seem to have been something which all his life he had had to carry alone by himself. He was constantly accused by his mother and never found any relief from it. In therapy he had hoped there would be somebody to listen to him and to understand what he had been experiencing all his life. In general this type of patient has a relatively good prognosis, if his appeal for help, through projective identification, can be listened to and responded to emotionally.

John did not accept any more treatment after he had been with Dr B. and said that he felt he had to carry his feelings of anxiety and guilt by himself. When the case of the accident later came before the magistrates, John was found guilty of severe neglect and lost his driving licence. He was then very anxious about not being able to carry on with his work and made another attempt at suicide. I don't know whether John managed to find his way back to treatment at a later date. If Dr B. could have allowed his counter-transference to link up the projection earlier he could have made much better contact by acknowledging how important it was for John to feel that the analyst was willing to experience deeply his overwhelming feeling of guilt and being a failure and that he felt he could no longer bear this awful feeling on his own.

Sidney

The second case I want to discuss illustrates problems of projective identification in a schizophrenic patient and how they can be successfully treated. Sidney, who was seen by me from autumn 1967, had been diagnosed several years before as schizophrenic, when he had an acute psychotic breakdown which was characterized by overwhelming panic, confusion, and fears of complete disintegration. He did not hallucinate during the acute phase, nor were the delusional aspects of the psychosis dominant at the beginning of the analysis, but he was unable to work or to maintain a close relationship with men or women in the outside world.

Sidney had been treated by another analyst for several years before starting analysis with me. The previous analyst's report to me emphasized Sidney's tendency to slip into a state of projective identification with the analyst at the beginning of each session, leading to his becoming confused and unable to speak in an audible and understandable way. The analyst interpreted to Sidney that he expected him, the analyst, to understand him even if he could not talk or think, since he believed himself to be inside the analyst; as a result of such interpretations he generally started to speak more distinctly.

During the analysis with me Sidney made further progress and at times felt more separate, so that the saner parts of his self were able to form to some extent a dependent relationship to me. However, from time to time, particularly after he had made some progress, or when there were long separations, he fell back to a parasitical relationship of living inside me by projective identification, which led to states of confusion, inability to think and talk, claustrophobia, and paranoid anxieties of feeling trapped by me. When envy was aroused through experiences in the real world, for example when he met a man who was successful in his relationship with women or in his work, after a short conscious experience of envy Sidney would frequently become identified with him. This was followed by severe anxieties of losing his identity and feelings of being trapped, rather than leading to the delusion that he was the envied man, or that he was able to function in the outside world similarly to the man with whom projective identification and confusion had taken place.

In the autumn of 1968 I had to interrupt Sidney's analysis for a fortnight, which disturbed him considerably. Consciously, he seemed unconcerned about my going away, which I had of course discussed with him several months before. However, two weeks before the interruption he became acutely anxious and confused and for a day he feared that he would have another breakdown and have to go into hospital. The disturbance started with Sidney's complaint that he could not drag himself away from the television screen, where he was watching the Olympic games. He felt forced, almost against his will, to look at it until late at night. He complained that he was drawn into the hot climate of Mexico, which made him feel that being there would make him well. He was also compelled to look at the athletes, wrestlers, and weightlifters and felt he was, or ought to be, one of them. He asked me questions: 'Why do I have to be an athlete? Why can't I be myself?' He felt that this looking at television was like an addiction which he could not stop and which exhausted and drained him. At times he felt so strongly 'pulled inside the television' that he felt claustrophobic and had difficulty in breathing. Afterwards during the night he felt compelled to get up and see whether the taps of the washbasin in his flat were turned off and ensure that the plugs in the basin and bath were not blocking up the drainage. He was terrified that both his bath and basin might overflow, and eventually he confessed that he was afraid of being drowned and suffocated.

I interpreted to him that after he felt that he was making progress and feeling separate from me he was suddenly overcome with impatience and envy of me and of other men who were able to move about and were active. I suggested that it was the envious part which drove him into the identification with other men and myself in order to take over their strength and potency, and in this way the omnipotent part of himself could make him believe that he could be mature and healthy instantly. He agreed with the interpretation without any difficulty and started to speak very fast; he said he knew all this and was aware of it, but he also knew that this belief was false and that it was a delusion, and he was angry at having to listen to a voice in him which was very persuasive and stimulated him to take over the mind and body of other people. I also interpreted to him that I thought that the threatening separation was stimulating his wish to be suddenly grown up and independent in order not to have to cope with the anxieties of being separate from me.

Sidney then told me that he was falling every night into a very deep sleep from which he could not easily awake in the morning and so he had arrived late for his session. He compared the feeling of being pulled into the television screen, which seemed to have become the delusional object, to being pulled into this deep sleep. He now spoke fairly fluently and more distinctly and conveyed that he now felt more separate from me. He said he felt disgusted with

176

himself for being a parasite and he also complained that the television experience and his bed were draining his life out of him, so that he had a strong impulse to smash both; he was glad that he had been able to control this in reality.

I acknowledged his own observation that his looking at television and being pulled into a deep sleep were experienced by him as parasitical experiences where he felt he was getting into other objects. I pointed out that he felt angry with that part of himself which stimulated him to get inside external objects, such as the athletes, representing me as a successful man who was travelling abroad during the break, and also into internal objects which were represented by his bed. I stressed that at first he felt he probably could control and possess these objects entirely when he got inside them, but very soon he felt enclosed, trapped, and persecuted, which roused his wish to destroy the bed and the television screen which had turned into persecuting objects. I thought that this fear of being trapped and his anger related also to the analysis and the analyst. Sidney's obsessions about the plugs of the basin and bath were also related to his fear of being trapped and drowned. It seemed that he had constantly to find out whether after his intrusion into objects he was trapped and was in danger of drowning and suffocating inside, or whether there was a hole through which he could escape.

Simultaneously with the projective identification related to the delusional television experience, Sidney was violently pulled into relations to prostitutes. He explained to me that there was a part of him which persuaded him whenever he felt lonely or anxious that he needed to have a lovely big prostitute for nourishment and this would make him well. During the session he assured me that he realized the falsity of the voice, but in fact he very rarely could resist. He felt he wanted to get inside the prostitutes in an excited way in order to devour them, but after intercourse he felt sick and disgusted and convinced that he had now acquired syphilis of the stomach. During this session Sidney asserted many times that he knew now quite well the difference between reality and the delusional persuasion and he also knew what was wrong. But it was apparent to me that in spite of this knowledge he was again and again put temporarily into a deluded state by a psychotic omnipotent and omniscient part of him which succeeded in seducing and overpowering the saner part of his personality and forced him to deal with all his difficulties and problems, including his envy, by projective identification. During the session the saner part of the patient seemed to receive help and support from the analyst's interpretations, but he felt humiliated and angry that he could not resist the domination and persuasion of the psychotic part when he was left on his own. In attempting to examine the reason for listening so readily to the internal voice, I found that he was promised cure and freedom from anxiety and from dependence on me. I was then able to interpret that the separation made him more aware of feeling small and dependent on me, which was humiliating and painful and increased his envy of me. By omnipotently intruding into me, he could delude himself that from one moment to the next he became grown up and completely all right and could manage without me.

I shall now briefly describe the relationship between ego splitting, projective identification, and the persecutory anxieties related to these processes in this patient. In the following session he reported that he felt much better, but in the middle of the session he became very silent and then admitted with shame that he had been intensely anti–Semitic some time before for a period of over six months. He had regarded the Jews as degraded people who were only out to exploit others in order to extract money from them in a ruthless way. He hated exploiters and wanted to attack and smash them for it. I interpreted that while he was aware that this happened in the past, he now felt awful towards me because after the previous day's session he had got rid of the greedy parasitical exploiting part of his self but had pushed it into me. He felt now that I had become his greedy exploiting self and this made him feel intensely suspicious about me. He replied that he feared that I must now hate and despise him, and that the only thing which he could do was to destroy himself or this hated part of himself. I interpreted his fear of my retaliation because when he saw me as a greedy, exploiting Jew he attacked and despised me, and feared that I would hate him because he believed I could not bear that he had pushed his own greedy self into me, not only as an attack but because he could not bear it himself and wanted to get rid of it. I suggested that it was when he felt that I could not accept his bad and hated self that he attacked himself so violently. In fact, the greatest anxiety during this session was related to violent attacks that were directed against his bad self which built up to a crescendo, so that he feared he would tear himself to pieces. He calmed down considerably after the interpretations.

The next session showed progress in so far as it seemed the splitting processes were diminishing, followed in subsequent sessions by some experience of depression. In the beginning of the session the patient reported that he had some difficulty in getting up, but he was glad that he remembered a dream. In this dream he was observing a group of Olympic runners in a race on the television screen. Suddenly he saw a number of people crowding on to the track and interfering with the race. He got violently angry with them and wanted to kill them for interfering and deliberately getting in the way of the runners. He reported that he had been looking at the television screen for only a short time the night before and had been thinking about the last session in which he had been afraid of damaging himself when he tried to cut off and destroy bad parts of himself. He was now determined to face up to whatever was going on in him. He had no associations to the dream, apart from the fact that the interfering people looked quite ordinary. I pointed out that in this dream he showed in a very concrete way what he felt he was doing when he was looking at television. The interfering people seemed to be the parts of himself which he experienced as worming their way into the track in Mexico when he was greedily and enviously looking at television. In this dream it was clear that people representing him were not competing by running, but were simply trying to interfere with the progress of the race.

I was then able to show him another aspect of the extremely concrete form of projection which related not only to the Olympic runners but to the analyst. I interpreted that he felt when the analysis was making good progress he experienced my interpretations and thoughts as something which he was watching with admiration and envy, like the athletes on television. He felt that the envious parts of himself actually could worm their way into my brain and interfere with the quickness of my thinking. In the dream he was attempting to face up to the recognition that these parts of himself existed and he wanted to control and stop them. I also related this process to Sidney's complaints that his own thought processes were often interfered with and I related this to an identification with the analyst's mind which he often enviously attacked. Sidney's co-operation during the last week had in fact been very positive, which had led to considerable unblocking of his mind, so that a great number of his projective identifications and splitting processes had shown themselves clearly in the analysis and could be related to the transference situation. In the dream he had succeeded in what he announced he tried to do – namely, to face up to the processes by bringing them into the transference rather than attempting to destroy and get rid of them by splitting and projection. This also enabled him to face up to his acute fear of damaging both his objects and his self through his projective identifications.

My interpretations seemed to diminish his anxiety about having completely destroyed me and my brain so that I could be experienced as helpful and undamaged, and for certain periods I was introjected as good and undamaged, a process leading gradually to a strengthening of the ego. One of the difficulties of working through such situations in the analysis is the tendency to endless repetition, in spite of Sidney's understanding that very useful analytic work was being done. It is important in dealing with patients and processes of this kind to accept that much of the repetition is inevitable. The acceptance by the analyst of the patient's processes being re-enacted in the transference helps the patient to feel that the self, which is constantly split off and projected into the analyst, is acceptable and not so damaging as feared.

I want now to describe briefly a short depressive spell in Sidney's illness which throws some light on his internal anxieties related to damage to objects and his self. A few days after the session just reported he was horrified about what was going on inside himself. For half an hour he experienced intense anxiety and reported that he was too frightened to look inside himself. Suddenly he saw his brain in a terrible state as if many worms had eaten their way into it. He feared that the damage was irreparable and his brain might fall to pieces. Despairingly he said how could he allow his brain to get into such an awful state! After a pause he suggested that his constant relations with prostitutes had something to do with the state of affairs. I interpreted that he felt that he had forced himself during the last weeks into people such as the prostitutes and the athletes and that he was afraid to see that damage outside. The damage to his brain seemed identical to the damage he feared he had done to external objects, particularly to me. He then began to talk about his brain as a particularly valuable and delicate part of his body which he had neglected and left unprotected. His voice sounded now much warmer and more concerned than ever previously, so I felt it necessary to interpret that his brain was also identified with a particularly valuable important object relationship – namely, the analysis and the analyst, which represented the feeding situation to him. This he had usually displaced on to the prostitutes, to whom he always went for nourishment. I gave him now detailed interpretations of the intensity of his hunger for me, his inability to wait, and I described his impulses and the self which he had experienced as boring himself omnipotently into my brain, which contained for him all the valuable knowledge which he longed to possess. Throughout the hour Sidney felt great anxiety and almost unbearable pain because he feared he could not repair the damage. However, he was clearly relieved through the transference interpretations, which helped him to differentiate and disentangle the confusion between inside and outside, phantasy and reality. I think it was particularly the interpretations about my brain – which showed him that I could still think and function – that both helped him to understand this very concrete phantasy in relation to his own thought processes and helped to relieve his anxiety about the damage he feared he had done to me.

Notes

1 Since Melanie Klein introduced the term 'projective identification' in her paper on schizoid mechanisms in 1946 it has been widely used by analysts to describe mechanisms and primitive narcissistic object relations which have been observed in patients suffering from neurotic or psychotic disorders. I want to use this note to compare and contrast some of the different ways the concept of projective identification has been used, starting with some aspects of the work of Dr Edith Jacobson, who describes psychotic identifications in schizophrenic patients which seem to me identical with the ones I observed but described as 'projective identification'. Jacobson frequently uses the term 'projective identification' in her book *Psychotic Conflict and Reality* (Jacobson 1967).

In 1954 Edith Jacobson discussed the identifications of the delusional schizophrenic patient who may eventually consciously believe himself to be another person. She relates this to early infantile identification mechanisms of a magic nature which leads to 'partial or total blending of the magic self and object images, founded on phantasies or even the temporary belief of being one with or of becoming the object, regardless of reality' (1954a). In 1967 she described these processes in more detail; she discussed (p. 54):

'the psychotic's regression to a narcissistic level, where the weakness of the boundaries between self and object images gives rise to phantasies, or experiences of fusion between these images. These primitive introjective or projective identifications are based on infantile phantasies of incorporation, devouring, invading (forcing oneself into), or being devoured by the object.'

She also said (1967: 84):

'We can assume that such phantasies, which pre-suppose at least the beginning distinction between self and object, are characteristic of early narcissistic stages of development and that the child's relation to the mother normally begins with the introjective and projective processes. . . . [The] introjective and projective identifications [of the adult patient] depend on the patient's fixation for early narcissistic stages and upon the depth of the narcissistic regression.'

181

In discussing clinical material of the patient A., Edith Jacobson described his fear that any affectionate physical contact might bring about experiences of merging, which in turn might lead to a manifest psychotic state. Her views that the introjective and projective identifications observed in the adult patient depend on the fixation to early narcissistic phases, where these identifications originate, seem identical with my own views, and there is nothing in her clinical and theoretical observations quoted above with which I would disagree. She stresses, however, that she differs from Melanie Klein and my own opinion in so far as she does not believe that the projective identifications of the adult patient, observable in the transference or acted out by the patient with objects in his environment, are in fact a repetition of the early infantile projective and introjective processes, but are to be understood as a later defensive process, as in her view early infantile processes cannot be observed in the transference. She also disagrees with my analytic technique of verbally interpreting the processes of projective identification when they appear in the transference, which I regard as of central importance in working through psychotic processes in the transference situation.

I have found that verbal interpretation in psychotic patients is dangerous only when the patient functions on a level where he expresses his own thoughts and words as concrete parts of himself which he can use to intrude physically into the analyst, a process which is likely to cause fragmentation of the self and confusion. During these times of the patient's concrete experiences the analyst's interpretations are also experienced as concrete intrusions which create confusional misunderstanding by the patient of what the therapist says and means. In such situations the patient has to become aware that he has lost his capacity for normal abstract thinking, which will return when the process of primitive projective identification for purposes of communication can be mobilized in the transference. When this process begins to function again the words and thoughts of the analyst begin to lose their concreteness, and with this the danger of verbal interpretation lessens. Edith Jacobson has apparently not been aware that the confusion is mainly caused by the appearance of concrete mental processes in the transference situation. In therapy she therefore avoids analysis of projective identification in the transference situation and concentrates on the defensive nature of the projective identification in her adult patients. She says that she has observed in her adult patients that they project the bad, unacceptable part of themselves into external objects. But she then avoids any attempt of the patient to assimilate the bad self into his ego structure but educates the patient to look for a suitable host for the bad self in the real external object relationship; in this way she tries to diminish the danger to the patient of his being involved with criminal or delinquent people in his environment. Here Edith Jacobson's description of her treatment of the patient A. is relevant; he had projected his own homosexual and delinquent self into a homosexual delinquent client whom he became very attached to and cared for as a dear friend, almost like a son, trying to help him to stop his homosexual behaviour and overcome his delinquent tendencies. However, when the patient's attempts to improve his friend failed because he again became involved in homosexual and other doubtful ventures, the patient became severely paranoid and confused. The paranoia was, however, not taken back to be interpreted and understood in the transference situation, as there must have been an avoidance of the paranoid transference to the analyst before, but Edith Jacobson tried to help the patient to find a more suitable, less disturbed 'friend' to act as the container or host for the patient's bad self.

Margaret Mahler described in 1952 symbiotic infantile psychoses and suggested that the mechanisms employed are introjective and projective ones and their psychotic elaboration. Her ideas seem to be closely related to, but nevertheless distinct from, what I have described as projective identification. She describes the early mother–infant relationship as a phase of object relations in which the infant behaves and functions as though he and his mother were an omnipotent system (a dual unity with one common boundary, a symbiotic membrane as it were). In 1969 she wrote that 'the essential feature of symbiosis is hallucinatory or delusional, somatopsychic, omnipotent fusion with the representation of the mother and, in particular, delusion of common boundary of the two actually and physically separate individuals' (p. 9). She suggests that 'this is the mechanism to which the ego regresses in cases of psychotic disorganization' (p. 9). In describing the symbiotic infantile psychosis she says that the early mother–infant symbiotic relationship is intense. The mental representation of the mother remains or is regressively fused with that of the self. She describes the panic reactions caused by separations which 'are followed by restitutive productions that serve to maintain or restore the narcissistic fusion, the delusion of oneness with mother or father' (1969: 73). It is clear that Margaret Mahler has introjective or projective processes in mind as the mechanisms which produce the symbiotic psychosis. I have, however, found no clear description of these mechanisms in her papers. She seems to see the symbiotic psychosis as a defence against separation anxiety, which links up closely with my description of the narcissistic object relation serving a defensive function. The symbiotic processes described by Mahler have some resemblance to the parasitical object relations I have described before. Projective identification which includes ego splitting and the projection of good and bad parts of the self into external objects is not identical with symbiosis.

For projective identification to take place, some temporary differentiation of 'me' and 'not me' is essential. Symbiosis, however, is used by Mahler to describe a state of undifferentiation, of fusion with the mother, in which the 'I' is not yet differentiated from the 'not I'.

2 In her paper on schizoid mechanisms Melanie Klein (1946) considers first of all the importance of the processes of splitting, denial, and omnipotence, which during the early phase of development play a role similar to that of repression at a later stage of ego development. She then discusses the early infantile instinctual impulses and suggests that while the 'oral libido still has the lead, libidinal and aggressive impulses and phantasies from other sources come to the fore and lead to a confluence of oral, urethral and anal desires, both libidinal and aggressive' (1946: 300).

After discussing the oral libidinal and aggressive impulses directed against the breast and the mother's body, she suggests (1946: 300) that

'the other line of attack derives from the anal and urethral impulses and implies expelling dangerous substances (excrements) out of the self and into the mother. Together with these harmful excrements, expelled in hatred, split–off parts of the ego are also projected into the mother. These excrements and bad parts of the self are meant not only to injure but also to control and to take possession of the object. Insofar as the mother comes to contain the bad parts of the self, she is not felt to be a separate individual but is felt to be the bad self. Much of the hatred against parts of the self is now directed towards the mother. This leads to a particular form of identification which establishes the prototype of an aggressive object relation. I suggest for these processes the term projective identification.'

Later on in the same paper Melanie Klein describes that not only bad but also good parts of the ego are expelled and projected into external objects, who become identified with the projected good parts of the self. She regards this identification as essential for the infant's ability to develop good object relations. If this process is excessive, however, good parts of the personality are felt to be lost to the self, which results in the weakening and impoverishment of the ego. Melanie Klein also emphasizes the aspect of the projective processes that relates to the forceful entry into the object and the persecutory anxieties related to this process, which I mentioned before. She also describes how paranoid anxieties related to the projective identification disturb introjective processes. 'Introjection may then be felt as a forceful entry from the outside into the inside in retribution for violent projection' (1946: 304). It will be clear that Melanie Klein gives the name 'projective identification' to both the processes of ego splitting and the 'narcissistic' object relations created by the projection of parts of the self into objects.

3 Felton (1985), working for more than ten years intensely with autistic children and their mothers, found that there exists a process which she has described as 'osmotic overflow' or 'pressure', whereby feelings, experiences, and memories existing in the mother but unbearably disturbing to her and which she wants to hide and not to know about are activated during pregnancy by the presence of the foetus and come under pressure. Unknown to the mother, these disturbing factors 'leak out' to the foetus. She describes this process as an antithesis to communication and projection, as there is no pressure to communicate but only an overflow of something which the mother is determined to hide for ever. The disturbing realization for the observer is the fact that the child has been deeply affected and overwhelmed by these processes. It is interesting that Bion observed similar disturbing processes, which he believed remained hidden and inaccessible in the foetus but suddenly overwhelm the adolescent or grown-up person in periods of crisis by emerging into consciousness.

As the foetus, and later on the infant, is completely helpless towards the 'pressures' which flow into him, which fill him with disturbing contradictory impressions, autistic patterns of behaviour can be noticed. The child feels a stranger to himself and different from everyone. He feels he is not allowed to know or understand what is going on because of the strong pressure of secrecy which overwhelms him. When his mother talks to the child he does not appear to hear, as if he is deaf, and he moves away from her or he turns round in circles or moves aimlessly; there is nothing in his body process which shows that he relates to her. In the posture of his body he often shows the signs of being oppressed, overwhelmed, as if he cannot hold himself up, as if he is not allowed to live. He looks flabby, sagging to the floor. The child also shows signs that he has no space inside him and he tries to create artefacts which help him to exist or to move. For example, a child collected tapes which had melodies lasting a certain time and when he moved from one part of the house to another he played the tape which lasted exactly the time he took to walk from one place to the other. Then when he went for longer distances the same process was noticeable, and without his tape-recorder and the carefully selected tapes he did not, or could not, move. To defend himself against the 'osmotic pressure' this autistic child used blocking mechanisms which prevented the pressure entering him. It seems that the child constantly anticipated the mother's disturbing reactions and shut them out because he recognized that the mother was dangerous to him and he had to shut her out. This blocking and shutting-out process does of course imply that only very little can be allowed to come into the child, but this is evidently necessary for the child in order to keep alive. Gradually the child became less defended. Some of this interaction between mother and child could more easily be observed. The mother had a deep feeling of guilt and responsibility towards her own mother, whom she felt she had neglected. She felt extremely embarrassed and ashamed about these thoughts which she wanted to hide and she had become very ashamed of the baby she had brought into the world because she felt these hidden thoughts were now connected with the child. At one point this autistic child, when he began to speak, expressed a constant deep fear of being disappointing to his own mother. He repeated again and again, 'I am not a disappointment to you. I don't want to disappoint you.' The mother didn't take much notice of it and didn't understand why the child continued all the time to talk to her like this, but he seemed to be so much under the pressure of the mother's guilt feelings which she did not acknowledge that apparently he could do nothing else but repeat endlessly that he did not want to disappoint her. I am able to report here only a few points of Mrs Felton's important work which I feel may help us to understand some psychotic patients better.

Steiner (1975) stresses his belief that there are different types of projective identification which belong to different stages in the development of the child including that of the prenatal state. In the same work (Steiner 1975) he talks about similar ideas, stressing that he does not believe that the baby of a few hours projects in the same way as a baby of three months, of six, etc. He argues that one should take into consideration the various senses through which the projection is made – smell, sounds, flavour – and also the velocity with which the projection works. He emphasizes his conviction that this pathological or even evacuative projection is a way of communication of a very primitive kind. In a later unpublished paper Steiner (1982) tries to show that the primitive projective process can work using the image of an 'osmotic system' of communication where contradictory feelings are communicated, and he postulates that this 'osmotic system' should help to understand what is going on *in utero*. He is convinced that the most primitive forms of projective identification are actually a relic of the osmotic system of communication *in utero*. It is interesting that both Felton and Steiner use the same descriptive term, 'osmotic pressure' or 'system', for these early processes. Felton is very emphatic and convinced that the osmotic pressure is only an overflow of disturbed feelings and thoughts of the mother that are meant to be secret and therefore are particularly anti-communicative in nature, while Steiner stresses the communicative value of the osmotic process. If Felton is correct in her observations, the child patient or adult using the 'osmotic pressure' in analysis will create a great deal of confusion in the analyst, who will feel constantly misled and misinformed if he tries to receive what comes from the patient as a form of communication. And the patient in his turn will feel also disturbed and overwhelmed by feeling that some of the analyst's secret mental processes come into him, creating enormous havoc.

Tustin (1972, 1981) using Hermann's (1929) suggestion that 'flowing over' is a precursor of projection, has suggested that flowing over and oneness are a process by which the illusion of primary unity is maintained; it is tenable that, in spite of the caesura of birth there is not an absolutely abrupt transition from the sensations associated with being inside the womb to being outside it. Tactile sensations of being in the 'watery medium appear to linger on and to be carried over into the child's earliest experience of the outside world' (1981: 80). In working with psychotic children, Tustin observed the importance of the overflow, the spilling over of psychological and physiological tension which the child experiences as tangible body stuff overflowing out of control.

Bion (1980: 104) writes: 'In carrying out an analytic investigation we should be aware of the fact that what Melanie Klein described as projective identification takes place even before birth – that is supposing that an embryo can be aware of primordial sensations.' He describes his 'imaginative conjecture' that even before birth the foetus becomes sensitive to what he calls 'happenings': events like the sense of the pulsation of its blood, physical pressure of a kind that can be communicated through a watery fluid such as the amniotic fluid or even extra-cellular fluid. He can 'conceive a situation in which pressure is transmitted to the amniotic fluid and can therefore possibly stimulate the optic and auditory pits. . . . I am guessing that even an embryo of three or four "somites" experiences something which will one day become what we call "sensations"' (1980: 100). He continues later (p. 100):

'I can imagine that even the embryo could much dislike the feeling of blood pulsating through its system. Similarly, that it might dislike the effects of the early stages of production of adrenalin or other developing functions. The more potentially sensitive or intelligent, the more it would be likely to be what could later be called aware of these sensations, dislike them and therefore get rid of them.'

The foetus may take a wrong turning in development, become incapable of having 'feelings' or 'ideas', and so be born lacking important elements of its equipment. However, the postnatal creature still retains its potential for intelligent activity. Bion attempts a few times to express thoughts of how this early antenatal situation could influence later development. It seems in this situation which he is discussing that the distinction of conscious and unconscious is not very illuminating. Because if the embryo tries to rid itself of unpleasant or unwelcome primordial sensations, it could have 'ideas' or 'feelings' that had never at any time been conscious. The nearest that one can get to describing it is that these ideas or feelings were available or not available; they have become out of reach of their origin. So when you are dealing with the grown-up you will have to distinguish between something that is conscious or unconscious and something that is inaccessible. He then describes patients who say they have no imagination, no dreams, and we have to consider the possibility that their dreams and their imagination are not accessible. Bion believes that the primordial antenatal germs of thought or feeling which are inaccessible can at periods of emotional turmoil such as at adolescence or latency come to the surface, and the child becomes suddenly incapable of understanding and has lost all his common sense. In other words, behaviour appears which we generally describe as psychotic. Bion gives a clinical illustration of an adult patient who struggles with something inside himself which he knew nothing about, a very severe asthmatic patient whom Bion saw in a hospital. After the first few sessions the asthma became worse, but nobody seemed to worry about this. As treatment proceeded the patient managed to create a very hostile attitude in the ward against the analyst while he himself maintained a strong admiration and idealization. Actually the patient, who had never experienced frustration, had never had any fear of insanity, and had never been physically ill, now began to be afraid of going mad, developed colds, and became unpopular. He even had an impulse – at times a very strong impulse – to commit suicide. This sudden appearance from the depths of these overwhelming anxieties is very alarming for the therapist and the patient. Bion feels that the state is remarkably reminiscent of that he described in which these primordial ailments are inaccessible because they have been got rid of at source. Now suddenly these inaccessible feelings, which have never been unconscious and which have never been conscious, now become both. Bion feels that these experiences which he describes throw a new light on the sudden appearance of psychotic illness.

4 I believe that the differentiation of the self and object representation is necessary to maintain normal symbol formation which is based on the introjection of objects experienced as separate from the self. Dr Segal (1957) also stresses greater awareness and differentiation of the separateness between the ego and the object in normal symbol formation. She thinks that symbolization is closely related to the development of the ego and the objects which occur in the depressive position (1957: 394):

> 'symbols are in addition to other factors created in the internal world as a means of restoring, recreating, recapturing and owning again the original object. But in keeping with the increased reality sense, they are now felt as created by the ego and therefore never completely equated with the original object.'

I have always found that the excessive projective identification in the psychotic process – which obliterates the differentiation of self and objects, and causes confusion between reality and phantasy and a regression to concrete thinking – produces the loss of the capacity for symbolic thinking.

The loss of the capacity for abstract and symbolic thinking by the schizophrenic patient, which leads on to very concrete modes of thinking, has been described by many writers such as Vigotsky (personal communication) and Goldstein (1985). Harold Searles (1962) in his paper 'The Differentiation between Concrete and Metaphorical Thinking in the Recovering Schizophrenic Patient' suggests that the concrete thought disorders depend on the fluidity of the ego boundaries when self and object are not clearly differentiated.

In one of his cases he describes 'abundant evidence of massive projection, not only onto human beings around him but also onto trees, animals, buildings and all sorts of inanimate objects' (Searles 1963: 25). Only when ego boundaries gradually become firmly established through treatment can figurative or symbolic thinking develop. Searles's observations have a close relationship to my own view that excessive projective identification, leading to fusion between self and object, always causes loss of the capacity for symbolic and verbal thinking.

5 In my paper 'On the Psychopathology of Narcissism' (1964b: 171) I stressed that 'projective identification was part of an early narcissistic relationship of the infant where omnipotent narcissistic object relations, particularly omnipotent projective identification, obviate both the aggressive feelings caused by frustration and any awareness of envy'. I believe that in the psychotic patient projective identification is more often a defence against excessive envy, which is closely bound up with the patient's narcissism, rather than a defence against separation anxiety. In my paper 'Object Relations of the Acute Schizophrenic Patient in the Transference Situation' (1964a) I tried to trace the origin of the envious projective identification in schizophrenia. The infant's experience of feeling small and in need of the breast may arouse strong omnipotent, *envious*, sadistic feelings. These often lead in the schizophrenic to a delusional *taking over of the breast/mother*, who in such situations is experienced as seductive, *tantalizing, and frustrating*.

6 Bion (1965) describes a more active case of parasitism. He emphasizes that such patients are particularly unrewarding. The essential feature is simultaneous stimulation and frustration of hope, and work that is fruitless except for discrediting analyst and patient. The destructive activity is balanced by enough success to deny the patient fulfilment of his destructiveness.

'A helpful summary of such a case is to describe it as "chronic" murder of patient and analyst, or, an instance of parasitism. . . . The patient draws on the love, benevolence, indulgence of the host to extract the knowledge and power which enables him to poison the association and destroy the indulgence on which he depends for his existence.'

(1965: 28)

I would add that it is important to differentiate the very chronic forms of parasitism from the massive intrusion and projective identification into the analyst which resemble parasitism but are of shorter duration and respond more easily to interpretations. These occur at times when separation threatens or when jealousy or envy is violently stimulated in the transference or in outside life. Meltzer (1967b) described a primitive form of possessive jealousy which plays an important role in perpetuating massive projective identification of a peculiar withdrawn, sleepy sort.

9
Projective identification and the problem of containment in a borderline psychotic patient

I drew attention in Chapter 8 to my view that projective identification, while sometimes taking the form of a violent and powerful expulsion of unbearable material, also provides the opportunity for communication between patient and analyst. If the analyst is functioning therapeutically, he should be able to contain the patient's communications (particularly in his counter-transference) and use them to increase his, and subsequently his patient's, understanding. On the other hand, projective identification is often confusing to the analyst and may prevent him from thinking and interfere with his capacity for judgement and assessment of the patient. From the beginning of treatment, especially with psychotic patients, powerful projective identification can take place and create an almost hypnotic atmosphere. In these circumstances the analyst's capacity to function therapeutically and to contain the situation depends upon his emotional resources and his theoretical understanding. It is important to realize that the two interact together, so that the analyst's emotional capacities can help him to empathize with what is happening, and his theoretical, conceptual capacity can help him to bear the emotions. The case I am now going to describe was first presented to me in a prolonged seminar lasting more than three hours. The patient, Clare, had been treated at that time by a psychotherapist, Mrs L., for four years.[1] The case illustrates how delicate the balance can be in cases involving powerful projective identification and how it can go wrong – leading to a failure of containment and a long-lasting therapeutic impasse.[2] I shall interpose Mrs L.'s report about the patient (in italic type) with my own comments in roman type).

'*Clare was thirty-five years old at our first meeting in 1975. She had recently given birth to a little boy who was then just over three months old. Exhibiting great anxiety, she told me that things had been amiss between her husband and herself since the baby's birth and that she had lost her appetite and her ability to sleep. Her husband would come home from work at some point in the afternoon, tell her to put on a miniskirt to excite him, and request her to make love immediately. There was a strong persecutory tone in her report, and her charges against the husband were very violent. In contrast to this was her description of the things her husband had obtained from her. She had agreed to his demands, which seemed to betray her need to share with him the illusion that she could do everything. She could learn how to play the piano for him; to play chess; to study mathematics, and above all put on weight. Her husband would bring home pastries and demand that she eat them; she had thus been able to put on 10 kilos.*

There was something very striking and powerful in her way of asking for help. She had two requests:

(1) 'It can't go on like that. The situation between my husband and me is intolerable.' This request was formulated in the register of 'doing': 'What must I do?' Moreover, she conveyed an absolute intolerance of the situation and an incapacity to wait and to reflect. The situation presented was one that seemed about to explode at any moment.

(2) 'The psychiatrist who treats my husband wonders why I married so late and thinks that I should try to understand why I chose my husband.' It seemed to me that she wanted an immediate answer. No postponement was possible; the request for help was pressing. I felt I could either say 'Yes' and be caught in the trap of a persecutory situation, or say 'No'.

'*I should perhaps explain why I did not decide against trying to treat Clare. I think I responded to a healthy part of her personality, which is full of vitality. This vitality had probably been stimulated again by the recent birth of the baby, of whom, however, Clare did not speak. I suspect that the non-verbalized part of the request was transmitted to me by her facial expression. This face has a capacity to change extremely quickly. Sometimes her slightly averted face closes itself, taking on a dramatic expression like a desperate attempt to escape an intolerable situation. I have thought subsequently that this may be the case, when she enters my apartment and when she leaves. Sometimes it also happens when she eludes a comment of mine. Her face has a strong impact on me. When she arrives with this expression I say to myself, 'What catastrophe is she going to report today?' On the other hand, sometimes her face opens up, and she is charming and cheerful. In taking on the patient, I felt concerned that I could not do anything for her obviously very sick husband.*

'*No sooner had I agreed to take her on as a patient, and no sooner had she left the first interview, than I was faced with a feeling of fright and terror.*

The predominating counter-transferential impression was the following: I had got on a train at full speed with her, and neither she nor I was allowed to think about this situation.

'Two months later she informed me that she had saved her husband's life. She had left him for some time but when she came home she found him inanimate on his bed. He had just absorbed a massive dose of antidepressant medication. She put down the baby and called the ambulance for him, and he was brought back to life at the point of death. He was eventually hospitalized in a psychiatric clinic and then sent to a convalescent home. At the same time his friends intervened on his behalf. They asked Clare to leave the apartment, and her husband found another woman a few months later. Clare moved to a new house.'

• This very lively report gives a clear picture of the difficulties which occurred in the preliminary interview with this patient. What strikes one first is that Mrs L. fell into a trap with her patient in the first interview but realized this only at the moment when Clare left. Only then did she realize that Clare had not allowed her any time to reflect whether she wanted to try to treat her or not. She also recognized that Clare had prevented her entirely from thinking. At that moment it was too late to do anything about it. What is important, however, whenever such pressure is felt in the therapeutic situation is that one allows some time to elapse so that one can recover the power of thought and try to understand what is going on. The very fact that Clare did not think and did not want Mrs L. to think either demands that the therapist must have some time to recover from this most powerful onslaught on her capacity to think. Otherwise Mrs L. is in danger of being taken over by a powerful influence and of not knowing what is happening. Mrs L. was aware that Clare wanted an immediate answer, but she forgot, under this pressure, that she also needed some time and distance to think things over. It was necessary to find a compromise. In such a situation, even half a minute's thinking can remind one that one is a therapist. Then it may be possible to tell the patient that you understand she is in a hurry and cannot wait but also that it is necessary to think over the question of the treatment for just one day. A patient will not like this response but she will certainly understand it, and then one can discuss with her what is happening in an unpersecuting way. One can say that one understands her anxiety and the pressure on her but that neither she nor oneself can think or make important decisions under such pressure. At such a time it is particularly important for the therapist to make it quite clear

193

what sort of help is available. In first sessions such as Clare's the urgent message to be understood is that there is an enormous amount of pressure to be contained. The analyst must realize this clearly herself and so contain it. But how did Clare put her therapist in such a situation? Understanding how this can happen is of crucial importance in containing it.

In listening very carefully to the description of this first interview I think it is clear that the power of Clare's projection was conveyed through what she said about her husband. She managed to stimulate Mrs L.'s anxiety about her husband so strongly that after the first interview Mrs L. was very concerned about him. Mrs L. recognized that he was in danger but was unable to do anything about it. It turned out afterwards that she was absolutely correct about this. This emphasizes how sensitive and perceptive Mrs L. is in receiving and perceiving Clare's projective identification, an important aspect of any therapist's capacity. Her difficulty was that she could not use the information gained from her counter-transference. She could not see how to bring what was being said and felt about the husband's obvious illness into the treatment. She did not know how to cope with this situation, and therefore, like Clare, was left very distressed. This is what Clare projected via an identification with her husband. As Mrs L. was not aware of Clare's projection into her husband she felt helpless and thought she could not talk to the patient about him. Yet, had she had some time to think about the problem, she might have been able to identify the patient's projection into her husband and she then might have been able to talk over the problem of the husband with the patient without feeling that she was interfering. Projective identification becomes less of a problem if it can be translated from a non-verbal communication into verbal thought. Only then can it be talked about so that the very powerful acting out of the patient and her husband can become accessible to the analysis.

In fact, Clare describes vividly how her husband sadistically overpowers her and how she becomes the passive victim, which she not only hates but enjoys. On the other hand, she has also described how she projectively identifies herself with her husband and so becomes the powerful dominator herself – something clearly seen in the patient's attitude towards Mrs L. during the interview session. Clare might consciously try to deny such links. She might say that it is all her husband's problem. In that case an analysis of the situation becomes impossible. Who can control the situation unless the analyst can bring the problem quickly into focus? So, diagnosing the projection into the husband is essential if Mrs L. is to be therapeutic. She has to become the container of these problems. Clare may not immediately feel capable of coping with the situation, but if Mrs L. can contain the problems then her husband would not be excluded from the therapy and can gradually be distinguished from the part of the patient projected into him. Once the projection into the husband has been understood, he would appear as a separate person, and the issues could be discussed between them and considered – something which is impossible while such powerful projective identification is dominating the picture. What is the consequence of Mrs L. not having recognized the projection into the husband? Mrs L. feels that she is not in control of what is going to happen and she is strongly affected by Clare's fear. Clare is terrified that either the husband, or those aspects of herself projected into the husband, will die. It is this that makes the whole problem so terriby urgent.

The way Clare conveyed the urgency of the situation is worth looking at in detail. First, she made her request, 'It can't go on like this. The situation is intolerable', and so conveyed absolute intolerance towards the situation that existed at that time and an incapacity to wait and to reflect. She seemed very insistent, but it isn't really Clare who is talking like that. The person who is being used by Clare to make this forceful request is her husband. This gives one the feeling that the husband is actually in the room. She is so completely identified with her husband that one feels that she is the husband and one should be fitting in with her and her husband's demands and submitting to her as she generally feels she has to submit to him. So in fact Clare, the husband, and Mrs L. are all together in the room. If one notices this, then one can suggest to Clare very clearly that all three are being included, and the husband is not left out. It is essential to see this in order to control the situation. If one is too much under pressure to observe what is happening and to think about it, one has to tell a patient that one will have to see her again, perhaps the next day. In this way one would prevent oneself becoming part of the collusive threesome.

Clare's second request is also significant: 'The psychiatrist who treats my husband wonders why I married so late and thinks I should try to understand why I chose my husband.' This provides the clue that she chooses her husband for a very important reason. At the present time it looks as if she chooses him for projection and identification in order to rid herself of all those

195

aspects of herself with which she does not want to cope, and at the same time she can feel justified in being so dominating. Why this is necessary is something one would have to consider by examining Clare's history.

Clare is the second of five children. She has a brother one year older and three younger siblings. She was separated from her mother at birth until she was four months old. Mother and daughter were in the same clinic, but the daughter was taken care of by nurses. Her mother said she had a haemorrhage. When Clare was aged one, her family went overseas. Her father went to war. News about the father was alarming, and her mother dreaded that he was dead. When she was two, her mother was pregnant and in mourning for her father. When she was three, her brother, Fabian, was born. The baby-sitter who had taken care of her for two years left also at that time. So Clare was left alone with a very upset mother and a newly born baby, who probably got all the mother's attention. Her father had gone away, as had her beloved baby-sitter. There were other disasters. Her father's only brother, aged twenty, died from tuberculosis, and the paternal grandmother had a breakdown. When she was five, her father came back, and her mother became pregnant again, giving birth to another brother, Guy.

The mother was severely depressed but strongly denied it. She managed to provide the family with food (in the difficult situation of the war). However, she did not apparently think anything of sending the children (aged four and five) unaccompanied very long distances to school or to visit acquaintances.

Clare had very painful and recurrent childhood bullous dermatitis. Fabian, the little brother, had severe abscesses of the leg and was in danger. When Clare was six, the family moved to Europe. Her father was present but persecuted her. He was severe, mocked her learning difficulties, and beat her frequently and violently. The family changed residence often (twenty two times in all). Her mother had two illnesses: a primary infection (tuberculosis) when Clare was twelve and gallbladder troubles when Clare was eighteen. Her father went back overseas.

Clare had married three years before the beginning of the treatment. She had lost a first baby. There was a mistake on the birth date. She gave birth to a dead child, a baby boy. Her husband could not understand why she was desperate, 'because he [the husband] was there and alive'. He did not allow her 'to weep for a dead child'. She wanted imperatively to have another baby and she became pregnant four months later. When she was six months pregnant, her husband wanted to commit suicide and forced her to agree to this. She thought she would be driven crazy.

- Clare's history underlines how essential it is when treating any patient to have detailed historical information. Listening to what

196

has happened to her, one is immediately orientated towards her communication in a specific way.

Clare completely lost her mother for four months from birth. As the mother was so ill, it is very likely that she did not see the mother at all. She did, of course, survive these four months, otherwise she would not be in therapy. But one has a very distinct feeling that there is a part of her which has not survived and which died in hospital but wasn't known to anybody, even to her mother. Where is this dead part of her? It must be somewhere. But where? In the interview she describes a husband who is dying or sometimes feels he is dying or that he wants to die. Things become clear. She has put the dead part of herself into her husband, and this dead baby part of her is hidden there. This understanding confirms the intuitive grasp of the psychiatrist who told her she had to find out why she had chosen her husband. The split between that part of Clare which survives and was alive and that part of her which is dead must have always been extremely important. She must always have been worried that, if these two parts come closer together, she would become very anxious or suicidal. The conflict was acted out with her husband. In some ways she wanted to help him to survive and in other ways desired his death as the only way out of her problems. As soon as this becomes clear it could be much easier to deal with both the patient and the husband, because you can now show them to what extent she uses her husband to get rid of the dead baby part of herself which she doesn't want. It was already clear that there was a part of her that she had projected into the husband; but with the advantage of the history, what kind of self she had projected into him could be seen. The patient and her husband cannot be helped to survive unless we understand this problem and by bringing it together in our minds gradually help the patient to understand it too. The violence and explosiveness can then be taken out of the situation, and the husband's problems can be understood as well.

The biographical notes also tell us something else of great importance. The patient lost her baby, her first baby. Given that we realize how upset the patient was about this death, we can understand why she immediately wanted to have another baby. She wanted to feel she had a live baby because a dead baby was too frightening for her. But what about the husband? He couldn't stand her talking about the dead baby. He wouldn't even allow her to weep. Obviously he wanted her to think of him as her only baby. Then, on top of it, when she became pregnant again and she was in the sixth month of pregnancy, her husband wanted to commit suicide, even wanted to force her to agree and to help him to do it. Why wasn't he pleased to have a live child? If one thinks about this situation it becomes clear that her husband was identified with the dead child, the first baby who could not survive. When his wife insisted on having another baby it must have felt to him that she wanted him to die and did not care whether he was alive or dead. She just wanted to have a live baby and that was all. So it was not only Clare who felt she was a dead baby. It was her husband too who felt he was the dead child. One cannot treat psychotic patients without knowing their history and without some empathic imaginative investigation of it. With this in one's mind, it would not be too difficult to interpret to a patient like Clare what she wanted to get rid of that she could not bear. What she was trying to expel was herself as her mother's dead baby. She had always wanted to do this because it felt so unbearable inside her.

By putting her dead baby part into her husband it was impossible for Clare to help either her husband or herself. In this situation she is entirely dependent on the understanding of her therapist. It is for this reason that it is so important for an analyst to understand what it means to treat a psychotic patient; it is the therapist who has to aim at making contact with all the split–off parts of her patient, and keep them in her mind. One does not control the situation by any external force; one just follows all the details of this situation which occur in one's mind so that one begins to understand what it means. One has to realize that the patient has no mind with which to think about the problems, and this makes it necessary that the therapist gather all the aspects of the patient's problems in his mind and think about them. If the therapist realizes that the patient does not want to take any of her problems back into herself he must not collude with this and do the same. The analyst has to look for the connections and links which help him to understand why she is so frightened of taking the problems back into her mind. Then, gradually, he should be able to make the patient aware of what has been going on. One must never overwhelm the patient with little bits of information and force this on to him or her. One must always relate whatever one interprets in some detail in a way which should be fully understandable. Then the therapist will find that it is at times amazing what the patient will be able to take from him and how grateful he is that he is willing to take over the role of thinking for him, until the patient can assimilate some of the problems which disturb him and what he finds so unbearable.

With the information we have so far about Clare it is much easier to understand her dilemma. In her view the only way out of her problems is to get rid of her dead baby self, which in this situation is confused with her husband. Her other dilemma is her difficulty in coping with the separation from her husband which has been forced upon her. She suffered through it but also felt relieved. On the other hand, she felt accused and responsible for her husband's suicide attempt, which implies that the responsibility for looking after this dead baby was entirely pushed back into her. The separation from her husband which is forced upon her creates an increase of the splitting of herself, now accentuated by the external environment.

The first two years

I shall now present some further reports about the progress of Clare's therapy, bearing in mind that the patient came only once a week, a problem created by the massive projection and manipulation which took place in the first interview and incapacitated Mrs L.

'*In the early sessions I was struck by Clare's psychological state. When she came to the sessions while she was staying in her parents' home, she was immobile and unfocused. She did not show her usual exaltation. It seemed that she was using her parents to project her exultation into them, which left her immobile and unfocused.*

'*The second year of treatment was saturated with disasters. In spite of the fact that her husband had chosen another woman, a triangular situation was soon set up between her husband, the other woman, and Clare. Clare became pregnant. A spontaneous miscarriage helped her to do precisely what she wanted to do: not to think about it. Then, a most traumatic event occurred. The patient's youngest brother died in a mountaineering accident (this was the brother who was born when she was six years old). Clare was in great pain about her brother's death, but as usual it was not possible for her to mourn for him.*'

- Here again we realize that Clare cannot keep any dead baby situation in her mind, a problem which we can now, through the knowledge gathered in our discussion, link with all the other dead baby situations, her own dead baby self, her husband's dead self, and so on.

'*After a year and a half of treatment I felt there was a calmer, and often even serene, period of about six months. Clare's material was more*

199

organized, and I noticed I was beginning to be more able to think about her. After a year and three-quarters, as Christmas was coming, Clare was able to cry because she felt lonely and abandoned by everyone, including me. I had been seeing her twice a week now for several months. At the beginning of the year I suggested to her that we increase the number of sessions to three, and in September of that year she also began to lie down on the couch. My suggestion that she increase the number of sessions seemed to be a response to a very alive and dynamic part of the patient's personality.'

● Mrs L. is here quite perceptive. But I want to stress another aspect of responding to an alive part of a patient. This is the danger of forgetting about the very dead part to which it is essential the therapist respond and with which he must stay in touch. Only by being aware of this part of the patient can it become alive and not feel abandoned.

The quiet period described above, which was characterized by a certain amount of elaboration on Clare's part, was terminated abruptly by a kind of tornado which broke out at the end of the second year. Before going into a description of the period of the crisis, I should like to present material from one particular session in which the dynamics between the different parts of the patient seem to be clear.

'Clare had just met a kindergarten teacher, with whom she had sympathized right away. This teacher is about to accept a subordinate position with the director of a day-care centre, although she herself is a director and is the same age. The teacher is entering a period of dependency which will last two years. Clare knows the director of that centre well. She has just served as a substitute for her and has met there the teacher, whom she immediately liked. She wonders how things will work out between them. It seems to me that there is a kindergarten teacher part in herself which will stop the experience with the director of the day-care centre after two years, and which does not accept, in the transference, the generational difference between mother and daughter. Another part of her merely wonders how the experience will unfold; this is the healthy part of her personality. Finally she explained that there is a good deal of affinity between the kindergarten teacher and herself but they will see little of each other; they will just say "Hello" to each other in the courtyard. They will not have their endless discussions any more since it appears that the other colleagues had felt excluded. I wondered:. was she telling me that she had to separate now from that part of herself which she had projected on to me until the last occasion, and that she will see me only once in a while in the courtyard because the

feeling of exclusion during the vacation, which she had projected on to the colleagues, has been too strong?'

- This is the first time Mrs L. reports that she is aware of a split in Clare's personality which is revealed in the material. It seems to me that Clare makes it clear that she is willing to accept the dependent role with Mrs L. (the teacher) for two years. There seems to be no hostility, and in fact there is an openly admitted affection, between the dependent part and the other parts of the patient's self. But she indicates there is not going to be any communication between herself and this dependent part. This is in line with our understanding of Clare so far. But in this description there is a definite lessening of the split between an infantile self and the more adult part of her. Nevertheless she is adamant that she will not communicate with the infantile part of herself (the teacher) in the therapeutic situation and informs Mrs L. about it. This is the aspect of the material I would have chosen to interpret as much as possible. In that way one must make Clare aware of what she is doing with herself and the dangerous game she is playing. She is coming so close to herself and yet still remaining so detached, which could easily lead to a disaster.

'When the fateful two-year limit arrived, tears, confusion, and a paranoid atmosphere prevailed, as at the beginning of the therapy. I wondered if the patient was about to re-experience:

(1) all the events of her second or third year of life;
(2) in the transference, the failure of her omnipotence: she is neither the mother, nor the director of the day-care centre, and has acted only as the substitute for her;
(3) her failed attempts to repair her depressed mother.

'Trying to gain some perspective of this period of confusion, at the end of which it looked as if there might be a rupture. I should like to describe some movements that I thought I could identify. There were two conflicts around trust. First, with regard to the damaged pregnant mother: Clare recovered memories of her mother when the latter was pregnant with her little sister and when she herself was ten years old. She associated this period with mother. Second, with regard to her father: when she was eighteen her father left for overseas. Her mother was then very ill with a gallbladder condition; the whole family had to help take care of her, and it came close to her needing surgery. The father telephoned her every day from abroad and had to be called back at some point. She described this period as a nightmare. In speaking of these two memories the patient doubtless referred to her mother's

201

*pregnancy when she was very little and in particular to the birth of Fabian.
She was also referring to how the mother deteriorated psychologically during
that pregnancy and then after Fabian's birth, and the father's subsequent
absence.'*

● I think this last point about her experience at Fabian's birth is
crucial. This is the event I would diagnose from Clare's history as
the most traumatic one.

*'There was also some acting out. She tried to make her husband agree to
share his time equally between Violet (his other woman) and herself. At that
time this seemed completely crazy to me, and I was at a loss.*

*'The demand which my patient made towards her husband caused Violet
to 'outbid her'; she left her formerly separate living quarters and came to live
with the husband. The following dream shows my patient's triumph over
Violet, who represents the mother. My patient dreamt that she saw "that
woman, Violet" and said to her, "You are fat, you are horrible"; Violet
rolled on the floor – which had an effect on my patient. Then she was with
three children – her son, her brother Fabian (the latter was four or five years
old, when they were still overseas), and a third, non-identified child. She
said to them, "Come now, we must leave." '*

● The dream implies that in spite of triumphing over Violet she
plans to leave her husband or the therapist. The importance of
Fabian in relation to the coming crisis is stressed by his presence in
the dream.

*'I am now going to describe the rupture which occurred while Clare and
Violet were competing for the husband. Clare became more and more acutely
aware of the pain her husband inflicted on her by using Violet as the weapon.*

*'One day in March, close to the date of the birth of her little brother,
Fabian, and to the third anniversary of the beginning of her analysis, Clare
told me on arriving at my office, "I had a dream; I understood that Violet
came to take away my huband or my apartment from me. For two days I
have been suffering terribly, a kind of pain that I have feared all my life. But
I felt it, and that was a relief. I wanted to kill Violet almost for real. I do
understand crimes due to jealousy." The patient continued, "I have the
impression that the therapy is finished. I have reached a certain level. I
cannot see myself continuing the therapy indefinitely. I have been told that
there are people who have themselves analysed for seven years." She said
goodbye, telling me at the same time that she would call me the next day. I
decided during the session to let her leave, because she was unable to hear*

what I was saying. After she left I then felt atrocious pain and I had the impression that I could not bear it.

'The following day Clare left a message for me by telephone, indicating that she would come the day after. On the second day she reported, "I realized that I could not terminate that quickly. I spoke of seven years, I thought I could manage up to three years. I am sure that I experienced something very profound and that I do not want to live with my husband any more. In three years I have changed so little that I have just taken this decision. The thought came to my mind that, if my husband took his own life, I would be relieved; but then I thought that one cannot wish other people's death. The blame would fall back upon me. Finally I thought, in reality, that I should have someone seize Violet at the entrance of her house and have her dragged to the forest. Fortunately I did not do it. I think about good and evil, about the Curé d'Ars, about St George killing the dragon, who represents evil, about Eve and the Serpent. I believe in the Evil One."*

'Before this session Clare had told me that her husband's mother was slowly becoming demented and also that he had a back problem and had to be laid up from his work. Then, two months later, she told me he had committed suicide after making a visit to his mother when she did not recognize him.*

'I find it difficult to know which of the two events, his mother's dementia or my patient's decision, carried more weight in his suicide. It seemed to me that Clare had intuitively anticipated that her husband was going to leave the responsibility for his demented mother to her.*

'In any case, after the husband's death, Clare was crushed with guilt feelings, which were projected into me. Her state began to worry me; she seemed to experience a terrifying fear of both herself and her son being pulled into suicide. However, this fear began to subside, and she was able to bring me books about suicide which had belonged to her husband, asking me to keep them for her.*

'I was also having increasing difficulties with the patient regarding the number of sessions. She had requested to cut down sessions to one a week. There were also difficulties with the length of the session. Clare did not accept the end of the sessions, I myself was unable to terminate them. I found myself again and again keeping her for twice the time of a regular session.'*

- It would, of course, be wrong to say that Mrs L. was not prepared for the explosion. Even in the very first interview she had noted that the patient was overwhelmed with feelings which could at any moment explode when she said, 'It can't go on like that. The situation is intolerable.' Mrs L. also recognized later, when she narrated the material about the kindergarten teacher, that this was explosive material. It was at that time that she became clearly

203

aware of the split existing in Clare's personality. So, for a considerable time before this eruption, Mrs L. had been trying to bring order to her own mind to understand exactly what was going on. She was trying not to miss the crisis and anticipated it. However, I think that when it did occur it completely over-whelmed her at first and left her with the incredible pain which Clare had projected into her.

Mrs L. was not able to prepare herself correctly for the explosion because she did not understand the details of the complex projective identification that has been described. Even in the first preliminary interview Mrs L. had felt overwhelmed by noticing that Clare's problems could explode at any moment. What Mrs L. had missed then was Clare's identification with her husband, the projection of her dead baby self into her husband, and the recognition that her husband had been identified with the baby which died at birth. It is this situation which made the whole therapy so explosive and which the therapist had no chance to interpret clearly. The explosion arose when Clare had the dream that Violet had come to take away her husband or her apartment. There was no time to think what this dream would mean.

In this situation the therapist had to understand her patient's basic problems and how intricately mixed up they were with her husband. The dream indicated that she thought everything which was valuable and important for her was to be taken away by Violet. Because of its timing it was also clearly related to Fabian's birth. In this case two situations were constantly being repeated: Clare being left for four months at the time of her birth (expressed as having her mother and life taken away); and the situation later on when she was three years old – Fabian was born (again expressed as her mother being taken away from her and again leaving her with incredible pain and murderous feelings, which at three years of age she could not possibly cope with). The case material of this patient shows so clearly how important it is to formulate a model of the patient's experience and to understand the details of the projections and splitting mechanisms right from the beginning of treatment. This makes it possible to follow the events of the therapy much more closely. It also allows the therapist to be in control of the problems and to interpret the projections and the projective identifications of the patient. This in turn helps the patient to feel more contained and prevents the violent acting out which was so terribly dangerous in this case.

In Clare's case the first three years of her therapy were experienced by her as the first three years of her life, and it was essential this be understood. Almost from the beginning of the therapy she seemed to make clear by her projections that she was terribly frightened of the specific events connected with this situation and particularly of the raw feeling of murderousness and pain they exposed.

It is interesting that after the death of her husband Clare once more insisted again on cutting down the sessions to once a week. I understood this as her saying, 'We have arrived back again at the beginning of the therapy.' At the same time there is also an open accusation that she is no better than she was at the beginning of the analysis. None the less, she returned not just for one session but for two more sessions. Mrs L. also noticed that she could not terminate the session until they had one of double length. In other words, Clare made it clear that she needed the analyst for two sessions, and this should have been verbalized. I also wonder whether the unconscious request for two sessions in one isn't a communication about the need to understand the two situations in one: the death of her husband and the projected suicide of the dead baby felt inside her.

'In the following session Clare brought along a rather sizeable sculpture which her husband had made some years earlier. This sculpture represents a hand. A man, representing the husband, is sitting on the thumb, turning his back to several women lying in erotic positions and representing envy, greed, lewdness, avarice, jealousy, and laziness. Clare told me that she would not destroy this sculpture because the pieces would invade her. She would like to entrust me with it but could not accept that if she did this I would ever give it back. Halfway through the session (after forty-five minutes) she hid the sculpture in the bag in which she had brought it with the aim of preventing me from seeing it. That day I understood that there was a part of her which she felt she could not integrate and which one could only destroy or protect.'

- Mrs L. does not clarify here what she feels this sculpture represents or why Clare was hiding the sculpture from her by putting it back into the original bag after forty-five minutes. Clare seems very aware that the feelings which drove her husband to suicide still remain projected into him and his possessions, like the books and now the sculpture. Therefore, Clare now wants Mrs L. to understand the problem and asks her to allow her to project into her the suicidal part of her husband and, with this, the part of herself projected into him. However, Mrs L., as at the beginning of the analysis, now seems to refuse the patient's projection. She not only rejects the sculpture but does not interpret the meaning and significance of wanting to bring the sculpture concretely to the therapist. Using the second forty-five minutes for hiding the sculpture would mean that Clare shows Mrs L. that it is once more she who forces her to remain entangled with her husband and his suicidal problems. Clare is afraid that she has to keep this problem to herself and so make the analysis useless.

'*Gradually I was able to reduce the time of the session to normal length, reducing it by ten minutes each time, after having informed the patient of my intention and discussing her feelings with regard to it each time. My own internal experience was very violent. Once or twice I felt relieved but most of the time I felt the need, which I could hardly restrain, to act in order to evacuate this horrible experience.*

'*I felt from that time on that it was possible to understand that the splitting which occurred in Clare could not be analysed, because she feared that her precocious ego, which had experienced an abandonment during the first four months of her life, would become too confused. She would say, for instance, "It can't go on. I am afraid all the time. Take this out of my head."*'

• Mrs L. expressed a very strong feeling that something had been projected into her which she felt she wanted violently to evacuate. In this she could hardly restrain herself.

   Mrs L. now makes it clear that she began to to realize that a very important aspect of Clare, connected with her first four months of life, was related to that part of herself which she was afraid could not be analysed. It was also related to that part of her husband's sculpture which she had wanted to give back to Mrs L. but which she had been afraid to do because she felt the therapist did not understand and had rejected it. Mrs L. felt that she was afraid that this could not be integrated. In fact, however, this was a mistake on the therapist's part. From the very first session Clare had indicated that she had projected that part of herself into her husband and was not offering it to Mrs L., in the hope of integrating herself through the treatment. As soon as Mrs L. saw the case history she should have realized that it was the four-months–old baby self, which had not been able to cope with the separation from her mother, that had been projected into her. Since that time there had been many opportunities for the analyst to contain this part of Clare and to help Clare understand and so diminish her anxiety about it and assimilate it.

Clare's case illustrates the need for careful integration and interpretation in cases of projective identification and splitting. The therapist needs to use her own feelings and her knowledge and intellect to conceptualize what needs to be interpreted to integrate the patient. If this does not take place from the beginning of the therapy there is, at a later date, a danger that abrupt attempts at assimilation of the split-off part of the personality will cause not only acute anxiety but even disintegration. In treating patients of this type it is essential to study and familiarize oneself with the technique of analysing and understanding these projections. By careful under-standing and interpretation one can greatly reduce both the acting out and the subjective experiences which are bound to overwhelm both the therapist and the patient, if their explosive potential is not gradually reduced in this way.

The success that can be achieved if the therapist can be helped to recognize and conceptualize projective identification and so contain it is in fact illustrated by Clare's case. Several years later Mrs L. reported to me that she had been able to interpret the projection into her of her four-month-old baby self, and the impasse had been overcome.³

Notes

1 Mrs L. had a psychotherapeutic rather than a psychoanalytic training and saw Clare first on a once-a-week basis.
2 In fact six months after the seminar Mrs L. approached me for regular fortnightly supervision of the patient. In the course of our work together, as I describe, it became clear that Clare's analysis was in an impasse caused by the problems of containment in its early stages. The supervision concentrated on Clare's dread of her destructiveness and constantly flying away. To prevent this confrontation Clare would cling to her once-a-week session and no more. The supervision aim was to make Mrs L. aware of the enormous pressure which she had not been able to contain and to help her again to take responsibility for conducting the treatment and to face Clare with her responsibility as a patient.
3 After the supervision ended, Clare continued as a patient, although she broke treatment twice from the moment she agreed to a second session. Mrs L. later reported to me how she eventually managed to make Clare recognize that she could not cope with the separation any more and that as a patient she needed constant care during Mrs L.'s absence. Clare came to recognize her massive need to be the therapist as in the past she had 'been her mother', when her mother was depressed. Only then could she experience the violence of her murderous feelings during the separation

and re-enact (through the memories revived by her deliverance of her first dead baby) the awful experience of her first four months of life at the hospital. Clare was still in treatment at November 1985, but the impasse had been overcome.

10

Further difficulties in containing projective identification

A second case, illustrating the difficulty of treating projective identification, concerns Charles, a hypochondriacal patient treated by Dr A., a psychoanalyst, who attended one of my seminars over a two-year period. Dr A. had helped Charles improve during his analysis but at the time his case was presented was having great difficulty. During the two years before 1983, with the help of presenting in my seminar, the analyst felt better about Charles because he began to understand the projective process in the analysis. The patient made remarkably good progress in his life situation. Only occasionally did Charles complain again about his disturbing pressure inside him.

The seminar in which the analyst had participated for two years prior to the time of the two sessions I will report had considered the development of impasses such as this. After presenting some basic information about Charles, in which I shall interpose reports from Dr A. given to the seminar (in italic type), with my own thoughts (in roman type) to describe the development of the case, I will describe some of the discussion in the seminar.

Charles started his analysis with Dr A. when he was twenty-four He stammered so much that he often distorted his face into grimaces. He was disturbed in contact with other people and had difficulties in studying medicine, because he felt he could not speak. He had no sensation in his mouth when he was eating; nothing had any taste, and he had to use a great deal of salt and pepper to establish any sensation at all. He also complained about pressure and pain in his abdomen. He had attacks of crying and screaming and he sometimes felt relieved after he screamed at his father. When the pressure in his

209

abdomen was relieved he felt relaxed, but this was rare, and he complained constantly to the analyst that he was trying to get rid of the pressure but did not succeed. Of his personal history I want to say only that the father was a successful medical practitioner, and Charles felt dominated by him. Also, from the early history it is significant that Charles had from birth a pyloric spasm, vomited explosively, and had to be operated on. For the first few years of his life he slept in the parents' bedroom. He had a very idealized picture of his mother but he constantly felt angry and critical towards his father.

There was over the years a great deal of improvement, but Dr A. had difficulties in dealing with Charles's main symptom, which was his complaint that he felt this great pressure inside his abdomen. Charles constantly fought against and tried to get rid of this feeling in the sessions by making noises or shouting. These very powerful attempts to empty himself out into the analyst led to severe disturbance in Dr A. over the years, and he had difficulty in knowing what to do with it. Dr A. became from time to time extremely angry and resentful and even thought of ending the analysis.

I shall now report some material of Charles as reported by Dr A. in the seminar.

'*At this time there were sessions in which Charles again put me under great pressure. He screamed at me and tried to prevent me from talking. I tried to resist him and managed to continue talking to him, which the patient accepted, and he seemed to be better. This led to an improvement in his relationship with one of his girlfriends. He described that she visited him, that they could talk much more intimately, and he was then able to confide to her some of his affection. During his girlfriend's visit a dead man had been found in the bushes of the district where he is working as a general practitioner, and he was asked to examine the body. He did so but was not satisfied with his examination and felt guilty because he had not noticed some of the pressure marks on the dead man's body which could indicate that the man had been murdered. In this connection he talked about a dream where there was a man who was found hanged. He could not give any associations, but I interpreted that it seemed to Charles that he was afraid that his passionate wish to take possession not only of his girlfriend but also of me could go so far that he could strangle me. Charles felt well understood by the interpretation and expressed his anxiety that his girlfriend might not wish to come to him any more because he had such strong feelings of possessiveness and wanting to capture her. He was nevertheless pleased that he had been able to describe his feelings to a woman for the first time. He then talked about a film by Chabrol. In it a man strangled his mistress in a passionate*

210

situation, and the police inspector did not really believe that there had been a murder. He tried to protect him to the extent that the man in the film was unable to convince the inspector of his guilt. He therefore felt that he had to carry his guilt on his back for the rest of his life. The associations seemed to confirm my interpretation of the patient's fear of his murderous possessiveness. Charles then spoke also of his difficulty in expressing his feelings towards me and his fear that his feelings could become too violent.

'I shall now bring some material from a session where some very intense transference involvement took place. The background of this problem is that Charles comes to the analysis from far away. He has to travel several hours but he never takes sufficient money with him on the journey even to buy a cup of tea. On the day in question I felt we had a very good session. The weather at that time was intensely hot, and I became concerned during the session that the patient was not able to buy any ice-cream or tea before beginning his return journey. Charles made no conscious complaint about this problem, but, as I was very concerned, I offered him 20 francs which would enable him to buy an ice-cream. The patient refused to accept the money from me.

'I thought that Charles's behaviour in never taking any money on the long car or train journey to the sessions was very obsessional. I had often interpreted to him that through this behaviour he wanted to exert pressure on me. I said that he wanted me concretely to give him some token of love in the form of some food or drink. Nevertheless, at the end of the session I still felt very strongly that I wanted to make this offer of money to the patient.

'In the next session Charles brought a picture of a fish which had been caught by an angler and was laid out on the floor. I interpreted that he had felt that I had tried to hook him during the last session. I had by then realized that my behaviour had been rather seductive. In his next associations Charles referred to a newspaper article about a child-murder, and I suggested that the murderer probably seduced his victim by offering him ice-cream. Charles then described that this child-murderer outwardly lived an apparently normal life. He was married and had children, and nobody could possibly believe that he had done something of that kind. I felt very strongly that in these associations he described me.'

- It was interesting that Dr A. reported the session with a great deal of amusement and that the analysts in the group responded to this rather manic attitude of the analyst by laughing.

Charles had become very restless during the session, and the disturbing pressure inside his abdomen, combined with the irritation in his anus, began again. He said, 'My real feelings are somewhere else, and what is coming up now has nothing to do with what I really feel. Dr A. explained that these *remarks are similar to what Charles had often said before when he accused the analyst of talking rubbish. Charles added that the murderer seemed to have had more experience of life than he. That made him feel very small. He complained that Dr A. would not take him seriously. Dr A. interpreted to Charles that offering him ice-cream had been like a seduction and had awakened murderous and frightening impulses. For that reason receiving the money for the ice-cream was so dangerous. Charles said, 'I want to smile, thinking about what has been doing on.' Dr A. replied, 'Whenever something seriously is being discussed between you and me, as in this situation, where there is a problem leading to some acting out on my part you adopt some kind of superior contemptuous attitude towards me.'*

● It is obvious here that Dr A. threw back Charles's unspoken complaint that he has not been taken seriously by the analyst by accusing the patient of never taking seriously what the analyst is telling him.

Dr A. then reported a session, just before the holiday, in which Charles said that he well understood why Dr A. wanted to take such a long holiday: because he was a difficult patient, and Dr A. must be exhausted by him.

Discussion in the seminar

At this moment I interrupted the seminar and asked those present whether they could make some comments on what had been going on so far. As nobody wanted to speak, I drew their attention to the fact that the analyst was quite cheerful about having offered the patient 20 francs to buy some ice-cream. When he said the patient had refused he was more serious. Everybody had laughed when the session was described. I felt that actually what was being described was a serious situation, and this could be clearly demonstrated in the material. I felt, through his apparent kindness in offering the money for the ice-cream Dr A. was at the same time risking the analysis. Charles must have realized this and so became greatly preoccupied with child-murder. In other words, Charles noticed that Dr A.'s 'kindness' in offering money for some ice-cream covered up very angry feelings which were experienced as murderous, out-of-control impulses – indicating that the analyst had failed to contain the patient's projections, communicated to him by the patient's description of pressure inside his abdomen. Charles is also afraid that he has damaged Dr A., particularly his capacity to understand and contain him, through his projection. He spells this out by saying that he must have exhausted Dr A. to such an extent that he was unable to work and could not analyse him any more. This was why he made the mistake of offering him money.

I also emphasized that Dr A.'s mistake meant that at that time he was not taking the analytic situation seriously. In fact, in that session it had been Dr A. who interpreted that Charles did not take analysis seriously – the opposite of what seemed to be true. It appeared that Dr A. had projected his problem into Charles and so created a great deal of confusion.

In the discussion, Dr A. became very defensive and minimized the importance of some aspects of what had occurred. He suddenly pointed out that he offered the money to the patient only at the end of the session; he said to Charles that if he really needed the money for the ice-cream he would give it to him. He didn't offer it to him too strongly. He also added that he had actually interpreted the danger which had threatened Charles by the offer of the money by referring to the incident in the following session. He was of course right that he did realize that the material about the child-murder and the other criminal material referred to in the session was interpreted by him in the transference. At the same time, Dr A. did not interpret clearly enough to Charles what had been going on between the two of them. In the seminar it emerged that Dr A. felt that, after all, the patient had always demanded too much from him and was tiring him out. There was some reality in this because the patient had been his most difficult patient for many years and he had in fact felt exhausted by the analysis. This showed how far the patient's concern that he had exhausted the analyst was a realistic perception, a fact which should probably have been made clear to him. There is a difference between a patient who has phantasies and fears that he has exhausted the analyst and one who has correctly perceived that he has tired out and exhausted him.

At this point another member of the seminar suggested that Dr A. had tried for a long time to understand and analyse the precarious situation in which Charles had put himself by coming without money. She suggested that Charles's repetitive behaviour eventually caused anger in the analyst because he had not succeeded in getting any further with it. As this went on and on, one could think that when the analyst suddenly offered some money to the patient he was trying to break through this deadlock by a kind of blackmail. Dr A. agreed with this suggestion and said he felt Charles put a great deal of pressure on him by not bringing any money and that he constantly produced this peculiar situation. It made Dr A. feel that it was always up to him to give Charles something: either money or an interpretation that would change the situation. As he had not been able to achieve great change so far, it created a very precarious feeling for Dr A., so that at that moment he could no longer cope with it. There were several other suggestions from the members of the seminar, and interestingly enough again a great deal of laughter occurred when the analyst's reaction was discussed. It was probably due to everyone becoming aware how angry and destructive Dr A. had been feeling and how he tried to deceive himself about it. During the seminar Dr A. suddenly became aware of his hostility and he said, 'It is easy for you to sit there and to talk about me and to laugh because you are not having to battle as I do with all these problems and having to feel awful about it.' After this brief outburst everything ended more constructively.

- It is not at all easy for an analyst to bear his mistakes and at first this creates a lot of anxiety and guilt in him. Even in a friendly discussion, as in the seminar, it can take some time to realize what has been happening and to feel more willing to accept it. I myself thought that Charles's behaviour was not so much an expression of his intense wishes, which he had wanted to have satisfied by Dr A., but an attempt to project into him the maximum of anxiety and frustration and so to make him experience how he, Charles, felt. At the same time, however, Charles had tried to make Dr A. feel incompetent about being able to satisfy his needs. His enforced abstinence on the journey to the analysis eventually created an enormous transference/counter-transference entanglement – a situation which in the end became unbearable for Dr A., who felt completely defeated.

In such a situation, I suggest, it seems necessary for an analyst to accept the frustrating behaviour of the patient. At first a patient will use all his strength and determination to maintain his behaviour and prevent the analyst from feeling able to change it or him. However, if the analyst can accept his behaviour, the strength of the patient's acting-out behaviour should gradually weaken. I have the impression that the situation with the money arose because Charles was experiencing considerable pressure before the holidays. He wanted to be close to his analyst and wanted a great deal from him. This need was probably recognized by Dr A., who recognized the heat of his desire and the tension of the session. Consciously Dr A. wanted to help and give Charles something concrete – the ice-cream – but in the circumstances this concrete offer of love could not be experienced by the patient as something good and satisfactory. It was experienced by Charles

214

only as an inability to bear the intensity of his needs. Charles, therefore, felt that Dr A. threw the feelings back at him in an aggressive way. This reaction completely overshadowed the apparent pleasantness of the offer. Charles was apparently not confused by the analyst's offer; he felt clear that he couldn't accept it and in this session was openly the little boy who felt seduced by a man who hated him and wanted to kill him. This was obviously an extremely powerful experience for Charles, and he must have felt that his own desires and wishes were unbearable to Dr A. Charles felt that the pressure inside him, which he had believed secret, had got out and caused damage.

When a containing relationship breaks down it is important to recognize that the patient feels that the container for his feelings has been destroyed, and therefore has himself to build up a very strong container. He needs a kind of wall or castle in order to keep the pressure from getting out of control. Such apparent self–containment is, of course, false. It cannot possibly work because it is associated with so much force and danger and constantly brings with it the fear that some kind of breakdown in his self–containing situation will arise. In Charles's case the patient was in danger of falling back to his previous state where he started shouting and trying to get rid of the pressure into Dr A., as he had done so disturbingly at the beginning of the analysis. One would predict that the relationship between analyst and patient would deteriorate for some time. I thought that the patient would now need to test very severely the analyst's capacity to contain him.

It is essential that when any analyst has made a big mistake in acting out, as Dr A. had, that he repair it. To do this he has to be able to face the deeper reasons for what has been going on between himself and the patient without too much resentment. Otherwise he cannot illustrate freely to the patient what has been going on between them. If this is possible the violent reactions related to the area of disturbed interaction between patient and analyst will diminish. In this way the patient has the ability to feel that the analyst's containing function is repaired. Unless this happens the feeling that the analyst as a container has been destroyed will remain, and nothing can be done to replace it. In this way, of course, a feeling of hopelessness and helplessness in both the analyst and the patient would be perpetuated. Even when the situation improves the patient often submits the analyst to several tests. These need to be understood and interpreted in a way to show the patient how this behaviour fits into the whole situation.

Further material

'*After the holidays Charles conveyed the feeling of timelessness in the analysis as if there had not been any holiday, implying that I should be always available to him, to bear his pressure, to be the container of his pressure. There seemed to be some kind of agreement between us that the pressure which had increased during the holidays, had at first gradually to be got rid of in my presence without being referred to. As a consequence it was very difficult to have communications on a verbal level during the first few days after the holidays. After some time, however, it seemed to be possible for Charles to acknowledge that he realized he wanted to torture me and also to make me feel what it was like to be left alone for such a long time during the holidays, and how bad he had been feeling about this. This acknowledgement seemed to be some improvement in comparison with earlier times when he had been unable to acknowledge what was going on in him. Charles then talked for the first time about the fact that he was a very slow eater in childhood and that he controlled the family with this and there was always tension in the room during the meals because of it. There had never been any mention of this problem before. His parents, particularly his father, seemed to be aware of this problem without ever mentioning it. Funnily, as I have said previously, when he once delayed his father using the lavatory by taking possession of it for a long time the father said something to the mother that the controlling attitude of his son seemed to be very destructive for the life of the family and he was angry about it, but Charles heard this only indirectly through the mother. This is the only time that the father expressed his fury about the patient's controlling attitude openly.*'

- The analyst seemed here to have the feeling that the damage which had been done before the holidays had healed and that the analysis was steering into quieter waters. However, as I have explained, there had not been sufficient work on the disturbance between the analyst and patient to be able to expect this.

At this point in the analysis, on a Monday session, Charles came feeling excited and enthusiastic because he had spent the previous night reading a book by Alice Miller. He had not been able to stop reading it until five o'clock in the morning. The book was called You Should Not Notice. *Generally Charles had great difficulty in reading any books and in taking anything in, but this book had absolutely thrilled him. Dr A. said he was touched by Charles's enthusiasm, which was unusual. Moreover, the pressure he generally felt was not noticeable during the session. In the next session Charles made some rather subtle critical remarks against orthodox analysts – criticisms which are very prominent in Alice Miller's approach.*

Then, in the following session, Charles made what the analyst felt was an intensely hurtful attack against him. Charles felt completely identified with Alice Miller's point of view. He said that during the eight years of his analysis there had been a lot of talking but that this was generally beside the point. He then stressed that he had always told Dr A. that what was really important in his analysis was the pressure in his abdomen and nothing else. Dr A. reported that he felt these critical attacks to be more and more unbearable. He thought he had tried so hard during the last eight years to understand the patient and to give him his best attention. He had struggled to stay in contact with Charles's feelings and anxieties, and now the patient regarded this achievement as absolutely nothing. *Dr A. found it too much to bear.*

In this atmosphere Dr A. first said something critical about Alice Miller. He felt irritated by Charles's extreme idealization of her. He said something along the lines that Alice Miller had given up working as an analyst to write books from which she made a lot of money. Dr A. reported to the seminar that he found his outburst against Alice Miller very revealing. He added that what he really wanted to tell the patient, who ridiculed him and put him down, was that by giving up analytic work what Alice Miller had really done was to give up dealing with the pressure that patients like Charles put on their analysts.

- In these comments Dr A. reveals how deeply hurt and resentful he feels towards his patient. He cannot contain Charles's behaviour.

Dr A. then explained that he felt Charles had used the analytic situation, where the analyst has always to control himself, to torture him. Charles probably thought that Dr A. had to grin and bear everything and could not say anything about how he felt tortured. So in this situation Dr A., the analyst, said to himself, 'As the patient does not respond to my careful interpretations and understanding, and in addition continues to belittle and ridicule me, I am going to give him what he really deserves, a beating up.' That was what Dr A. felt he had done through his remarks about Alice Miller.

Charles had responded to Dr A.'s comments about Alice Miller by asking how, as an analyst, he could lose so much control of himself. He was particularly annoyed about the remark relating to the money. He also added that he had never thought that Dr A. could be hurt by anything he said. He was astonished by his attitude. Dr A. then admitted to Charles that he was very hurt about some of his remarks. He also said that the patient had now to accept what the reality was, that he was also a human being, who could understand things and could be helped. This was the end of the session.

In the seminar Dr A. added a few points. He remarked that Charles had

217

said that very often he did not take seriously what he and the analyst were doing during the sessions. *Dr A.* had replied to this by saying, 'Now you tell me that you can't take seriously what you have been doing in analysis, although you have been coming for eight years. Surely this means we have to consider very seriously whether it is worthwhile to continue working together, because under these circumstances the analysis could not make any sense.'

Dr A. told the seminar that he decided it was necessary to stand by the way he had been expressing his feelings. They had accumulated too much. He could not cope and he had to express them. The members of the seminar were aware that he felt impelled to over-emphasize the importance of his behaviour and defend it. They remarked on this and were critical about his attitude, although mainly laughing about it. *Dr A.* stressed that he felt relieved that he had really been able to let go. He had let go his restraint and told Charles what an ass he was, how horribly he had been behaving. He even felt it was right to threaten that if he went on like that he really would have to stop the analysis. (Naturally this prompted a great deal of discussion in the seminar, but I will not repeat it here.)

In the next session Charles said that perhaps he should now attack the analyst and not come any more, but that would be going too far. He had now to acknowledge that he could hurt people and torture them and he could not simply say to himself that nobody would be hurt by his behaviour. *Dr A.* then reminded Charles that after an effective interpretation Charles often devalued him by saying that he was just showing off how good he was. He did not really care about his patient. *Dr A.* interpreted that it was now clear that Charles was envious of him and of his capacity to understand. It was for this reason that he devalued him and tried to ignore what he had been saying. Charles had been defending himself against having to admit his envy. (By idealizing *Dr A.* and telling himself that the analyst could not be hurt by any attacks.) However, through this idealization his envy had increased and with it the unpleasant feeling of pressure inside him. These he had tried to get rid of by his projections. Charles, who had evidently listened carefully to this interpretation, admitted that this was true. He said he felt greatly relieved that he had been able to take in and appreciate what the analyst had been explaining to him. This was the end of the session, and the seminar had to end at this point as well.

● It is very interesting that at this point (after his explosion) the analyst seemed suddenly able to recapture his capacity to understand and to function. He was now able to explain very carefully how Charles's envy related to the pressure in his abdomen. As soon as he was capable of interpreting the patient's attitude to him in analysis in detail, bringing in the defensive idealization which had prevented the patient from recognizing what he had been doing, a stronger picture of the analyst could be re-established in the analysis and in the patient's mind. The analysis now had a better prognosis.

Dr A.'s experience shows how projective identification can be both a great help as well as a great hindrance in analysis and always carries the risk that the analyst is overwhelmed by the projections. Containing the patient's projections is sometimes very difficult, particularly if the analyst or the patient is deeply disturbed about the process, as in this case. To deal with the situation it is essential for the analyst to clarify for himself what he feels about the patient. Then he can work the problems through by himself. It was Dr A.'s need to hide his overwhelming hurt and resentment against the patient which had led to the apparently positive acting out of offering Charles money for the ice-cream. Charles reacted to this incident by bringing material about being murdered, and this gradually led to the analyst having to admit to himself how violent his reaction to the patient had been. It was, however, only by the patient's idealization of Alice Miller that the analyst become aware to what extent he was overwhelmed by anger and resentment against the patient. He then suddenly realized to what extent Charles had idealized him, particularly when the patient complained of the pressure inside himself. Interestingly enough this did not lead then to a break-up of the analysis but to Dr A. recovering his therapeutic function and to increased co-operation between patient and analyst. It is important to realize that, when intense prolonged projective identifications dominate an analysis, some kind of acting out on the part of the analyst frequently occurs, as in Charles's analysis, and needs to be understood and utilized.

11

Projective identification and the psychotic transference in schizophrenia

As I mentioned in Chapter 1, the development of a psychotic transference in the treatment of schizophrenic (or similar) patients, and its interpretation to them, is the main road along which their successful psychoanalysis can progress. Central to the understanding of this psychotic transference is a full appreciation of the various ways in which projective processes can be involved.

In this chapter I shall attempt to examine the transference of the schizophrenic in detail and shall present some material gathered from colleagues with whom I have regularly discussed their schizophrenic patients. The theoretical formulations presented here are not meant to be a final statement, but before presenting two cases I want to discuss some background theory.

The technique used in the psychoanalytic investigation of the schizophrenic has not changed appreciably during the last twenty years, in so far as the patient has sessions five or six times a week in the analyst's consulting room or is seen regularly at a hospital or nursing home. The patient in the acute state generally does not use the couch. Not only his verbal communications but also his gestures and actions are used to help us to understand and interpret the relationship. Although the capacity of acutely ill schizophrenic patients to communicate in analysis varies considerably it is often astounding how clearly the analytic material develops. The language of the schizophrenic differs a great deal from ordinary language, particularly when the patient is deluded. Often it sounds more like a dream; in other words, it seems to be based on what might be called 'the primary process'. One has reason to believe that the patient himself does not understand his communications to the analyst, in the same way as people generally do not understand the language of their own dreams. Thus the patient needs the analyst's capacity for thinking and translating into ordinary words in order to make sense of his own communication. In more theoretical terms the analyst contains the patient's projective identification.

When the interpretation of what the patient is communicating is a correct translation even an acute schizophrenic patient is often capable of confirming it. I take the view, therefore, that even in the very disturbed schizophrenic patient there are remnants of the sane personality with some capacity for normal thinking which can be strengthened through interpretations. Interpretations help the transference to develop, and as it branches out I find it useful to consider that the schizophrenic personality is divided into many different parts relating to different objects and having diverse functions and meanings. One usually differentiates between the psychotic and the non-psychotic (or sane or adult) part of the patient, but in the acute psychotic state the latter is generally lost. The patient expects the analyst, if he is to be any help, to function as that part. To help him to do this it is necessary for the analyst to examine the transference of the psychotic parts of the patient in more detail. One then finds that some parts of a patient's personality are much more psychotically delusional than others.

I shall concentrate first on the most typical psychotic transference of the schizophrenic, based on 'projective identification', examining its origin in relation to normal processes. Secondly, I shall describe what may be called the delusional psychotic transference in schizophrenia, which will lead to an examination of the structure of the delusional schizophrenic process. I shall also attempt to differentiate certain less psychotic parts of the transference which appear in acute schizophrenic patients. This I shall call the infantile transference, because it refers mainly to relations of the baby self to a part-object, the breast.

The typical psychotic transference noted in schizophrenics treated by myself and some of the colleagues I have been supervising can be theoretically understood as a relationship in which projective identification predominates very powerfully. This transference is usually noticeable from the first session. It is often apparent that an intensely controlling relationship is in existence – whether this takes an active or passive form. Through projective identification the patient feels that he controls the analyst's mind and body, which in turn leads to fears that he has changed or driven mad the analyst and to paranoid anxieties related to his projected impulses. In particular he fears that the projected parts of himself, confused with the analyst, will re-enter him, leaving him deprived of his mind and self. It is this situation, which the patient believes very concretely, that gives rise to the psychotic transference becoming a delusional one. The patient feels delusionally that he is really trapped inside the analyst and/or the analyst is really trapped inside him, causing confusion and panic. The task of the analyst in this situation is, first, to help the patient to understand what is happening and, second, to get in touch with the infantile situation, revealed in the transference, which is the source of the trouble.

With these ideas in mind I shall now present two cases. The first patient, Iris, was treated by a psychoanalyst, Dr K., whom I supervised in 1962 and 1963. As before, Dr K.'s reports are in italic type, with my thoughts and comments in roman type. Iris developed a psychotic transference dominated by projective identification in the second session, which Dr K. dealt with very successfully.

Iris

At the commencement of the analysis Iris, a young unmarried woman of twenty-five, was in the throws of her third schizophrenic attack, which had been diagnosed as a combination of paranoid and hebephrenic schizophrenia. The hospital authorities were anxious that she was getting worse and might die in the third attack as she was beginning to refuse food and had become very restless. From the point of view of her infantile history it is interesting that Iris was hospitalized for pyelitis at the age of two-and-a-half, and this coincided with the birth of her sister; at that time she became almost completely anorexic in hospital, and was taken home and nursed back to health by the parents. Iris was transferred from a mental hospital to a private nursing home in order to be analysed and was seen by Dr K. regularly six times a week. In the first session she made contact with Dr K. and in the end asked him whether he was coming back, which he confirmed, explaining to her that he was going to see her regularly.

In the second session Iris, sitting in bed, greeted Dr K. with a burst of loud and inappropriate laughter. She then said, 'I can see a smile in your eyes. Do you think I am nuts in wanting to marry a man when I laugh like this at his letters?' In response, Dr K. said that Iris felt she was mad in thinking that he had kept his promise to be there. She believed that he was there only because of her smile, which had made him come and see her. Her smile was now inside him, in his eyes, controlling him.

- The smile seen in the analyst's eyes was clearly delusional omniscient material, and the analyst in response took up only the transference meaning of the remark.

Iris responded by saying, 'I liked Dr A. He had a funny sense of humour, that is why I liked him. He said he would come and never did.'

- This immediately posed the question, why did she like somebody who did not keep his promise and neglected her?

Dr K. had the impression that she was beginning to differentiate between him and Dr A. He interpreted that she was denying her belief that Dr A. had responded to her controlling wishes (which she felt to be cruel) by a cruel deception. Now she was afraid of controlling her analyst with her cruel magic. This Iris confirmed by saying, 'I am cruel to Tony' (the man who had written the letters referred to at the beginning of the session); 'he writes to me. My father wants to compel me to marry him. If I want to be married I don't need to be forced.' She made some spiteful remarks about Tony and laughed uproariously.

Iris continued, 'When I was ill, my father did something awful to me. I can't remember what it was; I think he said something about wanting to possess me. That is why I wanted to leave home. I got on well with my mother, who used to confide in me. I got on well with her.' Then she shouted, 'I am against psychoanalysis. My father's analyst' – this was a delusional phantasy – is eighty-three. He was familiar and rude on the phone; he shouted wild things into me.'

- At this moment it becomes clear that negative trends were emerging. The frightening, overwhelming father was pictured linked with an aged analyst who shouted intimate and wild things at her from which she had to escape. One can see here that a delusional transference was rapidly formed, with Iris fearing that just as she felt that she had forced her feelings into Dr K., he would force his feelings into her and overwhelm her.

Dr K. interpreted along these lines but did not take up Iris's fear of being sexually assaulted by him, who at this moment seemed to have become mixed up or linked with the father.

- Dr K. was taking the line that it is bad technique to interpret the rapidly emerging sexual transference to a schizophrenic. As I argued in Chapter 1, transference interpretations based on the classical Oedipal complex are not indicated with psychotic

223

patients. This was confirmed by the results. Dr K.'s interpretation of the projective identification successfully diminished the confusion and the concrete sexual transference. Suddenly the analytic situation became more manageable.

'After the interpretation Iris was quieter, but again idealized the mental hospital as a bad place to which she wanted to return. I could now relate this to the material of the session, her fear of controlling the good analyst by her feelings and her terror of being controlled in return. Later on it became clear that projective identification led also to fears of confusion with me. She once explained this by saying that she had to watch me very carefully in order not to do what I might be doing. She huddled away from me when she felt this was happening. On one such occasion she thought she saw a half-smile on my face and felt it appearing on her own. This frightened her, and immediately she would counter the situation by idealized phantasies of the mental hospital.'

Iris recovered from the acute schizophrenic state after three or four months' analytic work. However, the saner she became, the more she was afraid that madness and confusion would be pushed back into her by Dr K. This implied that she felt that Dr K. now contained some of her madness; this was particularly so at situations of parting such as before the holidays. There was some acute fear of this before the first holiday after four months' analysis. However, interpretations on this line brought relief and helped her to cope quite well with this holiday.

Iris's case illustrates the way the typical transference of the schizophrenic emerges very rapidly and can sometimes lead to a delusional transference. By the second session she seemed to believe that she had omnipotently gone inside Dr K.'s mind through her cruel smile. However, with this belief she distorted what had taken place with Dr K. (his visit to see her in hospital), turning it into a sexual advance. She believed that Dr K. (confused with her father) would attack her with wild things, from which she needed to escape. However, by concentrating on the delusion and the projective identification rather than the Oedipal material, Dr K. was able to contain this very fraught beginning to the analysis.

Sarah

I shall now illustrate a severe delusional state in which the patient, Sarah, experienced her infantile self as imprisoned in a world or object. This world was filled with sadistic cruel objects representing parts of herself which pulled her away from a dependent good relationship to the analyst/mother, particularly at weekends.

Sarah, also treated by an experienced analytic colleague, Dr O., whom I supervised, was a Jewish hebephrenic girl. She was sixteen at the beginning of the treatment, and had been manifestly schizophrenic for five months, prior to which she had been in acute psychotic depression for two-and-a-half-years, having been hospitalized and given ECT on two occasions. Sarah had been described as intelligent and amusing before her breakdown. No trauma had been reported, but it seems that (because the mother helped the father in the family business) there may have been some maternal neglect in early infancy. Some of the psychiatrists who saw Sarah during her acute schizophrenic state believed her to be hopelessly incurable. She did not respond to physical treatment and could not be spoken to using ordinary language. However, once in analysis things were different. She responded immediately to interpretations, and a very vivid transference appeared. At first her analyst, Dr O., represented a father or brother, but a predominantly mother/breast transference followed.

After steadily increasing co-operation in the first weeks of the analysis Sarah began to reveal a delusional system. She believed that she had been sold by her parents to a rich and powerful man. He was using her as the experimental animal in an elaborate research project into the cure of insanity. For this purpose she was confined to a cinema set where nothing was real. Most of the people on the set were contraptions, and the whole process was being simultaneously filmed and televised. The film set was defective because it was dull in colour, and the 'oxygen' she had to live on was not like fresh air. Dr O. was also described as a contraption, or actor, and Sarah's parents were discussed as imitations of the real parents. The only person Sarah saw as real in the outside world was a woman teacher she had loved.

When she had confided her delusional beliefs Sarah became more friendly but started to complain about Dr O. He was not real. Also colours were not vivid. Her grievances involved feeling imprisoned, which was expressed by remarks like, 'Why don't they cut the film?' and later a demand for leucotomy. But this oscillated with a suspicion that something good was being withheld from her, which was expressed by hinting that there was a drug that could cure her in a second.

This hint of the withheld breast increased before one particular weekend. She emphasized this by wearing a Jewish yellow star on her blouse. On the following Monday she revealed a dream of

Saturday night. In the dream she was in a car with others, and cars full of Nazi soldiers were in front and behind. It was all right until they had to stop, and then the Nazis got closer. She had previously revealed that she heard the voice of a Nazi boy. He told her cruel stories about concentration–camp atrocities which made her giggle, a delusion which could be linked to cruel masturbation phantasies. There seemed to be indications in the dream that Sarah felt that stopping the analysis during the weekends imprisoned her in her delusional system. Her compulsive sadistic masturbation got worse, as represented by the Nazis getting closer. This and a great deal of other confirmatory material suggested that Sarah's delusional world could be understood as a way of representing the imprisonment of her baby self in an object which seemed to be filled with cruel objects. There were the Nazis, representing sadistic parts of herself, who were in opposition to her need to depend on her analyst as the breast/mother.

Sarah's need for contact with the real world increased before the first analytic holiday. Her first experience of partial emergence from imprisonment was described by her as looking out from a bus window and seeing girls, probably twins, in bright scarlet coats for the first time in real colours. This experience implied that she still saw herself inside an object, the bus, but she was now able to see the real world in normal colour, as represented by the two breasts, the twin girls.[1] After this realization Sarah oscillated between the delusional transference relationship, in which she experienced her analyst as a persecutor who kept her imprisoned, and an infantile transference, in which she depended on him as a mother/breast. I will illustrate this phenomenon by summarizing the transference situation as it was reported by Dr O. over several sessions.

Sarah would start one session by saying repeatedly, 'You are a fool.' On being questioned about what she meant, she would explain it at first in a delusional way by saying that Dr O. was a very rich person with bad inclinations. He was wasting his time doing filthy work when he should be teaching at the university. At the same time, Sarah was implying that she, with her goodness, was protecting him. His bad ways were making him more and more enemies who would eventually overcome him. From previous material which had been worked through over and over, Dr O. decided it was unnecessary to repeat interpretations of the detailed projections in the delusional transference. Instead, he pointed out what was experienced at the level of the infantile transference. Sarah felt, he suggested, the analyst/ mother/breast was in danger by taking in the filth of Sarah's delusions and anxieties (particularly the despair which her mad self did not want to

226

acknowledge and which was always felt to be faecal). Sarah felt the analyst/mother/breast should have nothing to do with receiving such filthy faeces and should only be feeding her (teaching at the university). After this interpretation, to which Sarah listened intently, she seemed immediately to regain good contact with Dr O. She asked him why he covered his mouth and said she wanted to look at it when he spoke. After this experience, Sarah's relationship to Dr O.'s mouth became the regular expression of a good part-object relationship. It obviously represented the breast in the infantile transference.

- What, I think, was happening in these sessions was that Sarah felt her analyst was in danger. By allowing her to project all her anxieties into him, particularly her madness (the enemies), she thought he would be overpowered (he would get more enemies). She felt that her mad part was ruthless and interested only in continuing in the mad situation. The experiment, which she attributed to Dr O., involved no concern for the continuation of the analytic situation (mainly represented as the feeding/lecturing situation). By projecting madness into her analyst Sarah involved him in her delusional system, causing herself much anxiety. She then tried to deal with it by separating the projective and the introjective process: Why do you get involved with my projected delusions (filthy work) and why don't you instead give things to people who want to take good things in (lecturing)? What Sarah could not apparently bear to acknowledge was the fact that it was her analyst's acceptance of her projections, and his understanding of their meaning, that was such a relief to her. This is what made him such a protective and important person to her. It was her resentment at having to feel so small and dependent, in contrast, which caused her enviously to take over and identify herself with the analyst/mother in the protective role.

Before Christmas Sarah's anxieties increased, and she returned frequently to the hospital, where she was admitted whenever she wanted or the parents felt she needed it. Temporarily it seemed that the delusional process which overwhelmed her sane part had got the upper hand. She lectured Dr O. frequently. It seemed that her schizophrenic self was making enormous propaganda. The perverting influences of masturbation and withdrawal were recommended as the best means of coping with the loneliness of the Christmas holidays. Dr O. felt that through this state Sarah was making particularly cynical and omnipotent attacks on the psychic truth which had been acquired before. For example, she argued that 'what makes insane people happy is good for them'. The way she moved and some verbal hints and illustrations

227

gradually showed that what she was referring to was masturbation. So Dr O. could then interpret that she was arguing that masturbation was good for lonely babies. She insisted that 'people who have been in concentration camps emerged better people for having seen all the suffering'. These communications could gradually be recognized as an argument that the patient's anal masturbation and cruelty, combined with voyeurism, strengthened her capacity for love more than her mothers' milk (her analyst's help). Another argument, which sounded apparently sane, was that 'insane people are happier when visitors are introduced into the ward'. This could gradually be translated as meaning that the insane part of the patient would be far better off if the infantile parts of her, which had recognized the value of the analytic breast, would also become insane again.

Sarah's material illustrates the enormously persuasive power of the delusional schizophrenic part of the self and the way it sets out to seduce and pervert the more normal parts of the patient's personality. This is a very common feature in schizophrenic patients. It also illustrates the fight between the schizophrenic part of the patient and the saner infantile parts of the personality. For the purpose of the present argument, however, Sarah's case (like that of Iris) illustrates how, through projective identification, a delusional transference can be created which masks and is confused in the repetition of the patient's infantile experience. Sarah felt that sadistic parts of herself, 'her madness', could enter Dr O's mind as enemies which could overwhelm him.

There was also a gradual emergence of a positive more infantile transference to Dr O., representing an external object or part-object. She had to struggle to help the good infantile feelings separate from the bad delusional ones to receive something nourishing from the analysis.

The Erotic Transference

A second characteristic of the psychotic transference in the treatment of schizophrenic patients is that they tend to develop a strongly erotic transference from the beginning of the treatment. I mentioned in Chapter 10 how I learned from experience many years ago that, if this transference is interpreted early on in the treatment on an Oedipal level, the patient rapidly becomes more confused, hallucinated, and negativistic. Sometimes it may be almost impossible to continue treatment. As I mentioned in Chapter 1, I have taken the view that the reason for this difficulty is the concrete nature of the schizophrenic patient's thinking and feeling. He or she has the greatest difficulty in differentiating between phantasy and reality. Consequently the analyst's interpretations are felt to be concrete suggestions rather than interpretations of the patient's phantasies. I have described how in some of my early work I got quite a shock when patients responded to interpretations about their attraction to me as therapist as sexual invitations. I have found that in these circumstances, when patients feel a direct sexual advance has been made, they react in several ways. They may shyly decline, respond positively by making sexual advances, or respond in a persecutory manner by experiencing the interpretation as an actual sexual assault. This may explain why many schizophrenic patients have been driven into an acute schizophrenic state, within one or two sessions, by attempts to interpret the sexual Oedipal transference early on in the analysis.

In order to understand the erotic transference clinically and theoretically I believe it is necessary to examine, first, the psychopathology of the disturbance of symbolization which leads to concrete thinking. I have learned to interpret the processes of ego splitting and projective identification from the beginning of the treatment and that when this is done the interpretations are less likely to be misunderstood. Often no uncontrollable erotic transference develops. However, excessive projective identification (with its massive creation of objects fused with the self) interferes with symbolization and verbal thinking and makes interpretation no simple matter. It is projective identification which is responsible for the concreteness of the schizophrenic thought processes and which increases the tendency to develop an uncontrollable erotic transference. My understanding of the relationship of projective identification, ego splitting, and concrete thinking has led me to insist that the interpretation of processes of ego splitting must have priority in the treatment of schizophrenics over any other material presented; concrete thinking leads to constant misunderstanding of communications with the outside world, which is particularly serious if it includes the misunderstanding of the analyst's interpretations of the erotic transference.

The origins of the erotic transference of the schizophrenic are worthy of study. While it appears on the surface that most schizophrenics form an erotic transference which resembles an Oedipal situation, more detailed analytical investigation reveals that the analyst is usually experienced as a part-object, breast or penis. I have already demonstrated how this can happen in the hebephrenic patient, Sarah, discussed earlier in this chapter. Sarah would sometimes look at her analyst's genitals or at other times at his chest. Sarah's infantile relationship to the breast seemed to have been highly eroticized, a situation which would have been likely to interfere with her normal satisfactory breast experience and would be repeated in the transference relationship. When strong erotic sensations accompany the relation to the breast there is often a confusion between nipple and penis, a devaluation of the functional role of the breast, and delusional phantasies of a sexual relationship with the mother. On the other hand, the infant's experience of feeling small and in need of the breast may arouse strongly omnipotent, envious, sadistic feelings. These are accompanied by sexual feelings elaborated in masturbation phantasies. They often lead in the schizophrenic to a delusional take-over of the role of the breast/mother, who in such situations is experienced as seductive, tantalizing, and frustrating.

In fact, Sarah illustrates this contention particularly well. She would take over the role of the exciting mother particularly after weekend breaks in the analysis. She would then treat Dr O. as the baby, but taunt him with such questions as, 'How do you like my girlfriend?' (Referring to a woman she was in love with.) After this she would offer him her breasts to suck, mocking him at the same time with gestures and limiting Dr O.'s interpretations. At other times this was demonstrated by rubbing her breasts, or showing off her cubital fossae, which often stood for a sexually exciting breast, probably confused with the vulva. At the same time she could ignore and mock Dr O. with 'So you're still here?' In these circumstances slight mistakes on the part of the analyst seemed to increase the erotic excitement. Sarah, in the infantile transference, believed in the power of her omnipotent masturbation phantasies connected with entering Dr O.'s mind and body and controlling him entirely. For example, Sarah would explode in a flood of mocking and mimicry at any inadvertent expressive gesture or facial expression which Dr O. made as a deviation from his usual behaviour. She would try to make him laugh by behaving in a particularly funny way, or by attempting to evoke movements in the analyst by handing him things and asking him what they were, or by referring to objects behind him, trying to make him turn round. If Dr O. fell into the trap she would become excited and often showed her excitement by masturbatory movements with her body or her hands. Occasionally, in such situations, Dr O. seemed to occupy the role of the father in the transference as expressed by phallic joking and remarks such as, 'Doctor, you have a big staff.' But often it became clear that through this attempt at sexual seduction the mother/analyst was aggressively seduced out of her normal feeding role, probably as a result of the patient's frustration or envy.

To illustrate the way in which the erotic transference is bound up with projective identification, and the difficulties so caused, I want to bring some more detailed clinical material from Sarah's analysis. Dr O. had reported that, in spite of the delusional system, a transference had developed at an infantile level in which he represented mainly the breast or a person she could more rely on. However, he felt that the schizophrenic process seemed essentially concerned with masturbatory narcissistic excitement. This was aimed at replacing the need for dependence on the breast entirely, or delusionally taking over the exciting mother role, or at other reversals of the mother/breast/infant relationship. I shall now once again interpolate Dr O.'s report about a certain phase in the analysis (in italic type) with my thoughts about it (in roman type).

In the session before the one I want to report, Sarah said, 'They think they can rule the world, but it's the person who really has the thing who has the power.' On inquiry Sarah explained in her delusional language that the leader of the experiment planned to rule the world, but her own popularity was increasing and would give her the eventual power. Dr O. felt that this implied that Sarah was shifting from the situation of feeling persecuted to becoming the person who omnipotently took over the important role. As Dr O. felt that there had previously been evidence that some good feeling had been established towards him as the feeding mother, he interpreted that the baby part of the patient identified with the good breast and took over completely the role of the analytic breast. Meanwhile there was an increasing danger that Dr O. had an emptied outside breast and was felt to be made small, weak, and in her power. As the material occurred shortly before Christmas, Dr O. felt it implied that he would be completely dependent on her and unable to leave her. He added that this would lead to the danger that Sarah would break off treatment, as almost happened some time before. In taking over the breast entirely in the treatment, Sarah believed she could do everything for herself and would not need treatment. She replied that everyone knew that all men are equal. 'It isn't fair', she explained, 'to use me as an experimental animal.' Dr O. felt that he could interpret to Sarah that this comment was a protest by her baby part which was complaining she needed the analysis and did not often feel needed. In other words, he thought that the analysis at this point had made contact with her infantile resentment against the important, needed mother as represented by Dr O.

- What I notice here is that Dr O. concentrates his interpretations on the infantile transference. He does not refer to the delusional transference which the patient consciously addresses to him. I would have thought that at this moment Dr O. would have to remember that Sarah had complained that he was not caring

231

enough for her. He was using her for his own purposes to make himself important and leaving her small and unprotected. Yet he emphasized that Sarah had been successful in fighting against this feeling, which made her feel more lovable and stronger. I feel Sarah's statement that all men are equal and it isn't fair to use her as an experimental animal is a continuation of her complaint that she feels misused; she is not cared for and is made to feel inferior. She asserts her right to be loved and cared for. I would have interpreted along these lines, probably adding that if she feels she is lovable, but realizes that she still needs Dr O., she feels that he is important to her, and this increases her feeling of being small. In this way Dr O. would have made clear that he is aware that Sarah experiences him as superior, not caring, and using her for selfish purposes. I think that Sarah is resentful against him because she experiences his comments as rubbing in his own importance. He is felt to be showing off.

In the next session Dr O. reported that Sarah appeared for the first time with a hair-band but about which she was unable to give any information. He interpreted this hair-band as a representation of the good internal breast. Functioning with it, like the analysis, kept her thoughts in order. Dr O. reported that there had been other material before where the function of the analysis, as helping her mind, had been illustrated. He felt that the presence of the hair-band also showed that interpretations of the session before, about the threat to disrupt the relationship in the analysis, had helped to strengthen the good relationship. After Dr O. put this into words Sarah was at first silent. Then she said, 'Every step of cruelty is a step backwards, just as every step of kindness is a step forward.' Her hand gestured a masturbatory movement. She continued, 'A rich person who has grown up in wealth and wastes his time giving dope, like to horses, does not see as much of life and isn't therefore' – twisting her hair – 'as developed intellectually as the dustman. He at least meets people and does useful work.'

Dr O. remembered that in the past references to cruelty had been understood as some reference to cruel anal masturbation. Twisting her hair is also an expression of masturbation used before. Her response, therefore, seemed to imply that she wanted to illustrate with the hair-band that some forward movement had taken place. The rich person was generally a reference to the leader of the experiment in the delusional system, so Dr O. tried to show her, after acknowledging the ridicule in her speech of the leader of the experiment, that she still seems to make propaganda to the baby part of herself. She claims that her masturbatory finger can do more to develop her mind than Mummy's nipple in her mouth. This is implied with the masturbation; twisting her hair implied doing useful work. Dr O. confronted her with the falseness of this propaganda claim by showing her that at the moment she seemed, by hair hair-twisting fingers, to be again replacing the hair-band analysis, which seemed to be holding her mind together.

- I think Sarah was implying that she needed the hair-band to hold her mind together. However, she is obviously very uncertain about going forward or backwards. She seems to realize that the act of cruelty is going backwards. She wants to go forward. But I don't think she is clear how she can go forward. She probably feels she has to do it by her own masturbatory phantasy, because she is too uncertain about Dr O. at this moment. I think her speech about the rich person who wastes his time giving dope is an attack on the leader of the experiment who is an internal delusional figure but also the analyst. At that moment she feels that Dr O. is the one making propaganda speeches, which she calls giving dope but he would call doing useful work. She thinks that his proposition is driving her backwards to cruel phantasies, which she seems to be struggling against. She feels there is some possibility of going forward when she is able to feel and experience some kindness.

After Dr O.'s last interpretation Sarah adjusted her hair-band, adjusted her skirt, closed the slide-fastener of her pocket, and said, 'You are a fool.' On being questioned about this she explained that Dr O. must know that insane people do not know they are insane. Dr O. replied that he realizes this and agrees with it but suggested to her that the difficulty at the moment referred to the baby part of her. She does not wish to know that she is dependent on the analytical breast. It is his help outside which will preserve her sanity. He also linked this idea to Sarah's phantasies of good parents, which occurred in the last session as establishing good links. But, after some silence, Sarah said, 'But you are a fool for peddling dope, you could be outside doing it with oxygen.' Dr O. had established that this oxygen had for some time been a symbol for semen. He felt the material, therefore, indicated there was suddenly a confusion in Sarah's mind about the relationship of the breast, nipple, and penis. In the session before there had been references to oxygen and to the sexual relationship between the parents, so he tried to differentiate between the confusion in the baby's mind. Her baby self is centred between the nipple, which comes into her mouth and on which she feels dependent but which she confuses with her addiction to masturbation, and her father's penis, which is felt at the weekend to be going into the mother's mouth to feed and restore her. Her demand, 'You could be doing it outside with oxygen', therefore, refers to her baby self claiming that the penis could serve her in a much better way, without the dependence on the analytic

233

nipple. It would be better to be the Daddy/analyst's wife than the Mummy/analyst's baby.

● I think Dr O. had here become aware that Sarah was quite confused. He was trying to sort this out and help her with the confusion. But Sarah seems to have been insistent in pointing out to him that he has been a fool. She repeated this several times. In particular he has been a fool for peddling dope. In other words, Sarah must have been extremely aware that there was something false going on. She herself felt this was a propaganda situation which derived not just from her. She wanted Dr O. to face up to and to recognize this falsity. By her insistence that insane people do not know that they are insane Sarah also asks Dr O. for greater assistance. She wants to be helped out of her confusion so that she can become more able to distinguish between her insane phantasies and her sane ideas. She desperately needs this help. If this is right, the accusation of peddling dope is an accusation against Dr O. He is the one who makes propaganda which has a hypnotizing and confusing effect on her. It lulls her into a dopey state where she doesn't think clearly.

  Dr O.'s differentiation of the dope and oxygen seems to be right. It allows the confusion to be more clearly interpreted. But I think the frequent reference to dope and the accusations connected with it emphasize how important it is to listen to this patient's repeated accusations. She is complaining about something Dr O. seems to be doing. If he could understand this accusation he could be aware of his mistakes and confusion and interpret to Sarah more clearly. In fact, his interpretation of oxygen as something life-giving, but sexual in relationship to the parents, brings an erotic transference into the open.

After a silence Sarah said, 'You are a bore, a big bore.' On questioning she explained that it is 'the boring with this dope' but she kept looking at her own arms. On further questioning Sarah revealed that she had an injection there once. She asked Dr O. the name of the vein. He found himself telling her. 'Oh!' she said, 'I thought it was different', and got quite excited. Dr O., realizing his mistake, then interpreted that the baby part of the patient was now claiming that she was the Mummy receiving the penis, the big-bore needle, from the analyst Daddy. He acknowledged he had been mistaken to answer the question as if he were a nurse, and showed how in so doing he had concretely confirmed her idea. He also explained that behind this baby pretence of being Mummy lies the baby fear of being uninteresting to the analyst Mummy, who will leave her at the coming Christmas holidays

234

without any wish to return. At that moment very interesting material appeared. Sarah tied her shoelace, adjusted her hair-band, and explained, 'It keeps slipping.' Dr O. interpreted that she was saying he had made a slip which could be prevented if he could tie his own mind (representing both the good Mummy and Daddy) more securely together. Then she would be safer.

- I think that Dr O.'s interpretations now become more differentiated and are more helpful to the patient. None the less it is interesting that in adjusting her hair-band she explained, 'It keeps slipping.' This was interpreted by Dr O. that he had made a slip. However, Sarah referred not to one mistake but to a variety of mistakes he had made. The hair-band had kept slipping – as I have tried to clarify with my earlier comments. It would therefore have been helpful if Dr O. had referred to some of the other slips as well. He might particularly have mentioned Sarah's need constantly to repeat that he was giving her dope, referring to his confused interpretations, which she experienced as propaganda on his part preventing her from thinking clearly. In any case, the material just described brought Dr O. more clearly into contact with errors he had made, and the remaining interpretations he made were very pertinent.

Sarah now became very quiet and sleepy like a baby. She seemed much more in contact with the baby part, having received a feed – she was yawning, eyes drooping. She also looked at her watch, stressing the importance of the session ending in time and not wanting to intrude by seducing Dr O. into making a further error. In leaving the consulting room Sarah laughed mockingly at her mother, both in the waiting-room and in the street.

- It is interesting that while the baby/breast relationship in this session could quickly be re-established by the interpretation of the lace-tying, hair-band-slipping material, some of the mocking reversal of the baby/mother relationship was still being acted out outside.

The material I have presented here contains many points which I cannot develop in detail. It mainly illustrates how easily in a frustrating situation, such as before a holiday, omnipotent masturbation phantasies relating to the schizophrenic process become confused with the infantile dependence on the breast/nipple. The confusion between the nipple and the father's penis was increased by the baby being angry about the need for the breast. This had reinforced a tendency to bounce into identification with the erotic mother and so escape dependence. The material illustrates how an analytic mistake can lead to severe acting out. Dr O. confirms, by answering the question about the vein, that the baby's omnipotent assertion of being the mother is a reality. This would imply that the normal baby part and the good relation to the breast would be completely lost. Masturbatory excitement would become violent. Actually Sarah noticed the mistake, as she was quite taken aback by the answer – 'I thought it was different.' Sarah's excitement in this particular situation was not so severe for two reasons. First of all, Dr O. immediately recognized his mistake and analysed in detail the delusional identification with the mother. Secondly, in the analysis to date Dr O. had made few mistakes and had handled the transference well. Some real security in relationship to a mother figure was developing. This also explains Sarah's surprise about his mistake.

After about fifteen months of treatment, Dr O. reported a transference situation developing which is very revealing.

After weekends, on Monday, there is usually giggling and joking relating to the sexual excitement over the weekend. It has always been the pattern that the withdrawal from the analyst – as an important external object – over the weekend leads to genital or anal masturbatory excitement. Instead of being reported by the patient, this is always demonstrated. By Tuesday she is usually calmer, often presses her lip in one spot as if to hold it, which looks like an attempt to press her mouth into closer contact with Dr O., representing the breast. By Wednesday she is usually busily knitting a hair-band, which is going to replace the lost one. The hair-band has from previous sessions, such as the one reported before, the meaning of holding the good internal breast securely in place, which would imply a greater clarity in thinking and returning sanity. However, as soon as better contact is established – and she shows this by wearing the hair-band on Thursday – depression becomes quite visible, and she almost shakes with some inner emotion. The hair-band begins to slip down over her ears and eyes until by Friday, when she is again concerned about the coming weekend, the hair-band drops over her face, making her look ridiculous. At the same time the fingering of the mouth changes; she starts stroking her lips and plays with them. This resembles masturbation so clearly that Dr O. is able to show her that the good contact with the analysis is changing again into a masturbatory one before the weekend. To this she replies, in a strong American accent (Dr O. is American), 'Over and out', acknowledging the message received.

• One had of course to expect that, in spite of the co-operation of the patient, the repetition of the situation would go on for a long time before any further movement could be expected. From the point of view of our discussion it is important that the erotic transference during the week is greatly reduced unless there are outside disturbances.

The erotic transference that I have described is a great disturbance to the development of a positive non-erotic breast relationship in the analysis, on which normal development and analytic progress are based. I have attempted to make clear that the erotic transference is mainly caused by turning away from the good breast relationship because of feelings of frustration, jealousy, and particularly resentment and envy. By quickly and omnipotently putting herself in the place of the mother or breast, the schizophrenic patient, repeating an early baby situation, deludes herself that she is the mother, is grown up, can get married, etc. As this is a delusional omnipotent phantasy of the baby, care has to be taken to show this to the patient again and again to bring her back into a non-delusional contact. This movement generally leads again to resentment about being made to feel small by the mother/analyst, which can easily lead again to reversal if it is not interpreted in detail. It is important not to confuse the delusional sexual phantasies of the schizophrenic with the real Oedipal situation which can develop only when a non-erotic breast relationship has been safely established.

The development of the psychotic transference in schizophrenia is always in danger. Even if the analyst manages to contain it there can still be all kinds of external problems. To illustrate the difficulty that can arise I want now to discuss some consequences of defects in the setting or management of the schizophrenic patient. I shall, again, use Sarah's case as an example.

Dr O. reported several disturbances of the analytic process as a result of defects in the setting or intrusion upon the process. However, they became less explosive as the therapeutic transference to the breast was more strongly established. Parental neglect or stupidity; difficulties of the non–psychotherapeutic-orientated hospital staff in co-operating in the treatment; technical errors by the analyst; new shoes; expressive movements and gestures of his, answering questions which need to be interpreted; encouraging the patient too strongly to lie on the couch; and world events (Profumo affair, death of Gaitskell and Kennedy) – all have all played their part. I want to give you two examples.

First, Sarah's parents at the beginning of the treatment were told to send the analytic fees to Dr O. by mail in order not to disturb the patient. However, her parents again and again asked Sarah to give Dr O. the analytic fees in an envelope, which always led to several disturbed sessions. Each time this happened delusional material was increased in the sessions. The leader of the experiment would be talked about, or Sarah would give a very convincing performance of being a prostitute who was counting the money received from her customers, lifting up her skirts, rubbing her thighs, etc. In those situations the baby part of her asserted that the analyst/Mummy did not treat her out of concern and interest but entirely for money's sake. So that she, in taking over the role of the prostitute/mother, demonstrated that she was interested only in money and had no time for babies, etc.

It is, of course, very difficult to convince parents, particularly rather uneducated ones, such as the parents of this patient, as to the importance of the analytic management of the schizophrenic patient. Very detailed advice should generally be given at the beginning of the treatment.

A second example was where the psychiatrist on the staff of the hospital where Sarah was occasionally treated inadvertently caused an upheaval in the treatment which lasted about a week. Sarah was often well enough to stay at home for several weeks, but when she was disturbed either her parents or she herself had the right to ask for admission into the hospital. On these occasions Dr O. would go to the hospital and see the patient at the same time as he would see her in his consulting room but, because of the time taken in travelling, for a slightly shorter period.

On a Thursday, previous to the incident that I am reporting, Sarah had entered hospital at her own request because of shaking and depression in her head. On the Monday after the weekend Dr O. was met at the door of the ward by the psychiatrist, who hurried him into an interview room, looking very worried. Dr O. was momentarily afraid that something serious had happened. But when he heard that the problem was that Sarah's parents wondered if the fees could be lowered, he cut the transaction short. The whole incident took about three minutes in all. However, Sarah was outside the interview room and saw both analyst and psychiatrist emerge. In the treatment room afterwards she was at first quite silent, looking very paranoid. The details of the situation were explained to her, without in fact blaming the psychiatrist. Her mood softened, some superior demeanour crept in, and in judicial tones she said, 'When you introduce something before someone's eyes that can't be seen, the result is bound to be that everyone becomes involved.' She explained this further in her delusional way. She believed this was a part of the television broadcasting of the experiment which would result in everyone becoming her friend and Dr O.'s enemy. However, Dr O. interpreted the infantile transference, namely that the baby felt itself to have witnessed, due to parental carelessness, the actual coming together of the genitals in intercourse. She, rightly, felt this had excessively excited every part of her mind and was a sight which babies cannot see without harm. Her behaviour in the session was quite provocative; she was sitting with her thighs exposed, looking roguishly at Dr O. 'What are you thinking? . . . You *are* wicked. . . . You are not bad looking, you know.' The entire hour was spent interpreting the effects of the incident and how it had increased the eroticization of the relationship to the breast, the return of the nipple/penis confusion, the projective identification with the prostitute/mother, etc.

The following session was in Dr O.'s consulting room (the patient having in the meantime returned home). It was preceded by Sarah marching her mother up the road, ten yards ahead of her, before the session. Similarly it was succeeded by laughing and tyrannizing behaviour over her at the end, behaviour which was typical when Sarah was sexually over-excited. At the end of the next session she came into the front garden of Dr O.'s house, looked into the window of the consulting room, and laughed excitedly. Through all these sessions, this incident with the psychiatrist, representing a primal scene to her, was worked over in many different ways in the transference. Contact with Dr O. was slowly restored, and she became more serious and started settling down again into looking at Dr O.'s mouth. At that time his mouth represented mainly the part-object relation to the breast, which stood for the good non-sexual contact with the breast. At the end of the week she was still scolding Dr O. a little. He, in spite of everything, seemed to have been blamed for this incident. She said, 'The first thing they will ask you in court is your name, and what can you answer if you aren't real? Anyone can sue you, especially for cruelty, because the evidence is everywhere in broad daylight.' These remarks were, of course, again and again taken up in detail in relation to what she had witnessed, showing both her sexual excitement and her paranoid feelings stirred up by this incident. Only gradually was the status quo re-established in the transference.

Sarah's case illustrates, then, two very important requirements in treating schizophrenic patients: first, the need constantly to be alert for and to interpret the delusional transference; second, the need to examine the material very carefully for criticism of the analyst and its relationship to the delusional transference. Premature interpretation of infantile or Oedipal relationships can have very detrimental effects, especially if the delusional transference is ignored.

Note

1 This representation corresponds to the dreams of our neurotic patients where breasts are frequently represented by twin girls.

12

Projective identification and counter-transference difficulties in the course of an analysis with a schizophrenic patient

In this chapter I want to illustrate the importance of understanding the analyst's counter-transference reaction as a central means of understanding a schizophrenic patient's communications expressed by way of powerful projective identification. Very violent emotions of love and hate, severe confusional feelings, and severely disintegrated states of mind can be transmitted through primitive forms of projective identification which are sometimes not registered in an easily understandable form by the analyst. When the emotions are particularly violent the analyst may feel overwhelmed and be unable to function as a container. At such times the patient communicates non-verbally by a primitive hypnotic force. The analyst may then develop defensive counter-transference reactions, perhaps feeling angry. Only later he may realize that what he is feeling is despair and depression related to a sense of failure. In the analysis I shall now report the analyst felt that the confusing projection was an attack on the analysis, a kind of anti-communication which could entirely destroy the analytic relationship. An analyst's depressive counter-transference is often perceived by a neurotic patient, but still more so by a psychotic one. Psychotic patients tend to exaggerate the extent of their analyst's depression and may delude themselves that the analyst is unfairly treated. Such delusions should be diagnosed early, because to protect the analyst the patient may go so far as to try to kill himself.

Dr N. presented Maria, a hebephrenic patient, at my seminar on a number of occasions. He first saw her in his clinic when she was twenty-one years old. She had become manifestly ill when she was sixteen. Until then she had been successful in school, and no abnormality had been noticed. At sixteen, however, she began to fail in school, and her relationship to her mother changed. She became obstinate and irritable, and this was combined with excessive childishness. She also talked about voices in her head. At first she was diagnosed as hebephrenic, but until it was established that she was hallucinating there remained some doubt. When the diagnosis was confirmed she was given neuroleptic drugs. During this time Maria made a determined attempt to throw herself in front of a train. No psychological treatment was arranged until three years later, when Dr N., an analyst working at the psychiatric clinic, was approached by the patient's mother, who asked him to treat her analytically. Maria had begun to burn herself with cigarette ends and to cut herself with razor blades. At first Dr N. refused to treat Maria analytically. He feared that a schizophrenic patient was unanalysable. But three years later, when her tendency to cut herself badly became even worse, he started analysis with her four times a week and joined my regular seminar.

About Maria's history I want to mention at this stage only that she has two younger siblings: a brother two years younger and a sister four years younger. At the time of Maria's birth her father was very ill. He had epileptiform attacks, and a brain tumour was suspected which subsided after a brain operation. It seems that during her pregnancy and the first year of Maria's life her mother must have been very preoccupied with her husband's illness. This was a fact which Maria herself reported to the therapist. Another traumatic situation for her was the suicide of an uncle, her father's brother, when she was ten or so. It seems that her mother and this uncle may have had a love affair. Her mother is rather dominating; she loves talking and she often floods people with the need to talk too much. Her father is affectionate but rather weak. Maria seems both to be very fond of her father and to despise him because of his weakness. I shall now interpose reports from Dr N. (in italic type) with my comments (in roman type).

When Maria was first presented at the seminar Dr N. stressed that her treatment was for him particularly difficult and tiresome. She talks in a very confused and very quiet way and it is difficult to listen or even to hear at all. In the beginning he occasionally asked her what she had been saying because he could not understand it. But she would then be silent for ten to fifteen minutes. Because of that he had to stop his questioning. Only very much later was it possible to ask Maria occasionally what she had been saying. In spite of this Dr N. felt that she was very intent on making herself understood. She was frequently very angry with herself because she made

242

herself so incomprehensible. Occasionally she handed something written to Dr N. In addition she would express herself towards him in a symbolic way with magic notions and presents. For example, she gave him painted pictures which often looked rather childishly naïve, little chocolate hearts, and beads.

Dr N. gave an example of her verbal communication: 'Everything which I do seems to be quite dangerous, as if I catch fire. Nonsense; that what I do has anyhow always to be wrong, otherwise things wouldn't be like they are now; somebody closes the door. That means that I and this place am not allowed to go on in this way. I should. I feel lost. This comes now a little bit. This is that my parents complained about my talking. Oh! And now I am again angry. This doesn't really exist. But that state does exist. But it cannot really exist in reality. But it exists somehow. But it is nonsense, illness or something like that. Of course it was like that. Yes. Actually for a long time I don't understand anything any more. Because of that there is for me no time, or something like that. And if somebody really observed, then there is only the reality of the being observed.'

- This is a telling and typical example of the communication of a psychotic patient who desperately tries to communicate how awful it is to live in a state of uncertainty as to what is real and what is unreal and what has meaning and what is meaningless. She feels condemned by others, for example the mother and father, to continue living in a world of apparent nonsense.

Dr N. continued his report by saying that only in certain periods of the analysis was it possible to decipher Maria's thinking and talking, which had become invaded by her symbolic utterances. He was able to understand her better when he realized that she generally thought in a very concrete way. While she was thinking she regarded certain noises which existed in external reality as meaningful in some specific personal sense; her state of mind was also influenced by the voices she was hearing.

- In spite of all the difficulties Maria made an obvious improvement through the analysis. It was possible for her to be outside the hospital for long periods. She was even able to complete her interrupted school education, to be able to study, and to take part in seminars on nursing and child care. Dr N. found this astonishing as she was still behaving in a rather psychotic way when she was with him.

In the analysis it was clear that Maria felt she was a very small child and wanted to crawl round on the floor of the consulting room. She regarded herself as being part of Dr N.'s family and addressed him often as 'Daddy'.

243

She actually used his name for her own signature. At that time Maria frequently did not sit on a chair. She placed herself on the floor in the corner of the room behind a very large chair. She also generally avoided looking at Dr N. and sat in a position so that she could not see him, but she also used her long hair to hide her face by letting it fall over her face.

Another difficulty in the analysis was Maria's tendency to hurt her head considerably by hitting it against the radiator or against the hard floor. Dr N. felt compelled to prevent her from damaging herself. He felt that Maria had a very cruel archaic conscience which constantly provoked these severe self-punishments. He also observed that the self-damaging behaviour occurred particularly when he was experienced by Maria as very friendly. This was communicated clearly to him in one session after she had knocked her head very violently against the floor. She was silent for a long time, but when she recovered from the shock of hurting herself, she said, 'Why are you so nice and friendly to me?' She had obviously expected that after she had been speaking in her confused and incomprehensible way Dr N. would become angry and reproachful and would want to hit her, as her mother sometimes did when she was exasperated with her.

In another session Maria was again able to throw some light on her behaviour. For example, she insisted that to sit on the floor in the corner was her right place; when she felt so bad she realized that she was really bad and nasty, and therefore she had to sit in such a low place. But she also admitted that she felt sometimes like a small child who could only just crawl, was not able to talk, and could only play around. In that situation she was pleased when Dr N. could accept her as she was.

Dr N. said that when he began to understand some of Maria's behaviour and interpreted this to her he noticed that she would become very responsive. She could often speak for five or ten minutes quite normally.

- This patient, Maria, has a number of features in her behaviour and reactions to the analyst that remind me of other patients who were also entirely dependent on the analyst's understanding to find access to their normal thinking and speaking.

Dr N. reported some material after three years' analysis. He told the seminar that he had heard from Maria, who had gone away for a fortnight's holiday after Christmas. She had unexpectedly telephoned him to say that she was doing very well. Would he agree that she could stay away an additional week? Dr N. said that he had agreed to this proposal rather too quickly and that Maria had rung off rather quickly as well.

Maria did not come back at the agreed time. Dr N. became concerned and then heard from a psychiatrist in a mental hospital in another town. She was interned there because she had tried to commit suicide, again by cutting her

244

wrists deeply. *The psychiatrist felt that Maria was too ill to leave the hospital, and this was why she had not come back to treatment. Dr N. reported some material from the last ten days* before *Maria had gone away for the holiday.*

Maria was still not looking at him, but they had understood quite a lot about it – for example, how dangerous she felt it was for them to look at each other. In spite of improvements, some of the symptoms which made the analysis so difficult came back again. Dr N. then reported some specific material from the beginning of a session: Maria looked rather dark and lost. Dr N. thought 'Oh! This will again be a very difficult and confused session.' There were a lot of silences and many incomprehensible, confused sentences in which Maria said that she again heard a number of different noises and particularly very loud doors being opened. These noises came from the house next to Dr N.'s. In her mind these noises were always related to her. They had a particular meaning, a delusional meaning that Dr N. gave her a sign that he was present. In an earlier situation it had become clear that she heard the noises after the death of her dog, to whom she was extremely attached. Then her only very good friend had to go to South America, and this also disturbed her very much. Because Dr N. knew that these hallucinations had something to do with reassuring her that he was present, he drew attention to the fact that he was, because something again seemed to worry her as she heard the noises.

● This interpretation was of course rather vague. One has the impression that Maria, as she was planning to go away on holiday, was already very concerned about the analyst's depressed state of mind when she went away. There is also a hint that she fears the analyst will die, because she heard the noises after her dog's death.

Maria reacted to Dr N.'s interpretation by remaining annoyed. She also spoke in the third person, which she did very often to create a greater distance. She mumbled something which sounded like a reproach, but it was not possible for Dr N. to hear what it was she said. He gradually began to realize that Maria was preoccupied with disappointments which she had experienced with him. He then confronted her directly and said, 'I believe that you are talking about me and you reproach me because of some disappointments in the past.' Maria immediately responded by laughing. She reminded Dr N. that quite a long time ago, in fact more than five years ago, she and another patient had invented a plot of thinking and cultivating suicidal thoughts. When Dr N. visited the ward they both related their suicidal phantasies to him in very great detail. (Dr N. explained that in this situation he had very often talked about this plot in a very jocular way. Once he had said, 'If things are as bad as all that, then we all three can commit suicide together.') Maria had realized at that time that it was a joke, but she also sensed correctly that she and the other patient were getting on his nerves. Underneath he was becoming impatient and angry and was feeling hopeless and depressed about them. Maria had picked this up. Dr N. told the seminar that it was amazing that Maria remembered things so far back, long before he started analysis.

When he began analysis with her he did not realize how much difference it would make to her that he had treated her at first differently, simply psychiatrically. He explained that he believed Maria now went so far back in order to clear up some of the misunderstanding which had accumulated previously. It was clear that she was extremely disturbed about his jocular behaviour, and it was therefore now brought up to remind him of her capacity to notice his negative reactions to her. Dr N. thought it was as if Maria was saying, 'Can't you explain to me why you behaved to me at that time in this way?' and wanted him to think about it and explain it to her. Dr N. reported to the seminar that, as Maria had been discussing suicidal thoughts, he said to her, 'I now know you so much better that of course I understand you much more easily now. But at that time, five years ago, I was obviously not always in contact with, or sensitive to, your feelings. I am quite aware now that I worried you a great deal with my jocular remark.' After this, Maria looked him straight in his face. He felt there was a much better feeling in the session because she then spoke quite clearly. She told him about a number of previous disappointments with him, all of the same type. For example, she asked, 'Why did you keep me so long in the closed ward when it was no longer necessary to keep me there? Why didn't you prevent the authorities from putting me into another hospital or ward?' All these grievances were put forward with the implicit question: was the reason he had behaved in this way because he was fed up with her? Couldn't he stand her any more? Was that why he behaved towards her in this unsupportive way?

- I think it would have been important for Dr N. to ask himself why this material was brought up by Maria at this time. He felt there was a very strong and positive element in bringing these old grudges to the surface and giving him a chance to sort them out with her. But in the way he discussed this problem he seemed to be unaware that certain aspects of what occupied her from so long before were still relevant now. They might be particularly important in view of the impending holiday. In other words, was she frightened now that he had become terribly depressed and fed up with her? Was that the most urgent question to discuss with her and to try to clarify?

  In the material mentioned, Maria's planning suicide and worrying Dr N. about it had of course played a very important role. At that time he had warded off his anxiety by making a joke of it. But was he now making the same mistake by not taking the material seriously enough. I think it was too reassuring to say that he now knew her and also understood her much better. I have the impression that Dr N. was also surprised that Maria had remembered and also been shocked about the way he had behaved in the past. It is for this reason that he had to offer her reassurance that things were better now – for himself. Hindsight is always easier, but it is always very important to ask, when such problems appear from a patient's past: what is the here-and-now situation which provokes these questions? I suggest that Maria was afraid that Dr N. was fed up with her and depressed about it. For that reason, reassuring Maria in the present must have increased her fear. Reassurance is generally felt by patients as hidden aggression. In thinking back five years before Dr N. was quite clear that underneath his jocular attitude there had been a feeling of depression, hopelessness, impatience, and anger with his patients which he realized that she had picked up.

Dr N. reported a later session from the same week before the holiday. He stressed that Maria talked again in her very obscure and incomprehensible way. He felt he almost had to draw the information out of her noise and he decided to allow her to go on talking in this way for most of the session. He thought he was giving her some rest and allowing her to talk as she wanted to. However, by the end of the session he was feeling very angry and expressed some of it. He said, 'Why do you always behave again and again in such a puzzling way to me?' She then lifted her head and looked him straight in the face, saying, 'But I have also constantly to puzzle out what is going on.' She continued, 'It is not only that somebody else makes me puzzle about things, but I feel very puzzled when I am on my own. There are several words and thoughts, and sometimes sentences, which seem to be entirely disconnected, and I can't make out what they mean. When I am trying to write something down it isn't possible to concentrate because words or thoughts come in between and confuse me.' Dr N. made some interpretation to try to link this together. She replied, 'My mother also talks some words like that. Yesterday we listened to television and my mother constantly interrupted it. She always had to say what she was thinking so one couldn't listen to the television.' He then interpreted that perhaps her mother also interfered in her mind when she was alone. Maria agreed with this.

Dr N. had no notes about the next session but he remembered that in the last session before the holidays there was quite a lot of talk but perhaps not enough about her going away on holiday and the way she may have felt very

247

afraid that she was a heavy burden for Dr N. Perhaps she was too much for him. He explained that this was also the reason why she so often asked how he was feeling, whether he was feeling all right. She mentioned then that she had dreamt something bad but she didn't want to talk about it. It might have been about him dying. Anyhow, there was distinctly a feeling that he could get ill if she exerted too much pressure on him. Dr N. thought that this interruption by the mother might be related to Maria's fear that her mother also interfered with her relationship with her father. But she explained that she still did not agree with this. She had such a good relationship with her father, who was quiet. It was her relationship to her mother that was both more important but also confusing.

- From the last two sessions before the holiday it seems clear that Maria did reveal a great deal of her anxiety that Dr N. was depressed about her progress. She was afraid that he would die. He concentrated in the last interpretation on Maria's mother and father but left out of his interpretation Maria's acute anxiety revealed in her dream that he could die. In such situations interpretations of the here-and-now transference are essential to prevent the patient's anxiety getting out of control. After all, the analyst had shown signs of depression by getting so angry with Maria. The fact that his depression and anger with Maria were getting out of control must have increased her anxiety about him dying during the holiday.

  Maria's talk about her confusing and interfering mother was, of course, interesting. But it seemed most likely at that moment to have the purpose of trying to interest and appease the angry analyst. The problem is, how can this difficult situation be approached analytically? In these situations I think it is essential for the analyst to understand that he has been taking the patient's muddling and confusing talk as an attack on him, which creates a considerable hostile counter-transference and feelings of wanting to get rid of the patient. However, from the material in the last session before the holidays, it is clear that Maria's confused and puzzling talk is more a communication to him, in order to get help from him, rather than an attack on him. It is essential to make such an interpretation to a patient like Maria, as this would diminish her terrible sense of guilt. She feared that her analyst was feeling just as depressed and destroyed through her puzzling and confused talk as she felt about her internal mother's confused talking to her.

I would like to emphasize that the negative counter-transference of the analyst, which emerged so clearly in the last session in response to Maria's confused talk, had a profound effect on her. It actually contributed to the formation of her delusions. It confirmed Maria's fear that Dr N. could not cope with her problems and would eventually become so depressed that he would kill himself. Her anxiety about him was still increasing. One felt that she was reacting with exaggerated intensity. Only later was there clear evidence that her delusion about Dr N. threatening her with suicide was related to her perception of his counter-transference. In the seminar he was able to express his intense irritation and anger about not being able to understand the deeper reasons for the patient's confusion. During the holiday Maria made a very serious suicidal attempt. The delusional reason for this suicide emerged only slowly in the analysis. But it was triggered off through his *too quick* agreement to her apparent wish to prolong her Christmas holiday. Dr N. realized that he was fed up with Maria at that time and was glad to have to have a few more days' holiday from Maria. Nine months later Dr N. presented Maria to the seminar once more.

'She has now been five years in analysis. She sits in a chair opposite me and no longer avoids looking at me. She has passed an important examination which will enable her to get a job. She lives in a room of her own but she still is in constant touch with her home, particularly with her mother. But she complains that her mother constantly rings her up and does not leave her alone.'

Dr N. reminded the seminar that the problems between mother and daughter still concentrated a great deal on Maria speaking incomprehensibly to the mother, who often exploded in anger. The mother was a teacher of languages, liked talking, spoke in a loud voice in very well formulated language, and demanded from her daughter that she talked as well as she herself did.

A great deal of the analytic work was done to help Maria to keep the image of the analyst separate from that of the mother. Maria expected him to understand her better than the mother did and at the same time she felt that Dr N. would allow her in certain ways to be a baby because he understood her communication, her baby attitude and baby language, which she expressed non-verbally by talking inaudibly. When he confronts Maria with her way of communicating, she speaks clearly and distinctly for a while, but then she still drops back again into her quiet, inaudible communication. The delusion that she is the analyst's daughter has recently been better, and she recognizes this as something sick. But whenever there is some tension and some pressure on her, the delusion comes back. The difference between now and earlier on is that the delusion now generally disappears within ten minutes' work in a session. Before, it was very persistent.

249

• I think one has to recognize that while Maria seems better her confused way of communicating still continues, and so do her hallucinations and delusions. So, after five years of treatment, one could be concerned that the analysis is coming to an impasse. There has been apparent improvement, but continuation of the delusions would really imply a bad prognosis.

Some of the delusional ideas Maria now has refer to a BMW car which is the make of car driven by both Dr N. and her mother. There was recently an incident where she saw a black BMW in front of the Clinic. On this BMW there were two letters, D and H, which worried her. It gradually became apparent that it was connected with death (D—h). Dr N. said he was aware that Maria talks a lot about death, but it is so complicated that he still finds it impossible to discover the meaning of it. He concentrates on her fear that he could die or that something could happen to him. He also realizes that she fears he will die because she believes she is so bad, which reminds her of the time nine months ago when she tried to commit suicide.

Dr N. mentioned that in one session Maria was thinking of a time when she was settled in a room with friends who have a number of records of Wagner. Wagner has something to do with Hitler, and Hitler is, of course, bad. She remembered that recently she had been reading Goethe's Faust. *Then she became against incomprehensible. Dr N. gradually understood that she was reading* Faust *aloud. It was when Mephistopheles appeared that she felt she was Mephistopheles and had suddenly become the Devil. She then went on talking in a rambling way. She said that she realizes that this is a kind of theatre. But perhaps it is not theatre. Perhaps she is, or becomes, her mother, when she speaks in the way her mother speaks and when she complains that she is aggressive like her mother. Then she suddenly doesn't know anything further. Is it she, the patient, who is so furious and complaining or is it the mother who is furious and complaining? This is not a harmless play any more. It is not playing Mephistopheles, she is becoming Mephistopheles. She is the bad aggressive mother. Dr N. understood this situation and interpreted it to the patient. She seemed to understand and spoke more clearly for a short time. But then she became very confused again and was uncertain in her way of talking. She said she fears that she really changes into the mother, or the Devil.*

Dr N. told the seminar a little about his technique. He explained that he says, for example, 'Why do you say immediately that you are the Devil? Why do your feelings immediately change into something as dangerous as being the Devil? Perhaps you can notice that there is quite a lot of hatred and aggression in you.' He reported that when he talked to the patient in this way she stayed thoughtful for a moment and then she said, 'Perhaps it connects with the fact that formerly I thought of everything in an absolute way. Good and bad, black and white. There is something black and there is something white, and the black is something connected with death.' At that moment she saw on the analyst's desk four ballpoint pens. The four ballpoint pens reminded her about the four members of the analyst's family, which she believes she belongs to. She said it was obviously not by chance that the analyst bought four of these ballpoints. Then, very painfully, she said that she still wants to be a member of the analyst's family and wants to belong to it. Dr N. said he does not feel good about interpreting this to her again; she realizes this problem now and it is very painful to her. He feels that he would only rub it in if he reminded her of it again.

- It is important to notice here that the analyst is sensitive in using his counter-transference intuitively, because he shows his awareness of how very easily the patient gets hurt by him. I think that, in discussing the problem of black and white, Maria focuses attention on an extremely significant point. When talking about black and white and then becoming the Devil, she immediately had to re-create her delusion of being a member of the analyst's family. This implies that she still splits her problems very strongly into good and bad, black and white, love and violent hatred. This prevents any normal reparative thinking. It is only when the good and bad feelings are able to come closer together, through a lessening of splitting, that depression, and with this normal thinking and reparative impulses and function, can develop. If this is not successful, manic reparation takes place and manic reparation creates the danger of delusional reparation, which explains the reason for the patient's delusional belief that she is a member of the analyst's family. This problem has to be understood and has to be taken up in the analysis again and again in order to help the patient to create links. By such very detailed interpretations the patient will be gradually assisted in overcoming the serious gap in her thought processes, particularly in a situation when she feels well understood and cared for by the analyst.

Dr N.'s lack of understanding of this problem at that time was in my opinion not a counter-transference problem. He seemed insufficiently aware theoretically that in psychotic patients there is a fixation of the personality on an early level of development. Good and bad objects and thoughts have to be kept strictly apart, split off from one another. If this problem is not worked through in the analysis, the analysis will come to an impasse. In the analysis it is the analyst's capacity of integrating and bringing things together and showing this to the patient – his containing function

– which is essential for helping the patient to overcome the faults in her or his early development.

Patients who discover this problem of splitting in themselves are generally afraid that it is an insoluble process. They therefore easily fall back on manic reparation (delusion formation). This in turn increases their anxiety that the problem is irreparable. One has to show a patient like Maria that she has become concerned about this problem and to help her to realize that it is her concern as well as her analyst's help that can gradually assist her to find a better solution. One of the conscious difficulties is that, when she feels bad about herself, she feels completely bad, instead of being able to recognize that the feeling of guilt can also be helpful in trying to make something better.

The analyst then talked about the patient's fear of being left alone, which was so great that she sometimes wanted the neighbours to knock at her door so that she could realize that somebody was there. This was because when she felt alone she felt so terribly bad.

In the seminar I pointed out to Dr N. that I thought it was not only that Maria felt bad when she was alone. She also felt that she was going to be left alone because she was so bad. It was this that made it so terribly frightening for her to be left alone. One could also say that the patient feels that if she were good then of course nobody would ever leave her alone. It is likely that in this situation of being left alone she easily feels persecuted and then becomes very aggressive. There is also the danger that she can't bear to feel good *and* bad because her good and bad feelings are either split off from one another or have become confused. If she then feels in doubt about what is good or bad she probably will make herself entirely bad. It is easier to be wholly bad than to feel doubt about whether she is good or bad. So when Maria defends herself against confusion there is the danger that she may be feeling all bad again.

When good and bad feelings come close together confusional states frequently arise where good and bad feelings cannot be differentiated. It is this confusional anxiety which is such an important problem. Under these circumstances abnormal splitting may increase as the patient may feel that it is preferable to be the Devil than to be confused. It is therefore absolutely essential to understand confusional anxieties in the treatment of borderline and psychotic patients. They are one of the most frequent reasons why psychotic and borderline patients fail to make progress in the analysis. I want to stress that patients like this are unable, when they are alone, to experience anxiety and guilt in a way that enables them to work through this problem. It is essential for the patient, therefore, to have the help *in* the analyst's presence. The anxieties which the patient expresses have at first to be brought together *in the analyst's mind*, and he has to experience for himself what it feels like to be anxious, concerned, and depressed. It is also essential for the analyst to recognize the importance of first making the effort himself to bear the patient's anxieties and to remain in contact with both his thinking and his feeling. Only then can he gradually start to replay the problem back to the patient in a way the patient can understand and use. In the seminar Dr N. replied that he realized what I was explaining was quite true even if the patient cannot say it in words. His report then went on to reveal paranoid anxieties.

Dr N. gave an example of Maria's behaviour at that day's session. She had as usual quite a lot of messages and her notes in little paper bags. She dropped them with a great deal of noise on the floor. Then she lifted herself up and let herself drop into the chair from quite high up so that there was a big noise. Dr N. interpreted that this was an aggressive big bang. She was implying, 'All right, then I will do it aggressively and as noisily as possible.' Maria then turned round and looked at the analyst. He noted that he was in for a difficult session. He interpreted that she seemed to be annoyed and furious with him, and she replied, 'Why shouldn't I be angry, because I had to come yesterday and today at five o'clock in the afternoon because you changed my session?' Maria continued by developing a delusion that the change was intended by Dr N. to make her meet other patients. She then decided that these patients were his helpers. This, Maria felt, was typical of the way he directed and manipulated her.

- In other words, Maria believes that Dr N. cannot treat her on her own and needs helpers; she is an impossibly difficult patient to treat.

Dr N. then interpreted that she seemed to realize that she felt she was so difficult. Therefore, he needs additional helpers in order to make her better. Dr N. realized that in this situation he had always to cope with a very strong counter-transference feeling, because he always got very annoyed with her. He had to tell himself again and again that he was the analyst. He should keep quiet, and not get too upset.

- It is always very important as well as challenging to look at one's own counter-transference and to understand why one feels provoked by the patient. But I think provocation and the danger of being provoked are increased through having insufficient theoretical understanding as to why the problem repeats itself

253

again and again. (This is what I tried to explain to the analyst in the seminar.) In Dr N.'s description of Maria's behaviour it is clear that she tried by her behaviour to project her anger into the analyst. She was aware of feeling angry but she didn't know how to cope with it. In projecting her anger into him she wants him to feel her anger and to work it through inside himself. It also implies that she wants him to feel guilty because he changed the time of her session, which she doesn't like.

Maria went on to remind Dr N. of the time when she was an in-patient at the Clinic: 'Is it not true that in earlier times you brought chocolate bars and also records and put them on my bed?' Dr N. reported that this referred to a birthday when the patient believed that she found presents from him on her bed and was delusionally convinced that it was so. She still holds on to that view. Now she believes that Dr N. plays some kind of game with her. He said he remembers that at that time it seemed to be more possible for him to help the patient.

● From this material it appears that the patient feels that there is something going on in the analyst which he is not facing up to and will not explain to her.

Maria now became very silent and stayed silent for some time. Then she started to talk about her Uncle George, who was a younger brother of her father. This uncle had committed suicide when the patient was fourteen years old. She is frightened that the suicide had something to do with a tragic relationship between Uncle George and her mother, with which neither could cope. It sometimes seemed that her mother talked to Maria about this Uncle George and explained that George had been in love with her. At that moment Dr N. said he realized that Maria is also afraid that he will commit suicide, that he is becoming identified with this Uncle George, and this is of course related again to the question of death. He said that he felt that Maria fears that he could commit suicide because he is not sufficiently loved by the patient and that he would become desperate and would not be able to stand the situation. While this discussion was going on, Maria noticed that Dr N. apparently moved his head, as if he was nodding. He admitted this was so and that he was very interested in this material because Maria had never been able to talk so clearly about his counter-transference.
Maria then made it clear that she believed that Dr N. was in love with her. He interpreted that in that case he now understood the situation with Uncle George. It was now also understandable why Maria believed that he could not give these presents openly. He just put them on her bed in order to hide his love for her. He also explained that he now understands why she

wants to feel that she can end the treatment. It means that she wants the analyst to survive, to ward off the analyst's suicidal depression which she feels is related to it. She is convinced that death might occur because he cannot cope with his conflicting feelings for her.

Dr N. added that he realizes now that Maria's delusion that he is in love with her was related to her suicidal attempt nine months ago, during the holidays. He reminded the seminar that she rang him up to tell him that she was very well, obviously in order to make him happy. But he now realizes that he agreed too quickly with the patient's suggestion to stay away longer. He confesses that he felt relieved *at that time that she wanted to stay away longer because he had been feeling burdened and resentful about the patient's behaviour, particularly her being so often incomprehensible. He realized that he was not containing the patient's projection when he was in collusion with the patient's suggestion to stay away longer and this created an impossible situation for her. Her conscious reason for wanting to kill herself was to protect the analyst from herself and to save his life.*

- It is evident that Maria's delusion that her analyst is in love with her is a reversal, a projection into the analyst of her intense needs and frustrations. When Dr N. became clear about what was going on he realized, correctly, that he should not interpret the projection at that time and he also realized that there were still a number of confusions related to this which he did not understand.

  At this stage of the analysis it seems that Dr N. is in much better contact with the patient and himself. He is containing her better, which means that the patient will be able to reveal more of her confusion. I think it would be important to understand whether the idea that the analyst is in love with her belongs to the paternal transference or the maternal one. I felt during the seminar that the important factor was that Maria never felt that she could satisfy her mother's need for a perfect child. She always felt that her mother had been very dependent on her and that she, the patient, had not been satisfying enough to the mother, e.g. by talking too quietly, and so had aroused her mother's constant anger and frustration. During the analysis the patient's more persistent repetitive behaviour was very similar to the way she related to her mother, particularly in the quiet, puzzling talking, which was incomprehensible to both the mother and Dr N. His annoyance and irritation with Maria and his need for clear information and understanding of her are still very similar to the relationship to the mother, who even now phones her up a great deal. This implies to Maria that her mother still needs help and information from the patient. So the delusion of the analyst being in love with Maria is probably not related to the Oedipal level but to the very early relationship to the mother. This is being re-enacted with the analyst in a confusing manner.

During the next session Dr N. reported that Maria was rather confusing and in addition very hypochondriacal. Her hypochondriacal anxiety was expressed in the form of reproaches against Dr N., namely that she has probably a very dangerous internal disease which has not been diagnosed.

- Maria's communication is very interesting and important because she states clearly that there is an undiagnosed internal situation. She makes the analyst responsible for it and also makes him aware that he should look for this unknown internal situation which is threatening her.

Dr N. said he realized that when a patient goes to a physician to be examined the patient believes that the physician will think, 'Oh, yes, you the patient are having this psychoanalytic treatment, and the psychoanalyst never examines a patient properly to find out what is going on inside him' — which implies that Dr N. is being devalued. Dr N. referred now to a session which he wanted to report to illustrate some of these obscure points.

Maria has a sister two years younger than herself, and a brother one year younger still. Apparently this brother is coming back to the family now, and Maria seems to be quite pleased about this. She now looks for a little piece of paper where she has made some notes and then she mumbles something which Dr N. cannot fully understand about dreams. She thinks there are probably two dreams which she wants to talk about. In one of the dreams there is water and fire. In the second dream there is a young woman and a boy and both are ill. They had to come into the hospital to be treated. The woman came into the medical ward, and the boy had to come to the psychiatric ward. Very soon the woman noticed that it wasn't very good for the boy to have to go to the psychiatric clinic. In the third dream there are two people and a ship.

Dr N. interpreted that in the dream about the young woman and the young boy it seems that Maria is apparently represented by both of them. In this way she becomes distant from her own hypochondriacal delusion because she says that she has a real internal disease. She agrees with that: 'I prefer to be bodily ill rather than have a psychiatric disease.' He replies 'You express more clearly that you want to say, "I am really physically ill, and that has been overlooked so far." ' However, in spite of these dreams nothing further seemed to come up in the session. Dr N. said it was an example of how quite a lot is lost to him and is not very satisfying: 'When we are in such a session, I try to ask questions of the patient, and then everything gets worse.'

- This is a typical situation in which the analyst is left in a state of confusion which is disturbing to him and he demands clarity for the patient. But he has to bear this confusion even if it is very difficult for him.

One member of the seminar suggested that it is important to clarify the confusion which the patient tries to get away from but is also afraid to exacerbate. He proceeded to explain: we as analysts say that there is something very dangerous internally in the patient which is not diagnosed, not acknowledged. But the patient says she prefers to have the physical medical treatment. This would mean there should be some access to this dangerous internal problem but there should also be some sane part of the personality where there is no madness but understanding. The patient must feel that when she is in the psychiatric ward then she feels that Dr N. is trapped, is crazy or mad as she is. Then they are both mad and confused, and everything goes on in a circle; they can't get any further, and you, as the analyst, just give in and cannot think clearly, which is torturing.

- I agreed with this formulation. It implies that the patient is in despair that she can't get out of her entanglement with the analyst and that she is always put back again into the confused situation. In other words, the hypochondriacal delusion that she is physically seriously ill would be created to counteract the confusional state and collusion with the analyst. The implication of this is not just that Maria wants to get away from being ill and would therefore be playing a defensive role, but that she is desperate and frightened that she is in a relationship to Dr N. where there is a serious collusive situation with him and hence no possibility to get any better. In fact, Maria is insistent that she wants to understand this inner situation, that she wants to approach it; and she also wants to tell Dr N. that he should also try to approach it as the analyst because it is so important.

Dr N. agreed with this attempt at clarification and stressed that Maria still draws attention to the fact that her confusion is very much related to his own confusion. She decides therefore to part from Dr N., who is so much wrapped up in the situation which is incomprehensible and which she constantly feels herself be pulled into again. But the problem now is transformed as she seems to know that there is something which has shifted away from the unknown psychiatric problem and changed into the bodily internal danger. If the problem is divided and split up in this way there is a danger that there is

257

nobody available who understands what it is about. This leads again
to a delusional situation similar to the delusion of being part of Dr
N.'s family.

In general, shifting away from some entangled state is enormously
important to understand, because it implies that confusional anxieties,
particularly if they are projected into the analyst and not clearly
diagnosed by him, lead to a great need for the patient to find a way
out. It is at that moment that delusions form. In Maria's case at that
moment the delusion took a hypochondriacal form. Previously it
had taken the form of insisting that she belonged to Dr N.'s family.
Dr N. said in the seminar that he realizes now that shifting
everything on to the physical sphere is not only a defence to help
Maria to feel better. It also includes a belief that it is better for Dr N.
and will save him from his confusion and depression. Dr N. then
went over the reasons for the hypochondriacal state quite clearly. He
now seemed to understand it well, and I thought that he was no
longer part of the confusion. An important danger had been
removed from the patient, even if the situation would take some
time to sort out.

*Dr N. now briefly talked about the next session. Maria apparently had
sent off many applications to become a nursing sister, but most had been
refused. She said if she doesn't get accepted as a nursing sister then in one or
two years she will go abroad and look for a job there. Dr N. interpreted that
this seems again to imply a need to get away from him. Before, it always
looked as if she wanted to get away from the mother, but here he thinks it
refers to him. Maria seemed partially to agree with this but suddenly asked
Dr N. whether he knows somebody who is doing music therapy. She had
read that music therapy was very good for the treatment of schizophrenia. Dr
N. interpreted that she obviously feels she needs a different treatment. Music
therapy means a therapy without words, which she expects at this moment to
be more helpful than what he can explain to her. She immediately replied she
is so afraid that something may happen to him. She fears that this something
will always happen to Dr N. when she notices that her thoughts become so
loud at home so that her friend who is living in a house opposite from her will
actually hear it. Dr N. interpreted that she feels that something which she
has been thinking has actually come into the open. She said, 'You said that
these thoughts are really the ideas which were formerly my voices which now
become so loud.' (When these ideas become very loud she describes that she
has to attack herself and says to herself, 'What is this? What are you thinking
about?') Dr N. interpreted that 'It looks as if the patient is angry with herself
but in fact it seems she is angry with him, and this reminds her of the way her
mother has always been complaining about her.' Maria said, 'Now, these are*

not always complaining words, but there is a confused feeling that if I have something against you I am not sure that it may not also be against myself and this is now not quite clearly differentiated.' She added that she may again have thoughts about Dr N.'s wife and about an aunt. Then she said she thought Dr N. was really tortured by her. She feels that she makes life impossible for him and makes him weak by her thoughts and complaints. It is these attacks on him which make her afraid that he will die or cannot cope with the situation.

While she was talking about this Maria became a bit confused. She felt she is now between two families, no longer clearly belonging to Dr N.'s family. She then mentioned a great number of different things and at the end of this session she feared that if she continues like this she might create a great confusion in her head and then everything will get confused and upside-down. At that moment she can think only about drugs; this would be the only thing that can help her and so avoid the danger not only to herself but to Dr N. Suddenly she feels it is quite enough even to think about the drugs and that helps her because she feels a little bit clearer in her head. This was then the end of the session.

- In this session the progress which the patient has been making is considerable. There is no doubt that Dr N.'s capacity to contain Maria's projections, particularly her confusion, has improved. He is helping her to get out of the entanglement with him. She is still afraid of her aggression but, as she said herself, instead of voices she has now aggressive thoughts which come out loud and clear. It still causes her confusion and anxiety, but even this has diminished because she illustrates that she is now more able to think about what is going on inside herself. This probably also means that she has become more concerned about what she was thinking, and therefore at the end of the last session she recognized that even thinking about the possibility of needing drugs to cope with her confusion helped her to be less confused. Thus she felt she did not need the drugs.

I have for many years recognized that confusional anxiety plays a very central role in many cases of psychosis, also in hypochondriasis. It is interesting in this case that the patient herself realized that the hypochondriasis which had become so predominant in the last few sessions was a defence against her confusional state.

As Maria's case was presented to the seminar it became clear that her central anxiety was her voices, which gradually became confusing, aggressive, torturing thoughts. They had the power of both dominating and confusing Dr N. and preventing him from functioning and understanding the patient. They were also believed to cause him so much pain and depression that he would die. The confusion was apparently caused by a primitive hypnotic form of projective identification where confused loving and hating feelings would overwhelm both the patient and the analyst. This made Maria feel uncertain what she was feeling and doing and whether she was directing thoughts against the analyst or against herself. Her fundamental terror in this state was of a complete entanglement with the analyst with no way out apart from death, leading to the delusion that her death could protect or save the analyst from dying.

Some of Maria's delusions such as her conviction that she was a member of Dr N.'s family seemed to be not only a protection against pain and frustration but an escape into an ideal situation, a delusion of oneness with Dr N. which magically could save him and her from the destructive confusing relationship. The hypochondriasis, the delusion of suffering from a serious internal disease, was also thought of as an escape from the hopelessly confused and entangled relationship with Dr N.

At the end of the seminar Dr N. said that most of Maria's problems now seemed much clearer and he realized that it was essential to repeat clearly to her what he had understood and how important it was to make the correct links in his interpretation. He needed to give her a feeling that he, Dr N., would no longer be overwhelmed by her anxieties and that he really was no longer confused. He could face up to it without being destroyed by the patient's problems. This implies that it is essential for the analyst to feel secure enough about his understanding to work out the problems of the patient through the patient–analyst relationship.

What is extremely important in situations like those I have just described is that the analyst realizes what is essential to interpret. If he goes into too many details, picks up separately all the points, and inquires about them because he doesn't understand them sufficiently, then the patient becomes very anxious. Immediately she will be aware that the analyst is uncertain and confused, and then her anxiety will increase enormously. This technique cannot work in analysis. To treat patients such as these successfully it is important to concentrate and to observe the central problem: in Maria's case the confusional anxieties, which could be recognized by the analyst's confusion. He had to be willing to bear the anxiety of not being clear. The next issue is to recognize how desperately anxious the patient feels about making the analyst confused. This is quite an unbearable problem for the patient because it implies that neither the patient nor the analyst is capable of coping with the uncertainties.

They can be clarified only by quietly thinking about them and so being gradually able to find a solution in a constructive way.

Nine months after the seminar Dr N. reported that Maria had made very good progress and that her delusions and confusing behaviour had disappeared.

PART FIVE

Conclusion

13

Afterthought: changing theories
and changing techniques in psychoanalysis

The ideas presented in the preceding chapters were developed over many years. I want to use the opportunity provided by this final chapter to emphasize some of the crucial aspects of my approach and some of the ways I have changed my opinions.

From the beginning of my interest in psychological medicine I was curious about patients who were difficult to treat and were thought to be incurable. From this grew my interest in schizophrenia and other psychotic conditions, which I discussed in Chapter 1. As my analytical work progressed I became more formally interested in the therapeutic action of psychoanalysis and simultaneously in the factors which may be responsible for treatment failures or impasse. I have had much opportunity to think about this problem because during the last thirty years I frequently accepted patients for analysis who had a number of analyses before consulting me but who had not improved or had even become worse after their analysis. I have also described two such failures of my own in Chapter 7. It has long been widely accepted, of course, that some failures will arise in a psychoanalytic treatment when it activates latent psychotic processes, and that great care will be needed to work through such situations, which can be a frightening development. In the case of an impasse developing in an analysis, however, I have come to accept the existence of several varied causes (not just the eruption of psychotic processes) and believe that in each case what has been going on in the treatment has to be examined in very great detail in order to understand as specifically as possible how the problem has arisen. It is with the prevention of impasses and their working through that

265

many of my ideas are concerned. I shall summarize some of my views under several headings.

Envy

Melanie Klein (1958) drew attention to the role of excessive envy not only in frequently causing negative therapeutic reactions but also in occasionally leading to an impasse in analysis bringing about severe deterioration of the patient. At that time I myself and other Kleinian analysts believed that through a detailed analysis of envy in the transference situation it would be possible to prevent an impasse in analysis. However, as time went by, my experience was that this was only occasionally true. Non-traumatized severely omnipotent narcissistic patients (like Adam in Chapter 4) did do well with this approach. But I also found that, while envy and fear of being envied indeed caused many difficulties by inhibiting normal development in childhood and by slowing down progress in analysis, it was only one factor among the many others that can cause impasse. Envy and fear of envy have to be seen in the patient's total situation. By this I mean not only the envy in the early infantile relation to the mother and the breast but also the envy specific to either men or women. In men envy of the female function and the capacity to produce children is important. In women it is the envy and rivalry of the female towards the penis and masculine strength and functioning which matters. It is inevitable that envy arises in human development and that the child, or the patient in analysis, is going to feel small or inferior at some times. I particularly have in mind situations when the child, or patient, feels put down and may actually have been put down by the parents or by other children or, in analysis, by the analyst. In my experience it is when a patient feels accepted and helped in analysis, and feels that he or she has some space to think and to grow, that envy gradually diminishes. For these reasons interpretations of envy should not be repeated too often. The emphasis should be on helping the patient to bear the pain, discomfort, and shame which envy causes because it inhibits the capacity to love. Severely frustrating situations inevitably stimulate envy. The main problem that arises in analysis is that sometimes the patient feels humiliated because the analyst understands the patient so much better than the patient himself. This problem has to be faced by helping patients to understand that their progress in analysis depends on a joint effort on the part of patient and analyst and particularly on good timing and sensitive interpreting on the part of the latter. An over-emphasis on the interpretation of envy or the over-valuing of the analyst's contribution as compared to that of the patient is a frequent cause of impasse.

Destructive Narcissism

A second cause of impasse arises from the way destructive narcissism comes to dominate some patients in a disguised silent way and blocks the progress of analysis (as I have described in Chapter 6). I want to emphasize that once such a force is recognized by the analyst the situation becomes much more hopeful. As the inner silent hypnotic influence of the destructive figure, posing as a benevolent figure, is interpreted to the patient he becomes gradually more aware of what is going on inside him, and the paralysing influence on him and his analytic progress gradually lessens. Awareness of the inner dominating force helps the patient to report what is going on inside him, and in this way the analyst is able to help the patient to feel less imprisoned because he feels less threatened by a more open internal attack than by the disguised hypnotic influence which is utterly confusing. The patient has gradually to distinguish between the threat of the murderous inner attack and his own angry, murderous feelings against external objects. When this is achieved there is still a great deal of analytic work to do, but the impasse in the analysis is overcome.

There is another point that has become clearer to me during recent years. This refers to the existence of the death instinct. I have always felt that there are aggressive forces which are fighting against the forces of life, a factor that became clear to me when I discovered the importance of destructive narcissism, just mentioned. However, more recently I noticed that some patients complained about something deadly in themselves which was clearly not identical with aggression. Another striking feature in these patients was their marked inhibition in thinking and talking about the factors which seemed to be inhibiting their capacity for wanting to turn towards life. When they were, occasionally, aware of their fear of death, they felt scared to talk about it! They acted as if it had to remain a secret. Thus when the deadly force appeared as a deadly monster in dreams they could not bear to look at it, and they did not want to know about it. I saw this phenomenon as strongly related to Freud's observation that there is a death instinct always working mutely and secretly. It is typical of all the phenomena connected with the death instinct that they create something mysterious, hidden, unspeakable, and yet incredibly powerful and dangerous, against which it is impossible to fight. However, I found that by interpreting a patient's destructiveness it was impossible to mobilize or make conscious this deadly force. It was only when I interpreted it as something inert or deadly that it became meaningful to the patient. I have never been able to mobilize deadly feelings like this very quickly but I have found that, by drawing attention to the peculiar paralysing behaviour, the secretiveness, and the terror of something unknown, I could gradually help patients to observe more clearly what was happening inside them. They could formulate in their mind the existence of something deathly or murderous. Eventually what happens is that the murderous force appears in a patient's dreams. Once exposed, it can be seen that this murderous force is mainly directed against the patient himself and it becomes much easier to deal with the problem analytically. The patient can feel more clearly what he is frightened about. It also becomes more obvious that he wants to be protected from this force. At the same time previously unclear associations about aggressive feelings and thoughts can now be understood. In other words, the patient becomes more able to acknowledge that he has aggressive feelings and that these have often been directed against himself. I am convinced that the analysis and acknowledgement in analysis of this deadly force are often absolutely essential if impasse is to be prevented.

Confusion, collusion, and the role of history

A third point about impasse that I want to stress concerns the complex way transference and counter-transference reactions can cause both the analyst and the patient to become confused or to collude with each other in anti-therapeutic ways. For example, when there is a chronic misunderstanding by the analyst of a patient's provocative behaviour it may gradually cause such an intense negative counter-transference as to produce a vicious circle which can lead to an impasse in the analysis. I illustrated this point at the end of Chapter 2. Here I want to add another example which is still more telling.

Recently an analyst reported a patient to me in supervision, whom she found so difficult that she was aware of a very strong negative counter-transference building up inside her. She felt that she couldn't stand the patient any more and wanted to get rid of her. The main reason for the negative counter-transference was the patient's inability or refusal to speak. She came four times a week for analysis but generally spoke only a few words in each session. When the analyst attempted an interpretation the patient generally replied with, 'No, no', or 'I don't agree.' But that was all.

The patient, a young woman of about twenty-two, had been diagnosed as psychotic, probably schizophrenic, and had been treated in two previous analyses. In the first analysis the analyst himself gave her up. In the second one the patient got so angry that she refused to come. The present analyst, the third, was approached by the patient's mother, who was very concerned about her and wanted to do everything possible to help. In an interview she told the analyst how much she had always idealized her daughter and said she was the most precious gift that she had received in her life. She described her as a wonderful, obedient child who never caused her the slightest bit of trouble. She really meant life to her. But five years before this daughter, who had been active and had excelled at school, started to deteriorate; she withdrew from school and studies, failed all examinations, and could not concentrate on anything.

At the first interview with the patient the analyst explained to her that she thought there was a sick part in her and that she thought she needed help with that. The patient was surprised. She followed the analyst's instruction to go for some time to a mental hospital where she was also under the care of a psychiatrist who gave her neuroleptic drugs. From the hospital she was brought by her mother four times a week for analysis. During the first year the patient spoke no more than a few words but in outside life she improved and even returned to her studies. However, the analyst was unsure what to do about this 'frustrating' patient.

When I listened to the analyst's report about the interview with the mother I had a very clear picture in my mind of a mother exerting pressure on her daughter through her enormous idealization. This must have made the child feel that she was not allowed to exist, and that she had to give up her life to her mother. So she had not had space to live and she obviously had not had strength to say 'no' to her mother. I thought, therefore, that it was extremely important for the analyst to change the picture *she* had of the patient in *her* own mind, a picture where she saw a sick child being very aggressive and hostile to her, which she greatly resented and which prevented her from having a space to function as the patient's analyst. I suggested that I felt the patient was bringing the *healthy* part to her analysis – the healthy part which now tried to be stronger, tried to say 'no' to her, tried to disagree with the analyst/mother who would tell her that she should be a good girl and do whatever the mother or analyst wanted, namely talk. I pointed out that if the analyst continued to treat this healthy complaining part of the patient as sick and aggressive there was a danger that she would develop a hostile, rejecting counter-transference attitude, and this is what had in fact happened. An impasse would also be inevitable. If, however, the analyst regarded the patient's behaviour as a natural response to what had happened to her, she might see that, by bringing the part of herself which was healthy and wanted to say 'no' and to fight against her mother's influence, the patient was actually co-operating in the analysis rather than the reverse.

I want to draw attention here to my attitude to cases of this kind; it is typical of the direction of my work, particularly during the last five or six years. I like to scrutinize the patient's interrelation with his family carefully and to try to understand the role which the analyst now occupies in the transference. In the case I am discussing the patient's behaviour in the transference situation, in the context of her past, is scarcely negative. It was only through the analyst's misunderstanding of the patient's problem (in its historical context) that her negative counter-transference grew so overwhelming. Given her situation, the patient was bound to recognize the negative feelings her analyst was developing. She must have felt the irritation in the analyst's voice, the lack of enthusiasm, and even perhaps the hopelessness. In the past I have made similar mistakes in misdiagnosing the patient's attitude in analysis. To avoid such errors I now try as much as possible to assess the patient's relationship to her or his past and present environment and so to lessen the possibility of confusing the healthy and sick part of the patient. Looking at the patient's problem, by assessing the patient's behaviour and communication both in the present relationship to the analyst and simultaneously in the early environment, makes it possible to understand the atmosphere which may be created in the analysis. I now regard such efforts as an important aspect of how to look at the psychic reality of my patients.

The analyst's flexibility

I think it is essential that the analyst is aware that the analytic situation and transference situation are both affected not only by the patient's past experiences but also by the analyst's views, behaviour, and counter-transference. My understanding of the analysis of negative transferences and aggression has altered significantly. I now take the view, for example, that to analyse aggression one has to assess the patient's vulnerability and defensiveness very carefully. Specifically, one must examine how deeply the patient feels afraid of rejection and therefore needs to idealize the analyst in order to create a benign atmosphere. If the analyst tries to break down such idealization too quickly, what the patient says may rapidly become appeasing, or he may defend himself against collapse by withdrawing or by being critical. Such reactions by the patient mean that the analysis gets distorted and stuck. In the analysis of traumatized patients the analysis of the negative transference is particularly complicated by such reactions, and one has to scrutinize the patient's material very carefully indeed. Too much confrontation can be a mistake because it creates provocative and confusing material, mainly caused by the patient's fear.

The paramount importance of the patient's psychic reality is revealed by the psychoanalytic process. It is clear that all analysts believe that they want to help the patient to find his psychic truth, in analysis. However, in practice the way they go about it varies considerably, and I feel that idealizations are often too quickly broken down. It is important not to interfere with a patient's idealization of the analyst just on principle. A patient may have to make considerable progress in the analysis before he can accept the ups and downs of the analytic relationship, the battles which have to be fought, and the despair and emptiness which often seem unbearable. It needs quite a lot of trust for a patient to open up, and before confronting idealization I try to assess what the patient can cope with and to see that he doesn't come too quickly under a great deal of pressure. When a patient moves into a crisis I feel that it is important for him to get as much insight into the situation as possible, and simultaneously as much help from me as possible. This is what he consciously wishes, and it is in a crisis that the psychic truth of the patient is most likely to be accessible.

The crucial point about my current approach is that analysis should not be carried out rigidly. It is important to feel involved with the patient and not to assume an artificial detachment. Assuming detachment, for example if one goes so far as to try to control one's voice so that it sounds unemotional, is detrimental to the patient.[1] I remember well the detrimental effect of the detached voice of one analyst on a patient. The latter felt deeply rejected by this analyst whom he greatly admired but whose attitude of detachment had thrown a deep cloud over the whole analytic experience so that one had to regard it as a failure, created simply through this artefact.

It is essential that the patient experiences the analysis as enlivening and that the analyst is aware of how the setting itself and his technique can exert a deadening effect. There are many patients who have difficulties, particularly in the beginning of the analysis, in accepting the analytic situation: lying on the couch; the interpretative communication of the analyst; the not-direct answering of questions; etc. Other frustrations related to the analytic situation stir up intense feelings which are often difficult to bear and where there is a danger that the patient then defends himself or herself by deadening their feelings. It is essential for the analyst to be always aware of this danger and help the patient not to be drawn into such a deadening experience. We as analysts must understand how strong an influence on our patients we can have, something which applies particularly to the way we conduct ourselves towards our patients, for example in our way of speaking to them. There are many patients who listen very intently to the analyst's voice to assess its emotional quality, its warmth or coldness. Occasionally they are so entirely orientated towards taking in the analyst's voice that they lose the meaning of what he says.[2] As a final point concerning the analyst's contribution to impasse I want to re-emphasize the two-sided nature of the analytic process. I agree, of course, as many other analysts now feel, that our counter-transference is a very important aspect of our work. It helps us considerably to understand the difference between what the patient says and what comes across to us. We use our counter-transference to pick up the more hidden meaning of what is being expressed by the patient and to become aware that what the patient conveys in emotional experience is sometimes completely different from what he says. This is a very important aspect of our attempt to find the psychic truth. However, we should equally be aware that we as analysts may convey differences in what we are communicating by the tone of voice with which we speak. I want to stress again and again that the analysis is not a one-sided process but an interaction between two people.

Transference and delusion formation

The distortion of reality and the formation of delusions and hallucinations have always been a puzzling problem, but over the last ten years I found that when one succeeds in observing delusion formation in a psychotherapeutic setting it becomes evident that transference/counter-transference disturbances between patient and analyst play an essential part in delusion formation and can be clearly demonstrated, as I tried to show in Chapter 12. Such observations have important implications both for understanding the psychogenic basis for the development of schizophrenic conditions and for

improving the prognosis of the psychoanalytic treatment of schizophrenia.

I have often observed that the analyst's inability to understand
certain essential aspects of the schizophrenic patient's communication
can have a detrimental effect on the psychotic patient because it very
likely repeats the misunderstanding between infant/child and its
parents, particularly the mother in early infancy and later. This is
often clearly illustrated by the patient in relation to the mother,
although by itself such insight has very little influence on the patient.
It seems that it is essential to observe, understand, and overcome the
repetition of certain misunderstandings which appear very subtly in
the transference and create a very strong counter-transference
reaction which is frequently very confusing. In Chapter 12 I
described in detail the intense counter-transference reaction experienced
by Dr N. when listening to Maria's confusing communications. The
delusions and hallucinations developed in order to protect both the
analyst and the patient from the disastrous anxieties which the
analyst's counter-transference created. As soon as the analyst was
able to recognize his own counter-transference reaction and managed
to accept it, the detrimental influence of the counter-transference
immediately disappeared, and simultaneously the psychotic manifestations of the patient, such as her delusions and hallucinations,
vanished within a period of a few weeks. This remarkable change
was accompanied by an improvement in the patient's way of
thinking and understanding which ended her tendency to revert
constantly into psychotic thinking.

Confusional states

One basic problem, which is particularly essential if the treatment of
psychotic patients is not to end in impasse, is the need to understand
the infantile origin of confusional states and anxieties and its
implications for technique. In confusional states love and hate, and
good and bad objects, become confused, creating an overwhelming
and almost insoluble problem for the developing infant and one
which is invariably revived in most psychotic states. I believe that the
repetition of early infantile states is one of the most important factors
in creating transference and counter-transference entanglements
(such as many of those discussed in earlier chapters) which cause
confusion and then delusion formation as the patient tries to escape
the unbearable anxiety that pervades his analytical experience. The
repetition takes place, of course, via very intense projective

identification. In this way the unbearable anxiety is both communicated and projected into the analyst in the analysis. It is because these anxieties are at times so very violently projected that the analyst frequently reacts with the feeling of being attacked and may become irritated and resentful. Such counter-transference reactions may sometimes be inevitable as part of a successful treatment but they are perceived by the patient in an extremely exaggerated way and so frequently form the basis of delusions. For example, instead of the patient being afraid that the analyst has become depressed or anxious about him he will have an exaggerated conviction that the analyst is overwhelmed by suicidal feelings and will die. The analyst is therefore experienced as being completely unable to cope with the patient's projections. In this situation, as described in Chapter 12, the patient may feel entirely responsible for the life of the analyst and may communicate this predicament in very confused and confusing delusional forms.

Thin- and thick-skinned narcissistic patients

There are many narcissistic patients whose narcissistic structure provides them with such a 'thick skin' that they have become insensitive to deeper feelings. To avoid impasse these patients have to be treated in analysis very firmly and have to be confronted with their narcissistic attitude and their envy – particularly as their envy causes devaluation of the analyst and the analysis and of any need for help. With these patients the frequent repetition of interpretation and confrontation seems to be unavoidable, even if for a long time these repetitions do not seem to make any impact on the patient (see Chapter 4). When interpretations at last manage to touch them they are relieved, even if it is painful to them.

By contrast to those with a 'thick skin', some narcissistic patients are 'thin skinned'. They are hypersensitive and easily hurt in everyday life and analysis. Moreover, when the sensitive narcissistic patient is treated in analysis as if he is the 'thick-skinned' patient he will be severely traumatized. The analysis and the patient may be brought near to collapse, especially if the destructive aspects of a patient's behaviour are constantly repeated in the analyst's interpretations. Such patients can end the analysis very much worse off than before. In my experience the 'thin-skinned' narcissistic patients were, as children, repeatedly severely traumatized in their feelings of self-regard. They seem to have felt persistently and excessively inferior, ashamed and vulnerable, and rejected by everybody.

During puberty and later on, through their intellectual capacities and physical prowess, they often succeeded if not in overcoming at least in hiding their sense of inferiority, and thus often gained recognition and success in life. Generally, they have functioned quite well although with occasional breakdowns to indicate the precariousness of their narcissistic personality structures. Working with such patients the therapist realizes that there is a great deal of over-compensation and a tendency to feel superior in certain areas, with the result that the patient's sense of triumph and revenge against the parents or siblings (by whom he felt so belittled and humiliated) has been stimulated. When these patients gain some pleasure and pride in their achievements and work, or when they succeed in relating to their spouse, or in bringing up their family, one realizes that their positive narcissism plays an important part in keeping their personality structure stable. But if the destructive aspects of narcissism are over-emphasized in the analysis the narcissistic structure is not modified but simply becomes something bad, something to be ashamed of, and something to feel inferior about. For the 'thin-skinned' narcissistic patient an over-emphasis on their destructiveness is particularly dangerous if it inhibits or increases their difficulty in building up satisfactory object relations. I have found, therefore (as I mentioned in describing Eric's case in Chapter 7), that it is particularly important when treating such patients to help them to retain the positive aspects in their narcissistic organization by making them aware of the conflict with the destructive narcissistic part of themselves with which they are not identified.

I do not want to give the impression that these 'thin-skinned' patients are easy to treat, because fundamentally such traumatized and vulnerable people find it very difficult to cope with any trauma or failure. However, one has to be particularly on guard not to add to these traumas by making mistakes in our analytic approach which humiliate such people and put them down. These mistakes are very difficult to remedy afterwards.

Maternal projections before and after birth

As a last point I want to stress the importance of taking seriously some discoveries about disturbances in children and adults which have apparently been caused by projective processes coming from the mother before and after birth. The problem has been mentioned by several therapists and analysts such as Bion (1957), Steiner (1975, 1982) and June Felton (1985). As Felton's investigation of these problems seemed to be the most detailed one I shall briefly refer to her observations.

In examining autistic children and their mothers Felton found that there were areas in the mother's mind which she was intensely disturbed and embarrassed about, and which she had made brave efforts to exclude from consciousness. But it appears that the pregnancy activates these hidden processes which were never supposed to be known but which nevertheless in a mysterious way seemed to have seeped into the child. This process Felton calls 'osmotic pressure', although this is not a satisfactory term for a phenomenon that is predominantly a mental phenomenon, which may be accompanied by some intra-uterine physiological process not as yet investigated. The term 'osmosis' suggests a transmission from the mother through the placental bloodstream, which could of course be correct, but not necessarily. On the other hand, it is difficult to find a term to describe clearly a process which works like a physical osmosis but in the mental sphere.

The foetus seems to be completely helpless to ward off this 'osmotic pressure' coming from the mother, which dominates the foetus and later on the child. This process continues after birth and prevents the child from forming a normal relationship to the mother. By simultaneous observation of the mothers and the children Felton collected evidence of the child being overwhelmed and distorted in his way of thinking and feeling and unable to find a relationship to his self which would enable him to live and to function. It is hoped that Felton will publish her research on these processes in time.

My reason for emphasizing the importance of very early projective processes is related to my conviction that such antenatal influences do occur in varying degrees with patients who had to suffer *in utero* an atmosphere far away from the idyllic, harmonic, comfortable atmosphere often associated with the intra-uterine state. Children of mothers of this kind are from the beginning of life phobic about their mother. They are terrified that they may at any moment have to guard against something very frightening which is being forced into them. They need to block the mother's influence; this can be observed after the child is born but sometimes it starts immediately after birth and gives rise to severe feeding disturbances and the tendency to turn away from contact with the mother. This becomes even more pronounced when the child can walk. Felton points out that these problems may occur immediately after birth, but there is no reason to think, as Bion has indicated, that disturbances arising in the prenatal period cannot manifest themselves at later periods of life: latency, puberty, or even later on. He describes disturbances which suddenly overwhelm people and in which it is very difficult to understand the meaning of the sudden appearance of symptoms out of the blue. When children or adults communicate by projection something of this 'osmotic pressure', they often transmit something which they themselves feel is alien and confusing to them. If the analyst tries to confront them with what they transmit they feel persecuted and believe that the analyst is projecting his own problems into them, not diagnosing something coming from them. This is clinically of great importance because such children who are analysed as if they are very destructive and bad tend to feel more and more persecuted when one interprets in this way. It should be important to show them that they experience something destructive and disturbing which has happened to them and that they try to find in the analyst somebody who helps them to reach something more positive, good, and free from disturbing pressure. It is understandable when a child looks for help and understanding because of something inside him which he cannot recognize and understand that it increases the child's anxiety when the analyst fails to give him the space to find himself. With children particularly, one finds the increased need to find the good mother inside the analyst, and they are preoccupied with trying to find a good internal space to dive into but they feel terrified that it may again be poisonous and bad and that they will have to escape from this.

Some time ago a child therapist, Mrs K., presented to me the treatment of a child who from birth suffered from such severe diarrhoea that she had to be sent immediately to a clinic for several months so that her life could be saved. The baby nearly died in hospital but when the mother on a visit saw that the child became blue she was convinced that the child would die in hospital and she insisted on taking her home to look after her. However the diarrhoea and incapacity to control her urine, faeces, and even tears continued, and it was impossible to send this child to school (when she was four or five years old) because of the disturbing smell her continuous incontinence created. From the family history it was known that the mother had gone through terrible experiences years before in connection with her own family who were all wiped out in concentration camps. The thought of having a child who would be alive was almost unbearable to her. All during the pregnancy the mother was severely depressed. Afterwards she still seemed unable to recover, but nevertheless both she and her husband were devotedly trying to save the life of the child.

Mrs K. had a very difficult time with this child of six who could scarcely speak and was completely incontinent, but there was no question that she managed to provide her with a very loving atmosphere and acceptance although seeing her just once a week. Gradually the girl started to play. At first she was incontinent and seemed to be crying all the time with tears streaming from her eyes; her nose was running, and she also was inflamed on her forehead and looked quite awful. But gradually there was some improvement and it was interesting that for this child play with water became more and more important. After a year Patricia seemed to be very excited as she played. Throughout the first year she played with water but without ever lingering very much. Now she seemed captivated by the water. The play took place in a very small room with a basin and tap which she at last knew how to operate. One day she was letting water flow into the basin; then, suddenly taking notice of a big bowl which was under the basin, she filled it up and then dashed for a doll, plunged it into the water, which overflowed on to the floor, and cried, 'It's flowing, it's flowing', with a delighted look. From her facial expression Mrs K. had the impression that the child was suddenly conscious that something which she had experienced as 'frozen' no longer was so; now it flowed, and life flowed somewhere inside her. Mrs K. also thought that if she could let the water flow on the floor and rejoice about it, it was because she felt contained and at last capable of containing. Mrs K. was left with the impression that something very important had happened during this session. When Patricia came next time she was no longer drooling, and the incontinence had improved. When she started drawing in the session she drew a closed circle for the first time. In listening to this amazing experience I felt very touched. I think it meant that in this experience with the doll the child seemed to have discovered the place, the inside of the womb of the mother, standing for the therapist, where she could feel safe, and it is at the moment when she began to feel that she was safe, which meant life to her, that she actually found that now she could begin to live: to be born, to be alive. Before, with all the fluids running from all parts of her body, she was completely unable to find a space in which she could feel safe. Experiences of this kind are important for us to remember, and this also implies that for such patients the atmosphere of analysis must be one where a child gradually feels safe and accepted. Such children's experiences are also much more related to the inside of the mother than to the breast; and analysts who tend to interpret the positive and negative feelings only towards the nipple and the breast rather than to the inside of the mother may find difficulty in reaching children of this kind.

With this last example I have tried to draw attention to the importance of keeping an open mind about the influence of antenatal experience. Such experiences may be of great importance for understanding some of the entanglements which produce impasse. If we can keep an open mind we will probably find increasing evidence that such complex and primitive factors are at work in our relationships with patients.

Notes

1 I do not however think one should go as far as Greenson (1967) recommended, who stressed that the analyst should show his real feelings. I feel that one should neither disguise one's feelings nor exhibit them.
2 There are, of course, some analysts whose voice is more expressionless than other people's, which must be quite a problem in the analysis. They are probably not aware how damaging an expressionless voice can be in analysis.

On the treatment of psychotic states by psychoanalysis – an historical approach

During the last fifty years the psychoanalytic approach to psychosis has undergone very considerable change, and at the present time there is no unified theory of either the psychopathology or the technique of treating the psychoses. Many analysts working with psychotics have found it necessary to alter to some extent the classical technique of analysis developed by Freud in dealing with neurotic states, a technique which is based on a therapeutic alliance with the patient and on the capacity of the patient to come to treatment regularly and also to free-associate. Such a patient would be able to develop a transference neurosis and other transference manifestations which can be interpreted to a patient whose ego is sufficiently intact to co-operate in this way in an analysis. Freud himself thought that this technique was unsuitable for psychotics. The work of many analysts has been influenced by Freud's belief that psychotics do not develop a transference at all. However, an increasing number of analysts have tried to develop methods with the hope that eventually some contact with the psychotic, and with this some improvement of the psychotic condition, might be achieved. Freud (1933) discussed the intimate relations which exist in psychoanalysis between theoretical views and therapeutic treatment.

I believe that the changes in the therapeutic approach to psychotics have been certainly influenced by the theoretical views held by the therapist and by factors in the therapist's own personality. A clearly defined method of approaching psychotic states is important if we expect to conduct research to clarify the psychotic psychopathology rather than concentrating on symptomatic improvement. The therapist should ask himself whether he is inclined to change his psychoanalytic approach because he does not understand the psychotic patient or because he believes he has arrived at a better understanding of psychotic psychopathology, and alterations in technique are the outcome of his understanding. As it has turned out, in fact, many analysts have found that deeper understanding of psychotic psychopathology has made it unnecessary to change the usual classical psychoanalytic technique to any important degree. I shall try to indicate some aspects of the theoretical background of the therapies I am describing so that the theoretical reasons for any changes that there have been in psychoanalytic technique can be seen.

Modifications in analytic technique are particularly common in the approach to schizophrenics but not so much in work with manic-depressive patients. That is probably one of the main reasons why the number of descriptions of psychoanalytic therapy with manic-depressive patients is comparatively small compared with the extensive literature relating to the treatment of schizophrenia. In this Appendix, therefore, I shall concentrate mainly on the latter group.

I shall first attempt to give a picture of Freud's views relating to the treatment of psychosis. Freud made many basic contributions to the understanding of the psychopathology of the psychoses and undertook the treatment of some psychotic patients, occasionally with success. For example, as early as 1905 he reports an attempt to treat a manic-depressive patient in the symptom-free interval after the depression. However, the treatment came to an end after a few weeks when she became manic. In 1916 he reports that he has had two successes in treating similar states. In 1905 he states:

> 'Psychoses, states of confusion and deeply rooted depression are not suitable for psychoanalysis; at least not for the method as it has been practised up to the present. I do not regard it as by any means impossible that by suitable changes in the method we may succeed in overcoming this contra-indication – and so be able to initiate the psychotherapy of the psychoses.'
>
> (SE 7: 264)

Freud felt that analysts should limit their choice of patients to those who possess 'a normal mental condition'. By this he meant that the ego of the psychotic was in his view not sufficiently strong and integrated to maintain a therapeutic alliance and co-operation in an analysis. He particularly feared that the psychotic ego would be unable to control the patient's morbid impulses and behaviour. He believed that the strong ego was necessary since in the psychoanalytic method this (the ego) was used as a foothold from which to obtain control of the morbid manifestations.

This links up with his later formulations that some normal ego functioning was necessary in order to begin any psychoanalytic treatment. In 1916 he explained his views in much greater detail, tying them in with his developing ideas on the importance of narcissism. After discussing the narcissistic withdrawal of the libido from the object into the ego as an important factor in the psychopathology of dementia praecox (schizophrenia) and also the manic-depressive states, he says:

> 'Since we have ventured to operate with the concept of ego libido the narcissistic neuroses have become accessible to us; the task before us is to arrive at the dynamic elucidation of these disorders and at the same time to complete our knowledge of mental life by coming to understand the ego.'
>
> (SE 14: 422)

He continues:

> 'The ego-psychology after which we are seeking must not be based on the data of our self-perceptions but on the analysis of disturbances and disruptions of the ego. . . . But hitherto we have not made much progress with it. The narcissistic neuroses can scarcely be attacked with a technique that has served us with the transference neuroses. You will soon learn why. What always happens with them is that, after proceeding for a short distance, we come up against a wall which brings us to a stop. Even with the transference neuroses, as you know, we met with barriers of resistance, but we were able to demolish them bit by bit. In the narcissistic neuroses the resistance is unconquerable.'
>
> (SE 14: 422–23)

He continues a little later (p. 423) 'Our technical methods must accordingly be replaced by others; and we do not know yet whether we shall succeed in finding a substitute.'

He then discusses the material available from psychotic patients with the clear intention of stimulating research into the psycho-pathology and treatment of narcissistic states. But the pessimistic note constantly returns; for example, in 1916 he discusses how 'paranoiacs, melancholics, suffers from dementia praecox remain on the whole unaffected and proof against psychoanalytic therapy' (SE 14: 438–39) and goes on to discuss in detail the so–called transference neurosis in order to explain the lack of success with the narcissistic neurosis:

> 'Observation shows that sufferers from narcissistic neuroses have

no capacity for transference or only insufficient residues of it. They reject the doctor, not with hostility but with indifference. For that reason they cannot be influenced by him either; what he says leaves them cold, makes no impression on them; consequently the mechanism of cure which we carry through with other people cannot be operated with them.'

(SE 14: 447)

Freud then explained this lack of transference in terms of the patients having abandoned their object cathexes, and the object libido having been transformed into ego libido. Sixteen years later (1933), he again discussed the indications for and limitations of analytic treatment and issued a warning against over-enthusiasm about the results of psychoanalysis. Now, with his newer under-standing of the importance of instinctual conflict between the life and death instincts, he added: 'sometimes one special instinctual com-ponent is too powerful in comparison with the opposing forces that we are able to mobilize. This is quite generally true with a psychosis' (SE 22: 154). He again discussed the limitations of analytic successes due to the form of the illness and affirmed that the field of application of analytic therapy lies in the transference neurosis: 'Everything differing from these, narcissistic and psychotic conditions, is unsuitable to a greater or less extent' (SE 22: 155). It would seem that between the two series of Introductory Lectures (in 1916 and 1933) Freud had become more pessimistic about the possibilities of *analytic* treatment of psychosis. This pessimism may, however, have been connected with his increasing preoccupation with the problem of the relation between the suitability for analysis and constitutional excessive strength of instinct, and his awareness of the importance of the destructive (death) instinct, in severe mental illness, which he developed in greater detail in 'Analysis Terminable and Interminable' (1937).

In 'An Outline of Psycho-Analysis' (1940), Freud returned again to the discussion of the treatment of psychosis, now related to his greater understanding of the psychology of the ego. He explained that the psychoanalyst has to find in the patient's ego a useful ally. For this to happen the ego must have retained

'a certain amount of coherence and some fragment of understanding for the demands of reality. But this is not to be expected of the ego of the psychotic: it cannot observe a pact of this kind. . . . Thus we discover that we must renounce the idea of trying our plan of cure upon psychotics – renounce it perhaps for ever or perhaps only for the time being, until we have found some other plan better adapted for them.'

(SE 23: 173)

But later in the 'Outline' he added a further point to this when he described that in many 'acute psychotic disturbances there remains in some corner of the patient's mind a normal person hidden' (SE 23: 202). He then discussed 'the view which postulates that in all psychosis there is a splitting of the ego'. He continued:

> 'You may probably take it as being generally true that what occurs in all these cases is a psychical split. Two psychical attitudes have been formed instead of a single one – one, the normal one, which takes account of reality, and another which under the influence of the instincts detaches the ego from reality. The two exist alongside of each other. The issue depends on the relative strength. If the second is, or becomes the stronger, the necessary pre-condition for a psychosis is present. If the relation is reversed, then there is an apparent cure of the delusional disorder.'

(SE 23: 202)

Freud's description of the splitting of the ego in the psychoses into a normal and a psychotic part is of fundamental importance for the understanding of the psychopathology of the psychoses. As the 'Outline' was published posthumously (1940), Freud could not himself clarify whether this important observation on the splitting of the ego would have influenced his pessimism about the clinical psychoanalytic approach to the psychosis. The processes of splitting of the ego have been studied in detail by Melanie Klein. The division into a psychotic and non-psychotic part of the personality was studied by Federn, Katan, Bion, and Rosenfeld.

When one reviews Freud's contributions to the treatment of psychotic states one is impressed by his pessimism but also by his hope that eventually some way of approaching psychotic illness may be found. The pessimism is essentially associated with his belief that psychotics do not form a transference, based on his theory that in these narcissistic conditions, when object libido is withdrawn into the ego, the object presentations are completely given up. Freud attributed the extreme rigidity in resisting any change which he encountered in the psychosis to the same process: 'narcissism'. He regarded the omnipotence of the psychotic process – as, for example, in delusions and hallucinations – as an attempt at restitution designed to regain the objects of the external world. But this 'object libido' was similarly found resistant to any therapeutic analysis. Another important difficulty which Freud described was the ego deficiency in psychosis which he believed made co-operation in treatment impossible. Freud was aware that excessive strength of instincts played an important part in psychotic states but did not discuss specific psychotic conflicts between parts of the self, such as loving and destructive parts of self, based on his theory of the life and death instincts. He regarded the main conflict in psychosis as a conflict between the ego and reality.

Transference manifestations of psychotic patients as seen by analysts who have tried to treat psychotic patients by analysis

As Freud insisted that severely narcissistic patients – and he referred here frequently to psychotic patients – could not be treated by psychoanalysis principally because he thought that psychotic patients did not form a transference, it seems essential to compare Freud's findings with the experience of other analysts.

Brief summary of analyst's transference experiences with psychotic patients

Federn emphasized that psychotic patients form transferences but unstable ones. His most important finding in my view is the fact that he noticed that the psychotic is eager to make transferences with both the healthy and the disordered (psychotic) parts of his personality, which I shall describe later in greater detail.

Bullard stressed that in the psychotic there were profound swings of transference similar to those of the neurotic but so intense and so carefully concealed by a mask of indifference or hostile suspiciousness that many analysts believe that the analysis of psychotic patients is impossible.

Sullivan emphasized the capacity of schizophrenics to form a transference. He tried to communicate with patients by means of his interpersonal theory of schizophrenia and by understanding the patient's self system which, he felt, often collapsed in schizophrenia.

Fromm-Reichmann described the extreme suspicion and distrust of the schizophrenic patient towards the therapist who approaches him with the intention of intruding into his personal life and his isolated world. She first criticized other analysts' attempts to break through the patient's defence with interpretations but at a later period of her work she recommended that the investigation of the doctor–patient relationship and its distortions should be included in the therapeutic process.

A number of analysts talk of a narcissistic transference in psychotic patients. Abraham changed his view that psychotic patients do not form a transference, which he held until about 1912. He described the narcissistic grandiosity in one of his patients. From 1913 he observed transferences in schizophrenic patients, and in 1912 he noticed that melancholics were capable of establishing a sufficient transference to justify analysts treating them. If one scrutinizes Abraham's description of patients one feels that he must have interpreted the patient's narcissistic transference behaviour and gradually managed to release a more positive object-related response in the patient.

On the other hand Waelder – one of the first analysts to speak of a narcissistic transference – did not use the narcissistic transference for interpretations but as a vehicle for the directive influence which the analyst can bring to bear on the patient.

Pierce Clark was aware of the narcissistic transference in psychotic patients. But he suggested again no interpretation of this transference but acting out with the patient in so far as he advised that the therapist should lend himself fully to listening to and understanding the material being presented, but approach it not in terms of analytic interpretations but with emotional sympathy which would ensure the patient's complete harmony.

Stern described a transference based on the ungratified and ungratifiable narcissistic needs of his patients, who often view the analyst as godlike, omniscient, and omnipotent. He found that, when the analyst changed in the patient's eyes into a hostile and cruel object, the patient often came near to a psychotic state in the transference situation.

Cohn examined narcissistic transferences in great detail. He observed that in the narcissistic transference there is often a serious difficulty in distinguishing between subject and object which is due to projection. He described the narcissistic transference when the analyst was experienced by the patient on a part object level as if he were the patient's own stool.

Searles describes the transferences of the schizophrenic in very great detail and suggests that it is expressive of a very primitive ego organization comparable with that of an infant living in a world of part object experiences.

Stone emphasized that the transference love of the hysteric was different from the primitive phenomenon of the narcissistic trans-

287

ference. Sometimes the transference becomes particularly narcissistic when the analyst becomes confused with the patient's self.

Edith Jacobson stresses problems of intense transference feelings in depressed patients who live only in the aura of the analyst and withdraw from other personal relations. There is often an intense sado-masochistic transference at times of threatening narcissistic withdrawal.

Winnicott described that he was able to analyse psychotic patients at first without any change of analytic technique, and this meant that he analysed the psychotic phenomena appearing in the positive and negative transference situation. When he changed his views and felt that the psychosis was a kind of deficiency disease he simultaneously changed his technique and stressed that the analyst would have to make up for the failure of the early environment.

Bion, Rosenfeld, and Segal were encouraged through Melanie Klein's work on early schizoid processes such as projective identification and the paranoid anxieties related to them to approach psychotic depressed and schizophrenic patients by analysis. They have all described the psychotic transferences that they encountered in the analysis of psychotic patients.

Rosenfeld said in 1954 that the psychoanalytic manifestations attach themselves to the transference in both acute and chronic conditions, so that what might be called a 'transference psychosis' develops. He stressed that whenever an acute schizophrenic patient approaches an object in love and hate he seems to become confused with his object, a problem which has also been stressed by Stone, Stern, and Bion.

The contributions of all the analysts mentioned here to the treatment and the understanding of the narcissistic or psychotic transference will now be more fully described and discussed in the following pages.

Abraham made very important contributions to the treatment of psychosis, particularly to the manic-depressive states. As early as 1907 he discussed the psychopathology and treatment of dementia praecox, drawing attention to the similarities of the conflicts in hysteria and dementia praecox, for example, instancing 'the imaginary pregnancies' (1907a: 55). He also states that obsessive ideas constitute in their psychosexual genesis are entirely similar to hysterical pregnancies' (1907: 55). He also states that obsessive ideas constitute in many cases the most prominent characteristic of the illness. In 1908 he examined the differences between hysteria and dementia praecox and came to the conclusion that 'since we have traced back all transference of feeling to sexuality we must come to the

288

conclusion that dementia praecox destroys a person's capacity for sexual transference, i.e. for object love' (1908: 69). He regards

'the negativism of dementia praecox as the most complete antithesis to transference. . . . In attempting to psychoanalyse these patients we notice the absence of transference again. Hence psychoanalysis hardly comes into consideration as a therapeutic procedure in this kind of illness.'

(1908: 71)

Abraham describes the patient's interest or longing for an object but says that, if they get it, it has no effect on them. In discussing the general lack of interest in an object and the lack of sublimation he suggests that the psychosexual characteristics of dementia praecox indicate that the patient has returned to the stage of auto–eroticism and the symptoms of his illness are forms of auto–erotic sexual activity. Many of Abraham's observations, such as the preoccupation of the schizophrenic with auto–erotic masturbatory phantasies, have been confirmed by recent work.

In 1913 Abraham changed his view about the lack of transference in schizophrenia when he reported on the analysis of an undoubted case of dementia praecox, suffering from hallucinations: 'The patient during treatment soon proved himself capable of making a sufficient transference' (1913: 191). In 1916 he reported on another case of dementia praecox. He said that 'a psychoanalysis can be carried out with these patients just as well as with a psychoneurotic' (1916: 254). In both cases the work was facilitated on account of the abolition of many inhibitions: 'the material lies quite near consciousness and in certain circumstances is expressed without resistance' (1911: 152).

In 1911 Abraham reported on the investigation and treatment of six undoubted cases of manic–depressive illness. It is interesting to see how soon he began to discover transference phenomena in this group of patients. One of these cases had suffered from severe melancholia for twenty years. At the time of the report he had treated the case for only two months, but 'during this time no further state of depression appeared but there were two states of manic accentuation which were far milder than previously' (1911: 154).

In another case the effectiveness of analysis was shown in a striking manner. The treatment lasted for only forty sessions. In the sixth case the treatment could be successfully completed in six months. He commented that the treatment had a 'remarkably good result'. Six months after ending the treatment there had been no relapse. Abraham stated that it is usually extraordinarily difficult to establish a transference in these patients who have turned away from all the world in their depression, but he stressed that in one case, simply by the help of psychoanalytic interpretations of certain facts and connections, he succeeded 'in obtaining a greater psychic rapport with the patient than he had ever previously achieved' (1911: 153). In another case he was astonished that after overcoming considerable resistance he succeeded in explaining certain ideas that completely dominated the patient and observed the effect of this interpretative work. The initial improvement and every subsequent one followed directly upon the removal of definite products of repression.

During the whole course of the analysis he could most distinctly observe that the patient's improvement went hand in hand with the progress of his analysis. He commented that, with those patients who have prolonged free intervals between their manic and depressive attacks, psychoanalysis should be begun during the free period. Generally speaking, Abraham, though aware of the incompleteness of his results, felt very hopeful in this paper. He said: 'It may be reserved for psychoanalysis to lead psychiatry out of the path of therapeutic nihilism' (1911: 156).

In 1924 Abraham made further very detailed observations of manic–depressive patients. Particularly interesting and significant are his comments on the patient's behaviour in the analytic situation and his reaction to the analyst's interpretations. For example: 'We all know how inaccessible melancholic patients are to any criticism on the part of the analyst of their ways of thought: and of course their delusional ideas are especially resistant to any such interference' (1924b: 455). A patient once replied, when he had tried to make an interpretation, that he had not even heard him. He described the narcissistic transference in one of his patients who used always to walk into his room with an air of lofty condescension, displaying superior scepticism about psychoanalysis. In another patient this attitude used to alternate with one of chronic humility. He felt that melancholics are capable of establishing a sufficient transference to justify analysts in attempting to treat them and that important changes could not be effected in a patient until he succeeded in establishing a transference on to his analyst. He stressed, as in 1911, the patient's capacity to respond to interpretations and observed that in some cases the patient's narcissistic and negative attitudes towards certain people, or towards his whole environment, and his high degree of irritability in regard to them, diminished in a way which never happened before.

It is interesting, therefore, that Abraham, unlike Freud, found it possible to establish a transference in manic-depressive patients and that, in spite of the strength of the patient's narcissistic behaviour during the analytic sessions, he was able to produce a change simply by means of interpretations.

There were only a very small number of analysts who attempted to treat psychoses up to 1935. Their main preoccupation was the problem of the patient's narcissism. Waelder (1925) attempted to find a theoretical and practical basis for the treatment of the narcissistic neurosis. He developed a hypothesis concerning the conditioning factors by which the psychosis comes about or is avoided in those borderline personalities in whom the phenomenon of transition to the psychoses can be observed. He introduced the concept of the 'narcissistic repression', which seems, in his opinion, the basis of the withdrawal of the libido into the ego and which is also the basis of psychosis. He introduced a further concept which he called the 'union of instincts', involving the combination of narcissism and object libido, instancing people 'who succeed in linking the narcissism with object libido in a manner compatible with reality which prevents the formation of pathological psychotic symptoms' (1925: 269).

Waelder illustrated his theory with case material. He argued that if it were possible to use the libido which is flowing back into the ego at the outset of a psychotic disease in such a way that the instinct would be combined with sublimation in a manner compatible with reality, and if this union was related to object libidinal processes which are accessible to the analytic methods, we might hope to be able to find a way of curing the psychosis which has already broken out. The therapeutic task in these cases he described as 'sublimation of narcissism'. In discussing the transference, Waelder pointed out that the only form of transference which can be effectively established is the narcissistic one. He tried to make clear that the characteristic feature of the therapeutic intent that he advises implies an intervention into a healthy part of the personality which has not got a narcissistic fixation. He therefore depended on the existence of such a part of the personality. Practically the treatment must begin with an extremely passive period, which enables the analyst to find out what the possibilities are. The analysis is maintained with the narcissistic transference, and generally speaking one has to advance hand in hand with narcissism, avoiding frustration in regard to the narcissistic ideal and steadily aiming at affording narcissistic gratification compatible with reality. Waelder stressed the self-knowledge of the narcissistic patient and his capacity consciously to influence his mind:

'In psychosis of the schizophrenic typic, insight into the mechanism has a markedly greater power of assisting recovery than in neurosis. All self-knowledge consists in the establishing of communication between different tendencies which hitherto were cut off from one another. . . . This is a rare case in which the patient's understanding of the genesis of his illness suffices to cure him.'

(1925: 278, 275)

Waelder is one of the first analysts to speak of a narcissistic transference. This transference is apparently not used as a basis for transference interpretations but as a vehicle for the directive influence which the analyst can bring to bear upon the patient. When Waelder discusses psychotic mechanisms and tendencies cut off from one another, we are to some extent reminded of modern concepts of split-off parts of the self and of the interpretation of mechanisms of splitting in psychotics and borderline psychotic states which play an important part in modern techniques of treating the psychotic ego.

In 1933 Pierce Clark contributed to the treatment of the narcissistic neuroses and psychoses. He thought that it was the narcissism which constituted the first great barrier to any therapeutic approach and to possible readjustment in the narcissistic neurosis. He argued: 'In using the technique of ordinary analysis in such cases we may learn a great deal about narcissism, but we fail to help the narcissist' (1933b: 304). He developed in this paper his theory of the narcissistic fixation and how this might be approached and overcome by psychological treatment. He observed that the narcissistic ego has not developed beyond the infantile level of need for loving protection and support, and the patient is regarded as having a special individual requirement for a longer period of dependence than non-narcissistic patients. His theory is that, though the narcissist may need a longer time for development, there will eventually be a tendency to step away tentatively from his withdrawn position. He believed that the therapist should fall in with the narcissistic requirements of the patient; in other words, his role should be that of the 'tender, all-giving mother'. In practice, that would mean that the therapist would lend himself fully to listening to and understanding the material being presented, but would approach it not in terms of analytic interpretation but with emotional sympathy, which would ensure the patient complete harmony. The author noted that the relationship would later assume the conditions of ordinary transference analysis, but through this 'fortified technique' the ego is given a chance to resume its interrupted growth at a speed of its own choosing. At one point he asked whether 'such a passive all-giving analyst might not merely heighten the idealisations of the patient without increasing his testing of reality and his discharge of energy into sublimating activities' (1933b: 310). To counteract this difficulty Pierce Clark suggested that the narcissistic identification which the analyst provides must be gradually tinctured with reality requirements. He stressed that, once the narcissistic transference is established, the procedure is very similar to that followed in the analysis of the transference neuroses. 'The narcissistic shell must be broken through in order to expose the real weaknesses, the fears and dependent needs which lie behind' (1933b: 318).

Pierce Clark gave some case material of a psychotic patient but he did not report any significant clinical improvement by this treatment. His theories and approach have many points in common with those of later workers interested in dealing with psychotics, such as Fromm-Reichmann's early attempts at treating schizophrenic patients and Winnicott's later theories and recommendations for approaching psychotic patients.

Waelder and Pierce Clark seem familiar with the concept of the narcissistic transference, but they are not concerned with describing the narcissistic attitude or behaviour of the patient in the analytic situation, which was done successfully by Abraham. They both advise the analyst to change his behaviour and to fit in with the narcissistic patient's demands for love, support, and satisfaction in order to create and maintain the narcissistic transference.

Stern (1938) described the transference based on the ungratified and ungratifiable narcissistic needs of his patients, who often view the analyst as godlike, omniscient, and omnipotent. As a result of this they feel secure and happy in the analysis as if they were in a nirvana, but they remain without any insight. Stern stressed that a distorted perception of the analyst is quite real to these patients. The negative transferences have to be very carefully handled. When the analyst changes in the patient's eyes into a hostile or a cruel object, the patient often comes near to a psychotic state in the transference situation. Because of the omnipotence of the good or bad imago which the analyst represents, anything savouring of criticism has a most disturbing effect on the patient, as the analyst then changes into a bad figure, and the patient easily withdraws. Stern observed that in the narcissistic transference the patient never identified himself with the analyst but only with the concept of him produced by a process of projection of his own ego ideals. He particularly emphasized the sense of omnipotence with which the patient endows both the ideally good and the excessively bad imagos which he projects on to the analyst.

Cohn (1940) examined the narcissistic phenomena in the transference in greater detail. He believes that the transference in general may be regarded as a narcissistic phenomenon and he regarded the transference of the narcissistic neurosis as simply of a primitive and rudimentary type. He observed that in the narcissistic transference there is often a serious difficulty in distinguishing between subject and object, and that this problem is caused by the mechanism of projection. He relates the processes of incorporation, expulsion, and projection to organic fixations, which he thinks should be made conscious because they appear magnified as long as they are not evaluated by the conscious mental apparatus. He gives a number of clinical examples of the narcissistic transference; for example, with a depressive patient the analyst was treated as if he were the patient's own stool. This was one of the reasons why he could not distinguish between himself and the analyst. During the analysis it became apparent that the patient had projected not only his faeces and his anal sensations on to the analyst but also his own penis and in this way had lost it himself. In discussing a case of schizophrenia, he described a girl who seemed interested only in a book that she was tearing into little shreds. One day she suddenly attacked the analyst violently as if she were going to try to pull him to pieces. She said to him, 'You can't leave me. I have concentrated on you entirely.' Then she dropped back into her stupor and, he adds, the analyst into his ignorance. The analyst described that he had not realized at that time that the patient had been concentrating on him and not on the book. He is now aware that there had been a transference on a very primitive level. In most of his clinical examples he stressed the use of the mechanism of projection in the narcissistic transference. The importance of the mechanism of projection and the confusion of subject and object in the narcissistic transference was stressed by many later workers with psychotic patients (Searles, Rosenfeld, Bychowski, and others).

Bullard, Federn, Fromm-Reichmann, and others described very intense transferences in dealing with psychotic patients. Bullard (1940) said that in the psychotic there are profound swings of transference which are in a sense similar to those of the neurotic, but so intense and so carefully concealed by a mask of indifference or hostile suspiciousness that many analysts believe that the analysis of psychotic patients is impossible. Bullard stressed overt and concealed anxiety in psychotic patients and gave details of how to deal with this problem. When these anxieties were not clearly understood and brought to the surface, they threatened the continuance of the analysis and markedly affected the existing trend of rapport. He also mentioned that the intense, often paranoid hostility of the psychotic may be indicative of anxiety and may have a defensive purpose. He gave case material to illustrate a strong negative paranoid transference in which the patient threw things at him and insisted that the analyst was torturing him. He found that even such severe negative transferences can lessen markedly when the analyst is aware of the real cause of the patient's anxieties so that the patient feels better understood. Bullard (1960) described in greater detail the analytic approach to severely paranoid patients in a hospital setting. His patients appeared to have no insight and rejected therapy at the beginning. Bullard accepted the patient's paranoid attitude as a basis for starting treatment and did not attempt to create a positive transference artificially, which he feels would be a serious drawback to effective therapy. Bullard's contributions are particularly important because in contrast to many therapists dealing with psychotics he illustrated that the negative transferences of the psychotic can be understood and analysed in a therapeutic setting.

Federn treated psychotic patients from 1905 onward and made a very detailed contribution to the psychopathology and treatment of the psychoses in 1943. He found that psychotics form a transference, but this is quite unstable, and he therefore employed a different method from that with neurotic patients. He emphasized that in approaching psychotic patients we should remember that these patients are accessible to psychoanalysis because first they are still capable of transference; second, one part of the ego has insight into the abnormal state (but this is not a constant factor); and third, a part of the personality is still directed towards reality. The psychotic is eager to make transferences with both the healthy and the disordered parts of his ego:

'The transference of the psychotic part of the personality is dangerous and can lead to aggression and slaughter as well as to deification of the object. . . . Both aggression and deification can put an end to any contact with the analyst because of deeply rooted fears.'

(1943: 137)

In comparing the treatment of the psychotic and neurotic, Federn said that in psychosis normal resistances have broken down and have to be re-established by psychoanalysis. In order to re-establish the resistances in the psychotic, Federn advised that one has to abandon the usual psychoanalytic technique:

'First abandon free association, second abandon analysis of the positive transference, third abandon provocation of the transference neurosis, because it quickly develops into a transference psychosis

295

in which the analyst becomes the persecutor. Fourth, abandon the analysis of resistances which maintain repression. Phobias are left undisturbed because they protect against deeper fears and conflicts. . . . In analysing the psychotic regression must not be increased.'

(1943: 155)

He emphasized that the most important condition which should be considered in every psychoanalytic treatment of psychosis is the establishment of a positive transference, which must itself never be dissolved by analysis, and an interruption of the treatment when the transference becomes negative. Mainly for this reason Federn is emphatic that no psychoanalysis of psychotics can be carried out without a skilful and interested helper, preferably a woman, to take care of the patient between sessions and particularly during periods of negative transference. In discussing the ambivalence of the psychotic and the way this shows itself in the transference, Federn stressed that the analyst has to realize that ambivalence is replaced in the psychosis by two or more ego states. These split ego states alternate in their strength and with them alternate the positive and negative transference to the analyst. Federn advised that, in psychosis, the therapist should slow down and even try to stop the spontaneous delivery of still unconscious mental complexes, because one does not want to face any increase of the psychotic disorganization until the ego has been re-established within its normal boundaries. In his treatment of psychosis Federn relied on that part of the patient which is still in touch with reality and external objects, the remnants of the normal ego. In describing his attitude to the patient, he said:

'The psychoanalyst shares the acceptance of the psychotic's falsifications as realities. He shares his grief and fears and on this basis reasons with the patient. When convinced that by this procedure the patient feels himself understood the analyst presents the true reality as opposed to falsification. He then confronts the patient with his actual frustration, grief or apprehension, and connects this with the patient's deeper fears and conflicts and frustrations.'

(1943: 159)

An important factor in Federn's technique is the conscious education of the patient in connection with changes in his ego boundaries. He shows the patient, for example, that because of certain ego boundaries having lost their cathexis ideals, thoughts and memories are experienced as real and cease to be mere thinking. He stressed that the patient is able to learn to distinguish those ego boundaries with normal cathexis from those with cathexis withdrawn. He believed, contrary to Freud, that the loss of reality is a consequence of and not the cause of the basic psychotic deficiency. Federn made a detailed study of latent psychosis. He noticed that latent psychotic patients become openly psychotic during their psychoanalytic treatment. He was convinced that psychoanalysis often fosters the onset of psychotic depression and mania. In such situations he advised the immediate interruption of the free association method. He himself learnt to avoid the wakening of a latent psychosis and he became eager to take over those patients whose psychosis had been precipitated by the psychoanalytic work of other analysts, mentioning that many patients were sent to him by former patients and by Freud himself.

Federn's contribution to the treatment of psychosis is of particular historical interest for us as he was one of the first analysts to treat psychotics with psychoanalytically orientated psychotherapy. Another point of interest is Federn's concentration of psychotherapeutic effort on the psychotic ego, which he studied in detail, discussing in particular the splitting into healthy and psychotic parts, an observation which was taken up by Freud in the 'Outline' (1940). It is interesting that Federn held the view that neither the transference psychosis nor the negative transference of the psychotic could be influenced by psychoanalytic therapy.

It will have become clear that Federn made no attempt to treat the psychotic part of the patient's personality. His method of treatment was devised to suppress or, as he called it, to repress the psychotic productions which were overwhelming the patient's personality. It would perhaps be more appropriate to describe Federn's treatment as an attempt to help the patient to split off and to deny the psychotic parts of the self which had temporarily overwhelmed the more healthy part of the ego. The importance of this splitting process in the apparent recovery of the psychotic has been discussed by Freud in the 'Outline'.

Up to the mid-1930s interest in the psychotherapy of the psychoses was very limited, but after about 1935 this interest increased markedly, particularly in the treatment of schizophrenia from a psychodynamic point of view. In America this stemmed largely from the work of Harry Stack Sullivan and in England from that of Melanie Klein.

Sullivan (1947) studied the interpersonal relations of his schizophrenic patients by creating a psychotherapeutic treatment unit in the Sheppard and Enoch Pratt Hospital in Baltimore. He found that even severely ill schizophrenic patients responded to what may be called a treatment group, where all the workers – doctors, nurses, and helpers – aimed to assist the reorientation of the schizophrenic patient towards interpersonal relations. In fact, most of the patients seemed to recover in this setting and could be discharged. In many symposia and papers Sullivan stressed the psychogenesis of schizophrenia and the capacity of schizophrenics to form a transference. He disagreed with many psychoanalytic formulations. His basic developmental theory was expressed in these words:

'There is no developmental period when the human exists outside of the realm of interpersonal relatedness. From the very early post-natal stage, at which time the infant first learns to sense approval and disapproval of the mothering person by empathy, some degree of interpersonal relatedness is maintained throughout life by everyone, regardless of his early state of mental health: therefore its disruption in the schizophrenic is only partial.'
(Quoted in Fromm-Reichmann 1948: 162)

One of the analysts particularly inspired by Sullivan's work was Frieda Fromm-Reichmann, who continued her work with psychotics, which she had started in Germany, under his guidance and developed her technique of treatment while observing and treating severe schizophrenic patients in the Chestnut Lodge Sanatorium (near Washington, DC) over a period of more than twenty years. It is interesting to observe how her assessment of schizophrenic patients gradually made her change her technique in dealing with them. In her first paper (1939) she emphasized that the patient who later develops schizophrenia has been traumatized severely at an early period when the infant lives grandiosely in a narcissistic world of his own. In this state he feels that his desires are fulfilled as a result of his magical thinking. She thought that the early traumatic experience shortens the period of narcissistic security, which sensitizes the schizophrenic patients towards the frustrations of later life. As a result of this the patient escapes the unbearable reality of his present life by attempting to re-establish the autistic delusional world of the infant.

Fromm-Reichmann described the extreme suspicion and distrust that such a patient evinces towards the therapist who approaches him with the intention of intruding into his isolated world and personal life. It takes weeks and months of testing the therapist until the patient is willing to accept him, but after this his dependence on the therapist is very great, though he remains extremely sensitive about it. Whenever the analyst fails the patient, it results in a severe

298

disappointment which is experienced as a repetition of previous frustrations, and leads to outbursts of intense hatred and rage. Following these observations, Fromm-Reichmann recommended that the threatment of the schizophrenic must begin with a long preparatory period of daily interviews. As the treatment continues, the patient is asked neither to lie down nor to give free associations. Nothing matters except that the analyst permits the patient to feel comfortable and secure enough to give up his defensive narcissistic isolation and to use the physician for resuming contact with the world. The analyst's function is seen as trying to understand and to let the patient feel that he does, without attempting to prove this by giving interpretations, because the schizophrenic himself understands the unconscious meaning of his productions better than anyone else. The analyst gives evidence of understanding by responding cautiously with gestures or actions appropriate to the patient's communication. Altogether she recommends as a basic rule for the treatment of schizophrenics an atmosphere of complete acceptance. In this first period of therapeutic experimenting with schizophrenic patients, Fromm-Reichmann worked with a treatment approach based on the developmental theory of narcissistic injury which is identical to the one advocated earlier by Pierce Clark, and the positive relationship to the analyst is fostered to imitate an early omnipotent magical infant–mother relationship. This fostering of the positive relationship is reminiscent of Federn's recommendation of promoting a positive transference and the avoidance of frustrations leading to negative transference reactions.

In her later papers (1948, 1952, 1954) Fromm-Reichmann revised and criticized her earlier approaches. She said:

'Psychoanalysts used to approach the schizophrenic with the utmost care and caution. We assumed this to be the only way of making it possible for him to overcome his deep-rooted suspicious reluctance against reassuming and accepting any personal contacts, including those with the psychoanalyst.'

(1948: 164)

She now criticized this approach as this type of doctor–patient relationship addressed itself too much to the rejected child in the schizophrenic and too little to the grown-up person before his regression. She also felt that this approach of unmitigated acceptance may be experienced by sensitive adult schizophrenics as condescension or lack of respect on the part of the analyst and may be interpreted by the patient as a sign of anxiety on the part of the therapist. She now recommended that the investigation of the doctor–patient relationship

299

and its distortions should be included in the therapeutic process. In other words, the analysis of the transference which was formerly strongly criticized was now fully recommended. She also criticized the previous cautiousness in her therapeutic endeavours; she expressed the opinion that 'much valuable time had been lost by waiting too cautiously until the patient was ready to accept one or another active therapeutic intervention' (1948: 169). She also recommended more detailed investigation of the schizophrenic symptomatology and the schizophrenic productions; and thus follows Sullivan's direction, adding that, according to him, 'the psychodynamics of manic illness including the schizophrenic manifestations can be understood as the result of an expression of unbearable anxiety and at the same time as an attempt at warding off this anxiety and keeping it from awareness'. (1948: 170).

In 1954 Fromm-Reichmann discussed the devastating effect of schizophrenic hostility on the patient's own personality and connected it with states of autism and partial regression: 'This has led to a therapeutically helpful reformulation of the anxiety of schizophrenic patients as an outcome of the universal human conflict between dependency and hostility which is overwhelmingly magnified in schizophrenia' (1954: 194). She discussed the resentment or violence with which the infant or child ('the bad me', as Sullivan called it), and later the schizophrenic patient, responds to the early damaging influences of the 'bad mother' as he experienced her. This explains why schizophrenic patients are more concerned with their own status as dangerously hostile people than with the damage which may be done to others who associate with them. In describing the schizophrenic conflict about dependency, she discussed the tension between dependent needs and longing for freedom. The patient's fear of closeness is tied up with anxiety about their secret hostility against people whom they value and depend on. This, she emphasized, must be worked through in the transference.

In her paper 'Psychotherapy of Schizophrenia' (1954) Fromm-Reichmann stressed the importance of the non-psychotic part of the personality, arguing: 'we try to reach the regressed portion of their personalities by addressing the adult portion, rudimentary as this may appear in some severely disturbed patients' (1954: 195). This adult part is trained to join the psychoanalyst in his therapeutic endeavours. Even in her later work Fromm-Reichmann was reluctant to use more than minimum interpretations. Her therapeutic work relied greatly on guiding and directing the patient to a dynamic understanding and insight into his illness. It is interesting that Fromm-Reichmann was able to correct her 'fallacy' of concentrating in the treatment of schizophrenia on becoming a kind of ideal mother to the regressed schizophrenic patient. In her later work she concentrated on examining the conflicts and psychotic productions of the schizophrenic patient in the transference situation, which brings her work in many ways closer to the researches of analysts in England (see Segal, Bion, Rosenfeld, and others).

Searles, another member of the Washington group of analysts, made very detailed contributions to the treatment of schizophrenic patients while working for more than thirteen years at the Chestnut Lodge Sanatorium. Some of his papers, such as 'Dependency Processes in the Psychotherapy of Schizophrenia' (1955), were written in close co-operation with Fromm-Reichmann. He stressed that difficulties arise in the transference situation through projections. The analyst is perceived as hostile and rejecting because of the patient's own frustration and anger. He described the resistance against dependence because it means giving up phantasies of omnipotence. The patient defends himself against his dependency by projecting his dependency needs into the analyst. As a result of this he fears the therapist's demands on him and becomes competitive and contemptuous. In a later paper (1963) Searles described the transference problem in more detail. He believed that 'the transference of the schizophrenic is expressive of a very primitive ego organisation, comparable with that which holds sway in the infant who is living in a world of part objects' (1963: 661). He described three tasks which the therapist should perform. First, 'the therapist must become able to function as a part of the patient' (p. 667). Secondly, he must be able to foster the patient's individuation out of this level of relatedness, the level which has been described 'by Kleinian analysts as being a transference phase dominated by projective identification on the part of the patient' (p. 661). The therapist's third task is to discern and make interpretations concerning the patient's now differentiated and integrated whole object. This gradually transforms the patient's transference psychosis into a transference neurosis. Searles stressed the importance of a phase of therapeutic symbiosis where he regards verbal transference interpretations as contra-indicated. He explained that the patient deep in chronic schizophrenia is not able to employ or even to hear verbal communications. In this phase the patient uses the analyst as his own ego and has not sufficient ego functioning to understand interpretations, and he projects into the analyst a variety of part-object transference roles, which the therapist must be able to endure and eventually enjoy. Through identification with the therapist who can endure his primitive object relations, the patient ultimately develops ego strength. In examining the transference in this symbiotic phase, Searles said that it is astonishing to discover to what extent the patient is relating to himself or, more accurately, to a part of himself as an object. Searles does not discuss the splitting of the ego or self in detail, but his remarks illustrate to what extent he has observed processes which have been described by other analysts either as narcissistic transferences or as splitting and projections of part of the self into objects. He also studied the concreteness of the schizophrenic patient's thought processes which lead to transference difficulties; for example, the therapist may be experienced by the patient not as like his father or mother, but concretely as the father or mother.

Searles examined the schizophrenic transference in admirable detail and has become aware of the importance of projection and projective identification in the transference. I think, however, he is seriously mistaken in his belief that the analyst should enter into the symbolic transference as a state of mutual dependence, in which the analyst feels as dependent on the patient as the patient on him and often expresses his feelings of love and hate quite freely to the patient. I feel that Searles, who has trained himself to make elaborate use of his counter-transference feelings, is sometimes carried away by them and does not sufficiently acknowledge or recognize the patient's projected desires for a mutual relationship with the analyst which eliminates the differences between child and adult. I would regard Searles's behaviour as acting in with the patient, instead of analysing this most important conflict in psychotic patients, their difficulty in depending on an adult who is then felt to be superior, and their resentment and attempts to reverse the infant–parent relationship or attempts to seduce the analyst into a mutually dependent position or push him out of his legitimate role. In my experience this acting in does not lead to ego strengthening, but increases the existing ego weakness of the psychotic patient.

It is, of course, impossible to discuss all the contributions to the treatment of psychosis, and I shall now only briefly discuss Stone's view of the psychotic transference and Edith Jacobson's work with psychotic patients. Stone (1954), in contributing to the treatment of psychotic conditions, emphasized that the transference love of the hysteric is different from the primitive phenomenon of the narcissistic transference. The psychotic's transference is liable to invade or overwhelm his personality, just as his psychosis threatens to overwhelm his ego. Stone is aware that sometimes the sheer fear of the primitive intensity of their feelings forces some patients to remain detached, but where the transference does break through, insatiable demands may appear, or the need to control and tyrannize the analyst, or, failing that, complete submission to him. Sometimes the transference may be literally narcissistic when the therapist is confused with the self or is like the self in all respects. He stressed both the primitive destructiveness and the need to experience the analyst as omnipotent and godlike, and he suggested that, in the patient's phantasy of the analyst's omnipotence, guilt about primitive destructive aggression plays an important part. From his own experience one may speak with justification of 'transference psychosis'. In discussing the analyst's attitude, he suggested that the decisive factor is the ability to tolerate, over long periods and without giving up hope, the strains of the powerful, tormented, and tormenting transference and the potential counter-transference situation. It seems that Stone advised only a minimum change in the psycho-analyst's attitude, in fostering the positive transference, so that the patient would stand the strains of the hostile transference when it appeared. He did not believe that analytic treatment could be harmful in basically psychotic patients, since he did not feel that there could be such a thing as a latent psychotic state liable to be uncovered. This, of course, is in contrast to the opinion of Federn. Unfortunately, Stone's views are not exemplified by clinical material.

Jacobson has contributed mainly to the treatment of manic-depressive states, but has also made an interesting contribution to the treatment of schizophrenic patients. She emphasized that, in the course of the analysis of the depressive, the analyst inevitably becomes the central love object and the centre of the depressive conflict. As the analysis progresses, the patient may develop even more serious depressive states, characterized by deep ego and id regressions. She suggested that depressives try to recover their own lost ability to love and to function through magic love from the loved object. When they fail to get such help from without, they may retreat from their love object and from the object world and continue the struggle within themselves. In her experience the treatment of the manic-depressive starts regularly in the depressive state because they usually do not come for treatment during the symptom-free interval, or in hypomanic or manic periods. The depressed patient tends to establish either an immediate, intense rapport or none. She felt that there is usually an initial spurious transference success lasting many months; then there is an ensuing period of hidden negative transference with corresponding negative therapeutic reactions; third, there is a state of dangerous introjective defences and narcissistic retreat; and finally a phase of gradual constructive conflict solution. The most difficult period in the transference relationship is when the patient lives only in the aura of the analyst and withdraws from other personal relations to a dangerous extent. The transference phantasies assume an increasingly ambivalent sado-masochistic colouring, and the author stresses particularly the patient's exhausting sado-masochistic provocations. The patient may unconsciously blackmail the analyst by playing on his guilt feelings, hoping in this way to get the longed-for responses. Failing to do so, he will try to elicit from the analyst a show of power, strictness, or punitive anger, serving the alternative purpose of getting support or relief from the relentless super-ego pressure. She believed that in periods of threatening narcissistic withdrawal the analyst may have to show active interest in the patient's daily activities and especially in his sublimations, as she illustrates in case material. She also stressed that the depressed patient needs a more understanding attitude on the part of the analyst, an attitude which must not be confused with over-kindness, sympathy, or reassurance.

In *Psychotic Conflict and Reality* (1967) Jacobson explained that her treatment of schizophrenic patients was mainly with an ambulatory type and was designed to avoid severe psychotic regression. Psychotics tend to use the external world to prevent the dissolution of their ego and super-ego structures. She believed that Freud's observation that psychotics give up reality and replace it by a newly created phantasy reality occurs only if reality fails to lend itself to the patient's purposes and to help them in their conflict solution. She described that, if psychotic patients are able to project a bad unacceptable part of the ego into suitable external objects by a process of projective identification, they manage to remain sane as long as they can control these objects.

Jacobson is aware of the regressive narcissistic nature of the patient's relations to these significant objects, and the weakness of the boundaries between the psychic representation of these objects and their own self. In describing her analytic experience with one of these patients, she said that she permitted the patient to use her as he needed and she adapted her emotional attitudes and behaviour to his wishes for warmth, or closeness, or distance: 'I let him "borrow" my superego and ego, regard and treat me as his bad id and his illness: project his guilt, his faults and weaknesses into me or turn me into an ideal of saintliness he needed' (1967: 57). From her description it is clear that the patient not only projected his problems into her, but was acting out in the outside world significantly during this time. She said that she avoided giving him deeper interpretations of his acting out in the transference or in outside life until he himself knew that the period of danger was over. She would then use for interpretations the material that he had previously brought; and at such times interpretation would be surprisingly effective. The treatment was not used to work through the patient's early narcissistic projective identifications in the transference situation, as she was afraid of the danger of provoking a psychotic breakdown. Jacobson's method, as described here, has a great deal in common with Waelder's earlier attempts at treating the narcissistic neurosis by producing a sublimation of narcissism by linking it with object libido.

In turning now to the history of the psychoanalytic treatment of psychotic patients in England we have to consider first of all the pioneer work of Melanie Klein, who through her analysis of seriously disturbed children and adults investigated the earliest infantile levels of development. In 1935 and 1946 she described details of the object relations, mechanisms, and defences of two normal developmental phases, which she called the 'depressive position' and the 'paranoid schizoid position'. The paranoid schizoid position takes up the first four to six months of life, and the depressive position follows on. The working through of these positions extends over the first few years of life. She suggested that, in the paranoid schizoid position, anxiety was experienced predominantly as persecutory and this contributed to certain defences, such as splitting off good and bad parts of the self and projecting them into objects, which through projective identification became identified with these parts of the self. This process is basic for the understanding of narcissistic object relationships. She said that if development during the paranoid schizoid position has not proceeded normally and the infant cannot, for internal or external reasons, cope with the impact of depressive anxieties which originate in the depressive position, a vicious circle arises. For if persecutory fear and correspondingly schizoid mechanisms are too strong the ego is not able to work through the depressive position. This leads to regression and reinforces the earlier persecutory fears and schizoid phenomena. Thus the basis is established for various forms of schizophrenia in later life. Another outcome may be the strengthening of depressive features, which may be the cause of manic–depressive illness later on.

Winnicott (1945), in discussing the treatment of a dozen adult psychotic patients, said that no modification in Freud's technique was needed for the extension of analysis to cope with depression and hypochondria. It is also true according to his experience that the same techniques can take us to still more primitive elements, provided of course that we take into consideration the change in the transference situation inherent in such work.

Winnicott was influenced by Melanie Klein's earlier work, particularly that related to the depressive position and the manic defences. In referring to primitive pre-depressive relations he clearly indicated that he interprets them as they appear in the transference. By 1959 Winnicott had altered his views considerably, both in theory and in practice. He emphasized that psychotic conditions were caused by early environmental failure, stating that 'failure of the facilitating environment results in developmental faults in the individual's personality development and in the establishment of the individual's self, and the result is called schizophrenia' (1959: 135–36). As he regarded psychosis as a deficiency disease, he believed regression to the state of early infancy, which he called dependence, had now to be seen as a part of the capacity of the individual to self-cure. In analysis, 'regression gives an indication from the patient to the analyst as to how the analyst should behave rather than how he should interpret' (p. 128). The analyst, through his behaviour, has to make up for the failure of the early environment. Winnicott's views are here identical both in theory and in practice with those of Pierce Clark and Fromm-Reichmann's early experiments and recommendations (1939). In discussing the analyst's attitude to the patient during a transference psychosis, Winnicott emphasized that it is dangerous if the analyst interprets to the patient instead of waiting for the patient to discover things by himself. He feels that when the analyst is experienced through interpretation as a not-me (a separate object) he becomes dangerous because he knows too much. Fromm-Reichmann shared Winnicott's reluctance to use interpretations with psychotic patients. However, as I have pointed out, she later criticized her early tendency to maintain a very careful waiting and protecting attitude to her psychotic patients. She found this not only unnecessary but damaging because of the over-emphasis on the patient's infantile helplessness.

While there were some analysts such as Winnicott who did not continue the application of Klein's work to the schizophrenic processes, others, such as Rosenfeld, Segal, and Bion, were encouraged, particularly by her work on schizoid mechanisms, to treat schizophrenic patients by psychoanalysis.

Rosenfeld (1947) described an ambulatory analysis of a schizophrenic state with depersonalization. For some time he found the patient's narcissistic withdrawal and ego disintegration an insoluble problem until he became aware of her using certain schizoid mechanisms to defend herself against any painful feelings in the transference situation. She often lost all feelings and believed she had lost herself, experiences which could be traced to a process by which parts of herself were split off and projected into the analyst. She also had feelings of intruding inside the analyst and losing herself there, which gave rise to paranoid anxieties of being intruded into by and overwhelmed by the analyst. The patient's narcissistic withdrawal had therefore been partly a defence against these paranoid fears and partly a defence against closeness because of her fears of intrusion.

In 1950 Segal made history by treating a hospitalized acute schizophrenic patient by psychoanalysis, which retained the essential features of the classical method. Even in the acute hallucinated state she interpreted the patient's defences and material with the emphasis on the negative and positive transference. In contrast to Federn, she analysed all the important resistances and interpreted unconscious material at the level of the greatest anxiety. She emphasized that progress in her patient was achieved only by making the patient aware of what had hitherto been unconscious. She found that schizophrenics often tolerate in their ego thoughts and phantasies which would probably be repressed in a neurotic, but at the same time they repress the links between phantasy and reality, and these links have to be interpreted. She also illustrated that repression often referred to later infantile material of a depressive nature, while consciously very primitive archaic material was being produced in the analysis. In describing the transference at the beginning of the analysis, she stated that the patient was full of persecutory fears and he needed an unchanging good figure, which he tried to believe he had found in the analyst. However, to preserve this belief he had to use all his defences: 'If I frustrated him he would deny that frustration and split me into a good and bad figure. The bad figure would be introjected as hostile voices or reprojected into the hospital doctors' (1950: 27).

At the beginning of the treatment the patient was detached from reality and unable to grasp the nature of the treatment and constantly demanded reassurance. Segal's aim was to retain the attitude of the analyst even without the co-operation of the patient:

> 'to achieve this I had first of all to make him accept my interpretations instead of the various gratifications he wanted. . . . I tried to show him in every interpretation that I understood what he wanted from me, why he wanted it at that particular moment. I also followed most interpretations of that kind with an interpretation of what my refusal had meant to him.'
>
> (1950: 272)

She gradually understood that the patient's constant need for reassurance was aimed at making the analyst an ally against his persecutors, which were particularly related to the doctors in the hospital. She gave illustrations of how she managed to bring the negative persecutory transference, split off on to the doctors in the hospital, into the transference situation. Segal discussed the controversy as to whether the analyst should reassure the very ill schizophrenic patient in a moment of crisis and when craving for reassurance, as many of the analysts whom I have quoted would do – for example, Fromm-Reichmann, Searles, Federn, Pierce Clark, and Winnicott. Segal is convinced that by giving sympathy and reassurance the analyst becomes, for the time being, the good object, but only at the cost of furthering the split between good and bad objects and reinforcing the patient's pathological defences so that later the negative transference becomes unmanageable. In this paper Segal pointed out some technical difficulties in the analysis of the acute schizophrenic patients due to their concrete thinking disorder, a process which she traced to difficulties in the patient's use of symbols. As a result of this, the patient often misunderstands interpretations as they are experienced as concrete threats and actions on the part of the analyst.

In 1952 Rosenfeld described the analysis of an acute hallucinated schizophrenic patient in hospital. He stressed the peculiarity of the schizophrenic object relation; 'whenever the acute schizophrenic approaches an object in love or hate he seems to become confused with this object' (1952b: 457). He observed that the schizophrenic impulses to intrude into the analyst with positive and negative parts of the self, and the defences against this object relationship, were typical of the transference relations of most schizophrenic patients. He also discussed the role of verbal interpretations. While acknowledging the importance of the analyst's intuitive understanding of the patient's communications, he thought that the analyst should also be able to formulate consciously what he has unconsciously recognized and to convey it to the patient in a form that he can understand:

> 'This after all is the essence of all psychoanalysts, but it is especially important in the treatment of schizophrenics, who have lost a great deal of their capacity for conscious functioning, so that without help they cannot consciously understand their unconscious experiences which are at times so vivid.'
>
> (1952a: 117)

Rosenfeld stressed that, in the acute schizophrenic state, the patient tends to put his self so completely into objects (during the analysis into the analyst) that there is very little of the self left outside the object. This interferes with most ego functions, including speaking and understanding words. It also inhibits the capacity to experience relations with external objects. The patient may have difficulty in speaking and may be confused, negativistic, or withdrawn as a result of the severe anxieties related to this process and he may not be able to understand ordinary conversation. Rosenfeld emphasized that if we use interpretations to approach the patient and if our interpretations touch upon his anxieties we shall get some response. There will either be a change in his behaviour or he will talk (1952a). In this paper Rosenfeld developed the concept of the transference psychosis which had been introduced earlier by Federn (1943). However, Federn had been emphatic that the transference psychosis had to be avoided because it was unanalysable, while Rosenfeld affirmed the importance of recognizing the psychotic transference and working through it by means of interpretation.

Bion made important contributions to the psychopathology and treatment of schizophrenic patients from 1950. He emphasized that he did not 'depart from the psychoanalytic procedure usually employed with neurotics, being careful always to take up both positive and negative aspects of the transference' (1954: 23). He looked for evidence of the meaning of the patient's communication but also of his own counter-transference reaction. He investigated both the language of the schizophrenic and his disturbances in thinking. He stressed, for example, that the schizophrenic uses language in three ways: 'as a mode of acting, as a method of communication and as a mode of thought' (1954: 24). He clarified that the use of words and thought depended on the capacity for verbal thinking, which is often lost in schizophrenia through processes of severe splitting and projection, so that the patient is left with only an embryonic capacity for it. In the analytic transference this capacity for verbal thought is often projected into the analyst, which leads both to the persecutory fears of the analyst, who is believed to have taken it away, and to the patient fearing that he has lost it at an earlier stage of development, which increases the need to regress 'to fetch it'. Lack of the capacity for verbal thought is felt by the patient to be the same thing as being insane. Bion gave a vivid picture of his analytic approach in describing the interchange of communication between patient and analyst. It illustrated the importance of the analyst's verbal interpretations in dealing with the schizophrenic's severe disturbances of speech and thought.

In 1956 Bion contributed in greater detail to the understanding of the schizophrenic transference. He stressed the preponderance of the destructive impulses in schizophrenia, which are so great that even the impulses to love are suffused by them and turned into sadism. He also emphasized that there is a hatred of reality, as Freud had pointed out, but Bion added to this the importance of the schizophrenic's hatred of internal reality and all that makes for awareness of it. Derived from these two basic difficulties there is an unremitting dread of imminent annihilation. In discussing the transference with the analyst, which he described as thin but tenacious, he said: 'The relationship with the analyst is premature, precipitate and intensely dependent' (1956: 37). When the patient broadens it under pressure of his life or death instincts, two concurrent streams of phenomena become manifest:

> 'First projective identification, with the analyst as object, becomes overactive with the resulting painful confusional states such as Rosenfeld has described. Second the mental and other activities by which the dominant impulse, be it life instincts or death instincts, strives to express itself, are at once subjected to mutilation by the temporarily subordinate impulse. Driven by the wish to escape the confusional states and harassed by the mutilations, the patient strives to restore the restricted relationship: the transference is again invested with its characteristic featurelessness. . . . Oscillation between the attempt to broaden the contact and attempt to restrict continues throughout the analysis.'
>
> (1956: 37; 1957: 44)

In 1957 Bion made important contributions to the therapy of schizophrenia by differentiating the psychotic from the non-psychotic parts of the schizophrenic personality. He emphasized particularly the role of projective identification in the psychotic part of the personality as a substitute for repression in the neurotic part of the personality: 'The patient's destructive attacks on his ego and the substitution of projective identification for repression and introjection must be worked through' (1957: 63).

Summary

After Freud's pessimism about the analysis of psychotic patients, due to his belief that they formed no transference, two main trends in the approach to the treatment of psychotics have appeared. There were those who believed that the narcissism of the psychotic patient presented a complete obstacle to analysis unless the analyst changed his usual analytic attitude. Analysts who held the view that the narcissism of the psychotic patient was caused by an environmental failure attempted to provide the patient with a new and better mother in the form of the analyst, to make up for the deficiency of the early environment. Exponents of this approach were particularly Pierce Clark, Fromm-Reichmann in her early period, and Winnicott in his later work. Searles's approach is closely related to this, as he recommends the analyst's intense involvement with the psychotic patient, particularly in the symbiotic phase of the analysis. Waelder and Jacobson have also altered their analytic attitude. They do not analyse the transference but maintain a predominantly positive one and use it as a vehicle to sublimate the patient's narcissism or psychosis by relating it to object libido and the external world. Federn similarly encouraged the positive transference and avoided any analysis of transference manifestations. However, he differed from Waelder and Jacobson by training the patient to repress or split off the psychotic parts of his personality. Searles and Fromm-Reichmann in her later work differ from others in this group in so far as they analyse both the negative and the positive transference.

The second group of analysts attempted to deal with the narcissism and other psychotic manifestations of the patient by the classical psychoanalytic approach with only minor changes. First came Abraham, who found that the narcissistic defences of his patients were markedly diminished by interpretations. Then Stern, Cohn, Stone, and Bullard described characteristics of the positive and negative transference of psychotic patients, which they felt could be analysed by verbal transference interpretations.

Segal, Bion, and Rosenfeld stressed that no change in the analyst's attitude and only minor changes in technique were necessary, and that the psychotic productions attached themselves to the transference, which could be interpreted in both its negative and its positive forms to the patient. They also relied almost exclusively on interpretations to deal with the serious language and thought disorder of the schizophrenic patient, and saw these difficulties as part of the malfunctioning of the psychotic ego with its disturbed relationships to both external and internal reality and objects. The development of the treatment of psychosis over the last fifty years suggests that Freud's hope that some approach to the treatment of psychosis might become possible is now justified.

References

Abraham, K. (1907a) On the significance of sexual trauma in childhood for the symptomatology of dementia praecox. In *Clinical Papers and Essays on Psychoanalysis*. London: Hogarth Press, 1955.

—— (1907b) The experience of sexual traumas as a form of sexual activity. In *Selected Papers*. London: Hogarth Press, 1950, p. 55.

—— (1908) The psycho-sexual differences between hysteria and dementia praecox. In *Selected Papers*. London: Hogarth Press, 1950.

—— (1911) Notes on the psycho-analytical investigation and treatment of manic–depressive insanity and allied conditions. In *Selected Papers*. London: Hogarth Press, 1950.

—— (1913) Restrictions and transformations of scoptophilia in psycho-neurotics. In *Selected Papers*. London: Hogarth Press, 1950.

—— (1916) The first pregenital stage of the libido. In *Selected Papers*. London: Hogarth Press, 1950.

—— (1919) A particular form of neurotic resistance against the psychoanalytic method. In *Selected Papers*. London: Hogarth Press, 1950.

—— (1924a) The influence of oral erotism on character formation. In *Selected Papers*. London: Hogarth Press, 1950.

—— (1924b) A short study of the development of the libido viewed in the light of mental disorders. In *Selected Papers*. London: Hogarth Press, 1950.

Asch, S. (1976) Varieties of negative therapeutic reaction and problems of technique. *Journal of the American Psychoanalytic Association* 24: 383–407.

Bion, W. R. (1954) Notes on the theory of schizophrenia. In *Second Thoughts*. London: Heinemann, 1967.

—— (1956) Development of schizophrenic thought. In *Second Thoughts*. London: Heinemann, 1967.

—— (1957) Differentiation of the psychotic from the non-psychotic personalities. In *Second Thoughts*. London: Heinemann, 1967.

—— (1962a) The theory of thinking. In *Second Thoughts*. London: Heinemann, 1967.

—— (1962b) *Learning from Experience*. London: Heinemann.

—— (1963) *Elements of Psychoanalysis*. London: Heinemann.

—— (1965) *Transformations*. London: Heinemann.

—— (1970) *Attention and Interpretation*. London: Tavistock.

—— (1980) *Bion in New York and São Paulo*. Perthshire: Clunie Press.

Bullard, D. M. (1940) Experiences in the psycho-analytic treatment of psychotics. *Psychoanalytic Quarterly* 9: 493–504.

—— (1960) Psychotherapy of paranoid patients. *Archives of General Psychiatry* 2: 137–41.

Bychowski, G. (1953) Personal communication.

Cohn, F. S. (1940) Practical approach to the problem of narcissistic neuroses. *Psychoanalytic Quarterly* 9: 64–79.

Eissler, K. R. (1972) Death drive, ambivalence and narcissism. *The Psychoanalytic Study of the Child* 26: 25–78.

Federn, P. (1925) Narcissism in the structure of the ego. *International Journal of Psycho-Analysis* 9: 401–19.

—— (1932) The reality of the death instinct especially in melancholia. *Psychoanalytic Review* 19: 129–51.

—— (1943) Psychoanalysis of the psychoses. In *Ego Psychology and the Psychoses*. New York: Basic Books, 1952.

Felton, J. (1985) Personal communication.

Freud, S. (1905) On psychotherapy. SE 7. (Strachey, J. (ed.) (1950–74) *Standard Edition of the Complete Psychological Works of Sigmund Freud*. London: Hogarth Press.)

—— (1911) Formulations on the two principles of mental functioning. SE 12.

—— (1914) On narcissism: an introduction. SE 14.

—— (1915) Instincts and their vicissitudes. SE 14.

—— (1916) Some character types met with in psycho-analytic work. SE 14.

—— (1916–17) *Introductory Lectures on Psycho-Analysis*. SE 15–16.

—— (1918) From the history of an infantile neurosis. SE 17.

—— (1920) *Beyond the Pleasure Principle*. SE 18.

—— (1923) *The Ego and the Id*. SE 19.

—— (1924) The economic problem of masochism. SE 19.

—— (1930) *Civilization and its Discontents*. SE 21.

—— (1933) *New Introductory Lectures on Psycho-Analysis*. SE 22.

—— (1937) Analysis terminable and interminable. SE 23.

—— (1940) *An Outline of Psycho-Analysis*. SE 23.

Fromm-Reichmann, F. (1939) Transference problems in schizophrenics. *Psychoanalytic Quarterly* 8: 412–26.

—— (1948) Notes on the development of treatment of schizophrenics by psychoanalytic therapy. In D. M. Bullard (ed.), *Psychoanalysis and Psychotherapy*. University of Chicago Press, 1959.

—— (1952) Some aspects of psychoanalytic psychotherapy with schizophrenics. In D. M. Bullard (ed.), *Psychoanalysis and Psychotherapy*. University of Chicago Press, 1959.

—— (1954) Psychotherapy of schizophrenia. In D. M. Bullard (ed.), *Psychoanalysis and Psychotherapy*. University of Chicago Press, 1959.

Gitelson, M. (1962) The curative factors in psychoanalysis. *International Journal of Psycho-analysis* 43: 194–205.

Goldstein, W. (1985) *An Introduction to the Borderline Conditions*. New Jersey: Aronson.

Green, A. (1984) Symposium on the Death Instinct held in Marseilles.

Greenacre, P. (1954) The role of transference. *Journal of the American Psychoanalytic Association* 2: 671–84.

Greenson, R. (1967) *The Technique and Practice of Psychoanalysis*. New York: International Universities Press.

Grotstein, J. (1981) *Splitting and Projective Identification*. New York: Jason Aronson.

Hartmann, H., Kris, E., and Loewenstein, R. M. (1949) Notes on the theory of aggression. *The Psychoanalytic Study of the Child* 3–4: 9–36.

Heimann, P. (1956) Dynamics of transference interpretations. *International Journal of Psycho-Analysis* 37: 303–10.

—— (1975) Obituary of Lois Munro. *International Journal of Psycho-Analysis* 56: 99.

Hermann, I. (1929) Das Ich und das Denken. *Imago*. 15: 89–110.

Horney, K. (1936) The problem of the negative therapeutic reaction. *Psychoanalytic Quarterly* 5: 29–44.

Jacobson, E. (1954a) On psychotic identification. *International Journal of Psycho-Analysis* 35: 102–8.

Jacobson, E. (1954a) On psychotic identification. *International Journal of Psychoanalysis* 35: 102–8.

—— (1954b) Transference problems in the psychoanalytic treatment of severely depressive patients. *Journal of the American Psychoanalytic Association* 2: 595–606.

—— (1967) *Psychotic Conflict and Reality*. London: Hogarth Press.

Jones, E. *Sigmund Freud. Life and Work*, Vol. III, Chapter VIII: 295–97. London: Hogarth Press.

Kernberg, O. (1970) Factors in the psychoanalytic treatment of narcissistic personalities. *Journal of the American Psychoanalytic Association* 18: 51–85.

—— (1977) *Borderline Conditions and Pathological Narcissism*. New York: Jason Aronson.

314

King, P. (1962) Curative factors in psycho-analysis. *International Journal of Psycho-Analysis* 43: 225–27.

Klauber, J. (1972) On the relationship of transference and interpretation in psychoanalytic therapy. *International Journal of Psycho-Analysis* 53: 385–91.

Klein, M. (1935) A contribution to the psychogenesis of manic-depressive states. *International Journal of Psycho-Analysis* 16: 145–74.

—— (1946) Notes on some schizoid mechanisms. In *Developments in Psycho-Analysis*. London: Hogarth Press, 1952.

—— (1952) The origins of transference. *International Journal of Psycho-Analysis* 33: 433–38.

—— (1957) *Envy and Gratitude*. London: Tavistock; New York: Basic Books.

—— (1958) On the development of mental functioning. *International Journal of Psycho-Analysis* 39: 84–90.

Kohut, H. (1972) Thoughts on narcissism and narcissistic rage. *The Psychoanalytic Study of the Child* 27: 360–400.

Langs, R. (1976) *The Therapeutic Interaction*, 2 vols. New York: Jason Aronson.

Limentani, A. (1981) On some positive aspects of the negative therapeutic interaction. *International Journal of Psycho-Analysis* 62: 379–90.

Loewald, H. (1970) Psychoanalytic theory and the psychoanalytic process. *The Psychoanalytic Study of the Child* 25: 45–68.

—— (1972) Freud's conception of the negative therapeutic reaction with comments on instinct theory. *Journal of the American Psychoanalytic Association* 20: 235–45.

Mahler, M. (1952) On child psychosis and schizophrenia: autistic and symbiotic infantile psychoses. *The Psychoanalytic Study of the Child* 7: 286–305.

—— (1969) *On Human Symbiosis and the Vicissitudes of Individuation*. London: Hogarth/Institute of Psycho-Analysis.

Meltzer, D. (1967a) The weaning process. In *The Psycho-Analytical Process*. London: Heinemann.

—— (1967b) *The Psycho-Analytical Process*. London: Heinemann.

—— (1968) Terror, persecution and dread. In *Sexual States of Mind*, Chapter 14. Perthshire: Clunie Press.

—— (1973) *Sexual States of Mind*. Perthshire: Clunie Press.

Miller, A. (1983) *You Should Not Notice*. Frankfurt: Suhrkamp.

Money-Kyrle, R. E. (1956) Normal countertransference and some of its deviations. *International Journal of Psycho-Analysis* 37: 360–66.

Nacht, S. (1962) Curative factors in psychoanalysis. *International Journal of Psycho-Analysis* 43: 206–11.

Olinick, S. (1964) The negative therapeutic reaction. *International Journal of Psycho-Analysis* 45: 540–48.

References

—— (1970) Negative therapeutic reaction. Reporter on Panel. *Journal of the American Psychoanalytic Association* 18: 655–72.

Pierce Clark, L. (1933a) The question of prognosis in narcissistic neuroses and psychoses. *International Journal of Psycho-Analysis* 14: 71–86.

—— (1933b) The treatment of narcissistic neuroses and psychoses. *Psychoanalytic Review* 20: 304–26.

Reich, W. (1933) *Character Analysis*. New York: Orgone Institute Press, 1949.

Riviere, J. (1936) A contribution to the analysis of the negative therapeutic reaction. *International Journal of Psycho-Analysis* 17: 304–20.

Rosenfeld, H. A. (1947) Analysis of a schizophrenic state with depersonalization. *International Journal of Psycho-Analysis* 28: 130–39.

—— (1950) Notes on the psychopathology of confusional states in chronic schizophrenias. *International Journal of Psycho-Analysis* 31: 132–37.

—— (1952a) Notes on the psycho-analysis of the superego conflict of an acute schizophrenic patient. *International Journal of Psycho-Analysis* 33: 111–31.

—— (1952b) Transference-phenomena and transference-analysis in an acute catatonic schizophrenic patient. *International Journal of Psycho-Analysis* 33: 457–64.

—— (1954) Considerations regarding the psycho-analytic approach to acute and chronic schizophrenia. In *Psychotic States*. London: Hogarth Press, 1965.

—— (1963a) Notes on the psychopathology and psychoanalytical treatment of depressive and manic-depressive patients. *Psychiatric Research Reports of the American Psychiatric Association*, November.

—— (1963b) Notes on the psychopathology and psychoanalytical treatment of schizophrenia. *Psychiatric Research Reports of the American Psychiatric Association*, November.

—— (1964a) Object relationships of the acute schizophrenic patient in the transference situation. *Psychiatric Research Reports of the American Psychiatric Association*, December.

—— (1964b) On the psychopathology of narcissism. In *Psychotic States*. London: Hogarth Press, 1965.

—— (1965) *Psychotic States*. London: Hogarth Press.

—— (1968) Notes on the negative therapeutic reaction. Paper read to the British Psycho-Analytical Society and to the Menninger Clinic, Topeka.

—— (1970) On projective identification. Paper read to the British Psycho-Analytical Society.

—— (1971) A clinical approach to the psychoanalytic theory of the life and death instincts: an investigation into the aggressive aspects of narcissism. *International Journal of Psycho-Analysis* 52: 169–78.

—— (1972) A critical appreciation of James Strachey's paper 'On the nature of the therapeutic action of psycho-analysis' (postscript). *International Journal of Psycho-Analysis* 53: 455–61.

Sandler, J. (1976) Countertransference and role-responsiveness. *International Review of Psycho-Analysis* 3: 43–47.

Searles, H. F. (1955) Dependency processes in the psychotherapy of schizophrenia. In *Collected Papers on Schizophrenia and Related Subjects*. London: Hogarth Press, 1965.

—— (1959a) The effort to drive the analyst crazy – an element in the aetiology and psychotherapy of schizophrenia. *British Journal of Medical Psychology* 32: 1–18.

—— (1959b) Integration and differentiation in schizophrenia. In *Collected Papers on Schizophrenia and Related Subjects*. London: Hogarth Press, 1965.

—— (1962) The differentiation between concrete and metaphorical thinking in the recovering schizophrenic patient. *Journal of the American Psychoanalytic Association* 10: 22–49.

—— (1963) Transference psychosis in the psychotherapy of schizophrenics. In *Collected Papers on Schizophrenia and Related Subjects*. London: Hogarth Press, 1965.

—— (1965) *Collected Papers on Schizophrenia and Related Subjects*. London: Hogarth Press.

—— (1975) The patient as therapist to his analyst. In P. Giovacchini (ed.), *Tactics and Techniques in Psychoanalytic Therapy*, Vol. 2. New York: Aronson.

Segal, H. (1950) Some aspects of the analysis of a schizophrenic. *International Journal of Psycho-Analysis* 31: 268–78.

—— (1956) Depression in the schizophrenic. *International Journal of Psycho-Analysis* 37: 339–43.

—— (1957) Notes on symbol formation. *International Journal of Psycho-Analysis* 38: 391–97.

—— (1962a) Symposium on the curative factors in psycho-analysis. III. *International Journal of Psycho-Analysis* 43: 212–21.

—— (1962b) *Introduction to the Work of Melanie Klein*. London: Tavistock.

—— (1977) Countertransference. *International Journal of Psychoanalysis and Psychotherapy* 6: 31–7.

Spillius, E. (1980) Clinical reflections on the negative therapeutic reaction. *Bulletin of the European Psychoanalytical Federation* 15.

Steiner, R. (1969–75) *Processo di Simbolizzione nell Opera di Melanie Klein*. Turin: Boringhieri.

—— (1982) Intonation and osmotic communication. Unpublished paper.

Stern, A. (1938) Psychoanalytic investigation of and therapy in the borderline group of neuroses. *Psychoanalytic Quarterly* 7: 467–89.

—— (1948) Transference in borderline neuroses. *Psychoanalytic Quarterly* 17: 527–28.

317

Stone, L. (1954) The widening scope of indications for psychoanalysis. *Journal of the American Psychoanalytic Association* 2: 567–94.

Sullivan, H. S. (1947) Therapeutic investigations in schizophrenia. *Psychiatry* 10: 121–25.

Tausk, V. (1919) On the origin of the influencing machine in schizophrenia. *Psychoanalytic Quarterly* 2: 519–56.

Tustin, F. (1972) *Autism and Childhood Psychosis*. London: Hogarth Press.

—— (1981) *Autistic States in Children*. London, Boston & Henley: Routledge and Kegan Paul.

Vigotsky, R. Personal communication.

Waelder, R. (1925) The psychoses: their mechanisms and accessibility to influence. *International Journal of Psycho-Analysis* 6: 259–81.

Weiss, E. (1935) Todestrieb und Masochismus. *Imago* 21: 393–411.

Winnicott, D. W. (1945) Primitive emotional development. In *Collected Papers*. London: Tavistock, 1958.

—— (1955) Metapsychological and clinical aspects of regression within the psychoanalytic set-up. *International Journal of Psycho-Analysis* 36: 16–26.

—— (1956) Primary maternal preoccupation. In *Collected Papers*. London: Tavistock, 1958.

—— (1959–64) Classification: Is there a psycho-analytic contribution to psychiatric classification? In *The Maturational Processes and the Facilitating Environment*. London: Hogarth Press, 1965.

—— (1960) The theory of the parent–infant relationship. *International Journal of Psycho-Analysis* 41: 585–95.

—— (1963) Communicating and not communicating leading to a study of certain opposites. In *The Maturational Processes and the Facilitating Environment*. London: Hogarth Press, 1965.

Name index

Abraham, K. 20, 85–6, 97–8n, 125–26n, 287–90, 311
Asch, Stuart E. 86, 102–04n

Bion, Wilfred R. 24n; on analyst's role 34, 160; on maternal projections 158, 185n, 187–88n, 276; on parasitism 189–90n; on projective identification and containment 17, 158–59; on psychotic transference 288, 309–11; on splitting 285
Bullard, D.M. 286, 294–95, 311
Bychowski, G. 25n, 294

Cohn, F.S. 287, 293–94, 311

Federn, P.: on death instinct 126n; on latent psychosis 297; on narcissism 20, 26n; on psychotic transference 286, 294–97, 309, 311; on splitting 285
Felton, June 158, 185–86n, 276
Freud, Sigmund: on analyst's role 34–5; on death instinct 86, 88, 97n, 107–09, 111, 125n, 127–32n, 267; on narcissism 19–20, 105, 283–84; on negative therapeutic reactions 85, 88, 96, 96–7n, 100n, 102–03; on trauma 44n; on treatment of psychosis 12, 20, 281–86, 297, 310
Fromm-Reichmann, Frieda 17, 26n, 286, 293–94, 298–301, 306, 311

Gillespie, R.D. 5
Gitelson, M. 34
Goldstein, W. 189n
Green, André 27n, 125n
Greenson, R. 279n
Grotstein, J. 160–61
Gutman, Dr 6

Hartmann, H. 131n
Heimann, Paula 11, 39
Hermann, I. 187n
Horney, K. 86, 98n, 100n

Jacobson, Edith 181–83n, 288, 303–05, 311
Jones, Ernest 138

Katan, M. 285
Kernberg, O. 22, 26n
King, Pearl 35
Klauber, J. 34
Klein, Melanie 10–11; on death and life instincts 101n, 127–28n, 130n; on envy 100–01n, 127–28n, 266; on hypochondriasis 82; on infantile development 13–14, 23, 124, 184n, 305–06; on narcissism 19, 26n, 185n, 305; on negative therapeutic reactions 86, 100–01n, 266; on projective identification 13, 23, 157–58, 163, 181n, 184–85n, 288; on psychotic

319

Klein, Melanie (*cont.*):
  transference 14; on splitting 23, 101n,
  128n, 163, 285
Knight, Robert 26n
Kohut, H. 22
Kris, E. 131n

Langs, Robert 31–2, 34, 37, 104n
Limentani, A. 104n
Loewald, H. 31, 103–04n
Loewenstein, R.M. 131n

Mahler, Margaret 183–84n
Meltzer, D. 27n, 112, 153n, 169, 190n
Meyer, Adolf 26n
Miller, Alice 216–17
Money-Kyrle, R.E. 12, 34

Nacht, S. 17

Olinick, S. 86, 101–04n

Payne, Sylvia 11–12
Pierce Clark, L. 287, 292–93, 299, 306,
  311

Reich, T. 125–26n
Riviere, Joan 86, 99–101n, 153n
Rosen, John 26n
Rosenfeld, Herbert A. 4–12; on
  destructive narcissism 88, 109–10; on
  hypochondriasis 83n; on narcissism
  20–2, 86–8; on projection 189n, 294;

on splitting 285; on transference
  psychosis 11–12, 13–14, 288, 309; on
  treatment of psychosis 25–6n, 288,
  306–09, 311

Sandler, J. 31, 34
Scott, Clifford 5
Searles, Harold F.: on communication
  32; on projection 294, 301; on
  psychotic transference 40, 287, 294,
  301–02; on schizophrenic thinking
  189n; on treatment of psychosis 16–
  17, 26n, 301–02, 311
Segal, Hanna 24n, 31, 161–62, 188–89n,
  288, 307–08, 311
Slater, Dr 6
Spillius, E. 97n
Steiner, R. 158, 186n, 276
Stern, A. 20, 287, 293, 311
Stone, L. 20, 287, 302–03, 311
Sullivan, Harry Stack 26n, 286, 297–98,
  300

Tausk, V. 5
Tustin, F. 158, 187n

Vigotsky, R. 189n

Waelder, R. 287, 291–93, 311
Weiss, Eduardo 126n
Winnicott, Donald W. 17, 35, 288, 293,
  305–06, 311

Index of case histories

Adam 63–82, 84n, 266
Caroline 134–37
Charles 209–19
Clare 191–207, 207–08n
Claude 119–20
Edgar 5–6
Edward 6–7
Eliza 6
Eric 140–52, 153n, 275
Iris 222–24
Jill 116–19
John 171–75
Lucy 41–3
Maria 84n, 241–61, 273

Michael 91–6
Mildred 11–14, 306–07
Patricia 277–78
Pauline 137–38, 139
Peter 88–90
Richard 120–25
Robert 113–15
Sarah 224–40
Sheila 133–34
Sidney 175–81
Simon 110–11, 131n
Sylvia 38–9, 45–59, 139
Thomas 8–9

Subject index

aggression 99n, 129n, 162; *see also* destructive narcissism

analyst, the: analysis of 11, 18–19, 33; anti-therapeutic factors in 33–43; anxieties of 18, 40, 173–74; attitude and role of 34–7; and breakdown of communication with patient 45–60; criticism of 32–3, 39–40, 139, 141; danger to 8, 18–19; dependence on 87, 90, 113, 163–64, 244; functioning of 31–44, 160; and interpretation 15–18, 37–9; and projection 14–15; and rigidity and flexibility 39–43, 270–72; *see also* techniques

anxieties: of the analyst 18, 40, 173–74; confusional 258–60; infantile 13, 17, 44n, 127n

attitude of the analyst 34–7

autism 185–86n, 276–77

breakdown, communication 45–60

collusion 36, 39–43, 102n, 268–70

communication 3–4, 32, 58–9, 161–62, 220–21; breakdown 45–60; verbal and non-verbal 14–15, 194

confusion 268–70, 273–74

containment 159–61, 191–207, 209–19, 241

counter-transference 12, 139; negative 39–43, 268; and schizophrenia 241–61

criticism of the analyst 32–3, 39–40, 43, 139, 141

death instinct 8, 88, 103n, 107–13, 125–31n, 267–68; Freud on 103n, 107–09, 111, 125n, 127–30n

delusions 168–69; paranoid 6–7; projection of 14–15; sexual 9–10; and transference 222–28, 239, 272–73

dependence on the analyst 87, 90, 113, 163–64, 244

depression *see* manic-depressive states

destructive narcissism 22–3, 27n, 105–25, 125–32n, 134–37, 146, 267–68; *see also* death instinct

devaluation 69–74

dramatization 16–17

ego 282–86; *see also* splitting

empathy 12, 17, 161

envy 19, 21, 125–26n, 163, 266–67; and devaluation 69–74; and negative therapeutic reactions 96, 97–8n, 100–01n; oral 65–9, 101n

erotic transference 228–39

flexibility of the analyst 39–43, 270–72

foetus, pressures on 184–88n, 275–76

fusions 108, 124, 131–32n

guilt 33, 174; and negative therapeutic reactions 96–7n, 100n, 102–03n

322

hallucination 46, 64, 168–69
hospitalization 60n
hypochondriasis 63–83, 83n, 209–19

identification 20–1; projective *see* projective identification
impasse 3, 12, 39–42, 133–53; diagnosing 139
infancy: anxieties 13, 17, 44n, 127n; development 13, 17, 23, 184n, 189n, 305; and identification 181n, 184n; symbiotic psychosis 183–84n; and transference 221; *see also* maternal projections, mother–child relationship
inflexibility 39–43, 270–72
insight 12
Institute of Psychoanalysis 11
interpretation 15–18, 37–43; inflexibility in 39–43; timing of 15–16, 37; verbal 16–17, 182n

life instinct 108, 127–29n

manic–depressive states 13, 282–83, 289–90, 303
maternal projections 185–88n, 275–79
Maudsley Hospital 4, 6, 25n
mother–child relationship 17, 33, 103n; and analysis 35, 107; *see also* infancy, maternal projections

narcissism 19–23; destructive (*q.v.*) 22–3, 27n, 105–25; Freud on 20, 283–84; and impasse 133–53; narcissistic omnipotence 21–2, 63–83, 87–8; narcissistic omnipotent object relations 20–1, 74–81; and negative therapeutic reactions 85–96; and projective identification 23; 'thin- and thick-skinned' patients 274–75
negative therapeutic reactions (NTRs) 22, 59, 74–81, 139; in narcissistic patients 85–96; theory of 85–6, 88, 96–104n
nirvana principle 131–32n
non-verbal communication 14–15, 33

object relations 23, 99n; narcissistic omnipotent 20–1, 74–81
omnipotence, narcissistic 21–2, 63– 83, 87–8

oral envy 65–9
'osmotic pressures' 185–86n, 276–77

paranoia 6–7, 13, 157–58, 295
parasitism 163–64, 184n, 189–90n
perversions 131–32n
projection 14–16, 36–7; maternal 185– 88n, 275–79; *see also:*
projective identification 13, 157–59, 181–90n; in clinical practice 157–81; and containment 159–61, 191–207, 209–19; and counter-transference 241–61; and narcissistic omnipotent object relations 23–4; and psychotic transference 220–40; recognizing 161– 69; and techniques 169–71, 191
psychoanalysis: of the analyst 11, 18–19, 33; theories and techniques (*q.v.*) 265– 79; and the treatment of psychosis 3– 24, 281–311
psychosis: analysts' experiences with 286–310; Freud on 282–86; latent 18– 19, 297; transference (*q.v.*) in 14, 20, 23–4, 220–40, 272–73, 286–310; treatment of, with psychoanalysis 3– 24, 281–311

rage, narcissistic 22–3
reality: denial of 164–65; and unreality 243, 297
resistance to analysis *see* negative therapeutic reactions
rigidity of approach 39–42, 270–72
role of the analyst 34–7; *see also* techniques

schizophrenia 5–7, 220–22, 282–83; and counter-transference 241–61; mobilization of 11–12; psychotic transference in 220–40, 286–89, 291– 310; withdrawal 6; *see also* splitting
self-idealization 105–06
self-observation 87, 90
sex: delusions 9–10, 65; and greed 71–2; and transference 228–39
Shenley Hospital 25n
splitting 23, 101n, 113, 127–28n, 135– 37, 206–07, 229, 285, 297; patient's awareness of 198, 201, 252
symbiotic processes 167–68, 183–84n
symbolism 51, 59, 161, 188–89n

Tavistock Clinic 4, 8–11
techniques in psychoanalysis 265–79; collusion 268–70; confusion 268–70, 273–74; destructive narcissism 267–68; envy 266–67; flexibility of the analyst 270–72; history of patient 268–70; maternal projections 275–79; negative therapeutic reactions 86, 90; projective identification 169–71, 191; 'thin- and thick-skinned' patients 274–75; transference and delusions 272–73
theory, psychoanalytic 19–23; negative therapeutic reactions 85–6, 88, 96–104n; and psychosis 281–311; and technique (*q.v.*) 265–79
'thin- and thick-skinned' patients 274–75

transference: analysis of 7, 65–9; counter- 12, 139, 241–61; delusional 222–28, 239, 272–73; erotic 228–39; infantile 221; narcissistic 291–94; negative 125n; and projective identification 220–40; psychotic 14, 20, 23–4, 220–40, 272–73, 286–310
transference psychosis 14, 288, 301, 309
trauma 36, 44n

United States of America 14, 25–6n, 297–302

verbal communication 14–15, 161–62; of interpretations 16–17, 182n

withdrawal 6, 131–32n